Work, psychiatry and society, *c*. 1750–2015

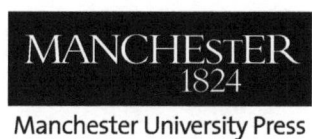
Manchester University Press

Work, psychiatry and society,
c. 1750–2015

Edited by
WALTRAUD ERNST

Manchester University Press

Copyright © Manchester University Press 2016
While copyright in the volume as a whole is vested in Manchester University Press, copyright in individual chapters belongs to their respective authors, and no chapter may be reproduced wholly or in part without the express permission in writing of both author and publisher.

Published by Manchester University Press
Oxford Road, Manchester M13 9PL
www.manchesteruniversitypress.co.uk

British Library Cataloguing-in-Publication Data
A catalogue record for this book is available from the British Library

Library of Congress Cataloging-in-Publication Data applied for

ISBN 9780 7190 9769 0 hardback

ISBN 9781 5261 2709 9 paperback

First published 2016

The publisher has no responsibility for the persistence or accuracy of URLs for any external or third-party internet websites referred to in this book, and does not guarantee that any content on such websites is, or will remain, accurate or appropriate.

Typeset by
Servis Filmsetting Ltd, Stockport, Cheshire

Contents

List of figures   vii
List of contributors   ix
Acknowledgements   xiii

    Introduction: Therapy and empowerment, coercion and punishment. Historical and contemporary perspectives on work, psychiatry and society   1
    Waltraud Ernst

1   The role of work in late eighteenth- and early nineteenth-century treatises on moral treatment in France, Tuscany and Britain   31
    Jane Freebody

2   Therapeutic work and mental illness in America, c. 1830–1970   55
    Ben Harris

3   Travails of madness: New Jersey, 1800–70   77
    James Moran

4   From blasting powder to tomato pickles: Patient work at the provincial mental hospitals in British Columbia, Canada, 1885–1920   99
    Kathryn McKay

5   'Useful both to the patients as well as to the State': Patient work in colonial mental hospitals in South Asia, c. 1818–1948   117
    Waltraud Ernst

6   'A powerful agent in their recovery': Work as treatment in British West Indian lunatic asylums, 1860–1910   142
    Leonard Smith

7	Work and activity in mental hospitals in modern Japan, c. 1868–2000 Akira Hashimoto	163
8	Patient work and family care at Iwakura, Japan, c. 1799–1970 Osamu Nakamura	182
9	Work and occupation in Romanian psychiatry, c. 1838–1945 Valentin-Veron Toma	194
10	Between therapeutic instrument and exploitation of labour force: Patient work in rural asylums in Württemberg, c. 1810–1945 Thomas Müller	220
11	The patient's view of work therapy: The mental hospital Hamburg-Langenhorn during the Weimar Republic Monika Ankele	238
12	They were 'improved', punished and cured: The construction of 'workshy', 'industrious' and (non-)compliant inmates in forced labour facilities in the First Republic of Austria between 1918 and 1938 Sonja Hinsch	262
13	Useful members of society or motiveless malingerers? Occupation and malingering in British asylum psychiatry, 1870–1914 Sarah Chaney	277
14	Work and the Irish District Asylums during the late nineteenth century Oonagh Walsh	298
15	From work and occupation to occupational therapy: The policies of professionalisation in English mental hospitals from 1919 to 1959 John Hall	314
16	Work is therapy? The function of employment in British psychiatric care after 1959 Vicky Long	334
17	The hollow gardener and other stories: Reason and relation in the work cure Jennifer Laws	351
Index		368

Figures

2.1 Sewing room, Willard Asylum, *c.* 1890. (Source: New York State Archives. Willard Psychiatric Centre, NY, Willard documentary images, 1880–1993, B1442.)   62
2.2 Men working outside, Willard Asylum, *c.* 1890. (Source: New York State Archives. Willard Psychiatric Centre, NY, Willard documentary images, 1880–1993, B1442.)   62
2.3 Women sawing, John Gehring's Asylum, Bethel, Maine, *c.* 1910. (Source: Courtesy of the Bethel Historical Society.)   69
5.1 Interior of the recreation hall with stage in the background, Madras, *c.* 1940. (Source: *Annual Report on the Working of the Mental Hospitals in the Madras Presidency for the Year 1940*, p. 22.)   124
5.2 Rope making, Government Mental Hospital, Calicut, *c.* 1938. (Source: *Annual Report on the Working of the Mental Hospitals in the Madras Presidency for the Year 1938*, p. 20.)   131
5.3 Embroidery class, Government Mental Hospital, Calicut, *c.* 1939. (Source: *Annual Report on the Working of the Mental Hospitals in the Madras Presidency for the Year 1939*, p. 19.)   132
5.4 Tailoring, Government Mental Hospital, Calicut, *c.* 1939. (Source: *Annual Report on the Working of the Mental Hospitals in the Madras Presidency for the Year 1939*, p. 19.)   133
5.5 Weaving section, Government Mental Hospital, Calicut, *c.* 1939. (Source: *Annual Report on the Working of the Mental Hospitals in the Madras Presidency for the Year 1939*, p. 19.)   134
7.1 Aerial photograph of Matsuzawa Byōin, *c.* 1935. (Source: Tokyo furitsu Matsuzawa Byōin ehagaki (picture postcards of Tokyo Prefecture Matsuzawa Mental Hospital). Byōsha kyūsai kai, *c.* 1935.)   169

8.1 Imai Inn, c. 1905. (Source: Image courtesy of Mr Hiroshi Imai.) 183
8.2 A patient with two attendants and a cook in front of the waterfall, c. 1910. (Source: Image courtesy of Mrs Suzue Sodeoka.) 184
8.3 Hojo, Nanzenji-Temple. (Source: Photo by Osamu Nakamura, 2010.) 185
8.4 Iwakura Mental Hospital, 1909. (Source: Image courtesy of Mr Ichiro Tamaki.) 186
8.5 Patients of Muramatsu Guest House walking around Iwakura, c. 1935. (Source: Image courtesy of Teruko Muramatsu.) 187
8.6 A patient at Muramatsu Guest House chopping wood, c. 1935. (Source: Image courtesy of Mrs Teruko Muramatsu.) 188
8.7 Patients at Muramatsu Guest House doing exercises, c. 1935. (Source: Image courtesy of Mrs Teruko Muramatsu.) 189
9.1 Map of Romanian territories between the First and Second World Wars. (Source: Keith Hitchins, *A Concise History of Romania*, Cambridge Concise Histories Series (Cambridge: Cambridge University Press, 2014), p. 157, map 7. Reproduced by permission.) 195
10.1 Zwiefalten Asylum, cobbler's workshop, 1912. (Source: Archives, Centre of Psychiatry Südwürttemberg.) 223
10.2 Zwiefalten Asylum, carpenter's workshop, 1912. (Source: Archives, Centre of Psychiatry Südwürttemberg.) 223
11.1 Piece of fabric, embroidered by a female patient in the Staatskrankenanstalt Hamburg-Langenhorn, 1920s. (Source: Staatsarchiv Hansestadt Hamburg 352–8/7, Sig. 1609 (Abl. 1995/2).) 246

Contributors

Monika Ankele, PhD, studied history in Graz, Vienna, and Berlin. She specialises on the history of German psychiatry, in particular the history of everyday life, patient's history, ego-documents, and material culture. Since 2012 she has been a researcher at the Department of History and Ethics of Medicine at the University Medical Centre Hamburg-Eppendorf. She is currently working on prolonged bath treatment and rest cure in psychiatry during the nineteenth and twentieth centuries (a project funded by the German Research Foundation).

Sarah Chaney is a Research Associate at the UCL Centre for the History of Psychological Disciplines. Her recent PhD thesis focused on the emergence of the concept of self-mutilation in late nineteenth-century psychiatry and psychology. She is currently expanding this into a monograph on the history of self-harm from 1850 to the present day. Her ongoing research interests include approaches to bodily damage and food refusal, patient narratives in mental health care and the role of art and art practice in the twentieth-century psychiatric hospital. She is the principal investigator on a Wellcome Trust People Award: 'Mansions in the orchard: Space, architecture and asylum in the "care in the community" era', exploring the twentieth-century Bethlem Royal Hospital.

Waltraud Ernst is Professor in the History of Medicine at Oxford Brookes University. She has published widely on the history of psychiatry, with a particular focus on nineteenth and early twentieth-century British India. She is the author of *Mad Tales from the Raj* (1991, 2010) and *Transnational Psychiatries and Colonialism* (2013). Her edited books include *Crossing Colonial Historiographies* (2010), *Transnational Psychiatries* (2010), *The*

Normal and the Abnormal (2006), *Plural Medicine, Tradition and Modernity* (2002), and *Race, Science and Medicine* (1999).

Jane Freebody is a postgraduate student in the Department of History, Philosophy and Religion, at Oxford Brookes University. Her areas of research include moral therapy, notions of well-being and occupational therapy, from *c.* 1750 to 1980. She is particularly interested in comparing French and English therapeutic approaches.

John Hall is a clinical psychologist by background. He has worked in Oxford since 1980, and was formerly head clinical psychologist for Oxfordshire and Senior Clinical Lecturer in the Department of Psychiatry at Oxford University. He then became Professor of Mental Health at Oxford Brookes University, where he is now a Research Associate in the Centre for Health, Medicine and Society. His main research interests are in the history of mental health in the twentieth century, especially changing patterns of professionalisation.

Ben Harris is a Professor of Psychology and Affiliate Professor of History at the University of New Hampshire, where he teaches courses in the history of psychology and history of psychiatry ('Madness in America'). His doctorate is in clinical psychology (Vanderbilt University) and he has held fellowships in the history of science and medicine at the University of Pennsylvania and the University of Wisconsin, Madison. His research lies at the intersection of the history of psychology, history of medicine and history of science. He is the former President of the Society for the History of Psychology and Executive Officer of the Cheiron Society.

Akira Hashimoto is a Professor at the Department of Social Welfare, Aichi Prefectural University, Japan. He received his PhD (Doctor of Health Sciences) from the University of Tokyo in 1992 and studied on a German Academic Exchange scholarship at the University of Dusseldorf, Germany (1992–94). He is currently researching the history of psychiatry in Europe and Eastern Asia in the nineteenth and twentieth centuries from a comparative point of view.

Sonja Hinsch graduated from the University of Vienna with a degree in sociology. Since 2010, she has been a researcher on the project 'The production of work', funded by the European Research Council. Her doctoral thesis is on the topic of work and non-work in forced labour institutes and workfare programmes in Austria, 1918–38. In 2014, she was awarded a postgraduate research fellowship at the Leibniz Institute of European History in Mainz.

Jennifer Laws is an interdisciplinary scholar at Durham University, where she enjoys an active membership in the Department of Geography and Centre for Medical Humanities. Her research interests include the relations between work and mental health; the philosophy of active therapies and, more broadly, the ethical and political constructions of active selfhood. Jenny teaches on a range of undergraduate and postgraduate courses in health and social theory, and currently holds an ESRC Future Leaders Award for the project 'The active patient: Energy and desire in active recoveries'.

Vicky Long is Senior Lecturer in Health History at Glasgow Caledonian University. Her research examines modern British history and the history of healthcare, and she has published on occupational health, work, disability, and mental healthcare. She is the author of *The Rise and Fall of the Healthy Factory: The Politics of Industrial Health in Twentieth-Century Britain* (2011) and *Destigmatising Mental Illness? Professional Politics and Public Education in Britain, 1870–1970* (2014).

Kathryn McKay is a PhD candidate in the Department of History at Simon Fraser University in British Columbia, Canada. Her research primarily focuses on the intersection between colonialism and psychiatry especially as it concerns the First Nations peoples of British Columbia during the late nineteenth and early twentieth centuries.

James Moran is Associate Professor in History at the University of Prince Edward Island, Canada. He is the author of *Committed to the State Asylum: Insanity, the Asylum and Society in Nineteenth-Century Ontario and Quebec* (2001). More recently, with David Wright, he co-edited *Mental Health in Canadian Society: Historical Perspectives* (2006), and with Leslie Topp and Jonathan Andrews, *Madness, Architecture and the Built Environment: Psychiatric Spaces in Historical Context* (2007). He is currently finishing a book called, *Non Compos Mentis: Madness and Civil Law in Trans-Atlantic Historical Perspective*.

Thomas Müller, Priv.-Doz. Dr med., MD, MA, is Head of the Research Unit for the History of Medicine at the University of Ulm's Centre for Psychiatry I/ZfP Südwürttemberg. He teaches the history of medicine at Berlin's Charité and at the University of Ulm. He is also curating the *Württemberg Museum of Psychiatry*. His main research topics are the history of psychotherapies and psychiatry, comparative history of medicine, international transfer of medical knowledge and science, 'Medicine and Jewry', and the integration of the history of medicine into current *curricula* of medical education.

Osamu Nakamura is a Professor of Philosophy at the School of Humanities and Social Sciences, Osaka Prefecture University, Japan. He has investigated the history of his home town, Iwakura, Kyoto, Japan, which has been famous for hosting mentally-ill patients since the middle of the eighteenth century. His doctoral thesis (Kyoto University, 2007) is 'Family Care of Mentally Ill

Patients in Iwakura, Kyoto, Japan – What Made Family Care of Mentally Ill Patients Possible and What Brought It to Its End?'

Leonard Smith is a Senior Honorary Research Fellow in the History of Medicine Unit, University of Birmingham. He gained his PhD in 1982. He has written extensively on the history of mental health institutions in eighteenth- and nineteenth-century England. In 2014 he published a monograph on the management of mental disorder in the former British West Indian colonies up to 1914. He trained as a psychiatric social worker and has worked professionally within the mental health field since 1972.

Valentin-Veron Toma, PhD, MD, MA, works at the Institute of Anthropology 'Francisc I. Rainer', in Bucharest, Romania. He is medically qualified, has done postgraduate training in social anthropology, and received his PhD in psychiatry at the 'Carol Davila' University of Medicine and Pharmacy. His research interests include medical anthropology, cultural psychiatry and the history of psychiatry.

Oonagh Walsh is Professor in History at Glasgow Caledonian University. Educated at Trinity College, Dublin and the University of Nottingham, she has published on a range of areas in modern Irish history, including Protestant women's social, political and cultural experiences, the development of the asylum system in the west of Ireland, and twentieth-century obstetrics. Current research interests include the impact of epigenetic change and the Great Famine in Ireland, 1845–1951.

Acknowledgements

Some chapters in this book are based on presentations given at the International Research Symposium on 'Therapy and Empowerment – Coercion and Punishment', held at St Anne's College, Oxford, in June 2013. Podcasts of some of the presentations are available at Pulse Project Podcasting, University Lectures & Science Education: www.pulse-project.org/node/549.

Thanks are due to The Wellcome Trust for sponsoring the event. Delegates greatly benefitted from discussions at the conference. Special thanks to Burkhart Brueckner, Wendy Bryant, Sally Denshire, Yolanda Eraso, Leisle Ezekiel, Tudor Georgescu, Catherine Lidbetter, Carol Mytton, Judith Pettigrew, Beryl Steeden, and Farzaneh Yazdani. John Hall's and Jenny Butler's intellectual and practical support of the programme was much appreciated. Without Emma Hallett's administrative help the event would have been much less productive and enjoyable.

Thanks also to those authors who did not attend the conference, but were willing to contribute chapters at short notice, enabling us to produce a book that is wide ranging in geographical and thematic scope.

Introduction

Therapy and empowerment, coercion and punishment. Historical and contemporary perspectives on work, psychiatry and society

Waltraud Ernst

Patient work was a major feature of lunatic asylums or mental hospitals during the modern period. It was considered not only therapeutic but also to contribute to the upkeep of institutions. Although many other aspects of psychiatric treatment have been focused on by historians, patient work has not received any in-depth, systematic assessment.[1] This can largely be accounted for by the enduring emphasis in the history of psychiatry on the medical ideas and administrative interventions that contributed to the transformation of lunatic asylums into mental hospitals and psychiatric care facilities. This book therefore constitutes the first attempt to examine patient work in a wide range of psychiatric institutions and to conceptualise the meaning of work in relation to its specific sociocultural, economic and political contexts. Due to the current dearth of studies on work and psychiatry, the closest thematic link with other historical literature exists in relation to the fields of industrial therapy (IT)[2] and occupational health.[3] The conceptual and methodological concerns connected with the central themes of this book therefore require further elaboration.

Labour, work and action

What kind of human activity counts as work has over time been subject to varied definitions. In its most basic, biological sense, human activity is essential to meet the need for sustenance and comfort. Beyond the satisfaction of basic necessities, its role in what makes man and woman human and enables them to realise their potential as social and political human beings has been a central concern for philosophers, economists and the general public. The amount of attention being paid to human activity, variously referred to as work, labour or action, tends to wax and wane with life's vicissitudes, relative economic prosperity, dearth and deprivation, and the cultural and ideological preoccupations of particular sections of society at particular times and places.

From his socially privileged position in fourth-century BCE Athens, the Greek philosopher Aristotle mused on the difference between labour and work on the one hand and political action on the other. He defined labour as activity that meets the basics of life, being connected with tasks of living that are necessary for survival (food production, shelter). Work entailed, in contrast, the creation of an artificial world of things that were of lasting value in the public realm and enhanced the quality of collective life. In this scheme neither labour (pursued by *animal laborans*) nor work (performed by *homo faber*) are considered free activities as they are shackled to the necessities of survival (labour) and the pursuit of a comfortable, collective or 'good' life (work). Both are also subject to prevalent social inequalities (such as slavery, social and gender stratification) within the household and the public sphere. Aristotle postulated a third kind of human activity that was situated in the public and political sphere and elevated above labour and work: action.

The fact that only full citizens, a minority of the population in ancient Greece, had access to the political arena does not, arguably, distract from the philosophical principles underlying the classical understanding of human activities. Inequalities and issues of power that frame labour, work and political action are recognised by classic philosophers, but not located at the centre of analysis in the same way that post-Enlightenment thinkers such as Marx, Foucault and Arendt have proposed. This underlines the complexity of dealing with the subject of work in relation to particular historical and cultural contexts and alerts us to the varied ways in which human activities have been classified. Despite various different emphases, modern authors tend to agree that the human condition entails more than the mere satisfaction of basic human needs through labour, insisting that all aspects of the classic tripartite scheme of human activity are required for a fulfilled and dignified life or *vita activa*. In other words, being alive as a complete human being, rather than merely as a fed, watered and exercised body is seen to entail the freedom to act and communicate freely. This premise should be an important ethical consideration in any investigation of people's work activities. In the case of patients such analysis is complicated by the fact that their activities take place within institutions that are expressly designed to inhibit the free expression of the full range of their inmates' physical, mental and emotional inclinations, and to segregate them from the wider public sphere and, and in some circumstances, to impose rather than merely encourage engagement in labour and work activities.

Other aspects of work and labour that require analytical attention are those highlighted by the political economists and their critics. While Adam Smith's distinction between 'productive' and 'unproductive' labour is now considered

Historical and contemporary perspectives 3

by mainstream microeconomics to be an outmoded aspect of his economic theory, its ambition to assess labour in relation to the wider context of capitalist production enables us to ask in what way patients' activities were productive and contributed to the generation of value and profit. According to the classical political economists of the eighteenth and nineteenth centuries, labour that produced value and was potentially profitable (as in the manufacture of a bed or chair) was considered productive, while labour that left no lasting result (such as domestic duties) was unproductive. What counted as 'productive' labour in institutional settings? Were the same criteria employed as in the world of manufacture outside the walls of the asylum? Were the goods resulting from productive work marketed outside the closed institution and hence part of the local economy and the wider cycle of economic production? Did patients' activities merely enable institutions to be 'self-sufficient' and, in Smith's reading, involve 'unproductive' labour in the shape of domestic tasks? Or was the labour performed in the asylum located outside the realm of modern market economies and hence its usefulness defined in terms of its contribution to a type of internal subsistence economy?

These economistic questions are important because, even if work in psychiatric institutions was not fully integrated into the structures of market-based economies and merely part of a mixed economy of subsistence and marketable labour, the monetary value attributed to patient activities in institutional financial accounts as well as asylum staff's perception of the social and economic value of particular types of work were ultimately anchored in and constrained by the premises of the wider economy extant at a particular time and place. For example, inside as well as outside institutions domestic labour did not count as a productive activity and hence was not entered into account sheets; nor was food produced for inmates' consumption. Surplus produce and domestic duties sold or performed by patients outside the asylum were, however, accounted for in monetary terms. The economic benefit derived from patients' labour and work, whether considered unproductive or productive, went well beyond what can be discerned from monetary value-focused institutional book keeping and superintendents' statements about the profit realised from the sale outside the institutions of goods and services produced by patients.

If the focus is shifted from work and labour to the person who pursues them, the issue of work satisfaction arises. Most prominently, Marx has dealt with this in depth. His notion of 'alienation' was developed in relation to labour performed in the mills and factories of industrial capitalism. It could be argued that this limits any applicability to patient work. However, some of its tenets help sharpen our focus on the varied ways work may have affected people, especially when their activities were not self-determined but dictated by others who, like Marx's bourgeoisie, held power over them within a highly hierarchical context characterised by inequality. Patients in the asylum lost the freedom to determine their life and destiny, and to direct their own actions. They may not even have been able to freely define their relationship with other people but have been ascribed particular roles (of patient *versus* staff; violent maniac; idiot). They were also usually not permitted to own the products of their labour and make use of the value of the goods and services they produced. Patients may therefore have been subject to one or several types of alienation that Marx has so deftly identified: the workers' alienation from, first, the product (no control over product, from design to its consumption); second, the act of producing (no choice of psychologically satisfying activity); third, themselves (being subjected to external demands imposed by others); and fourth, others (being forced to compete with others). All of these aspects require probing with regard to the very different institutional settings and conditions within which patients performed – mostly unpaid – work and labour.

However useful concepts such as alienation, unproductive labour and the tripartite systematisation of activity may be, we also need to consider that abstract categories and common meanings of work are not necessarily identical and that a great variety of understandings have prevailed and affected people's lives in different ways over time. The light-hearted 1960s British ditty that 'work is a four-letter word'[4] encapsulates sentiments and echoes the experiences of a generation of people that are worlds apart from, say, those who during the 1930s and 1940s put up gates at Nazi concentration camps that proclaimed '*Arbeit macht frei*' (work makes you free). Moreover, apparently identical definitions of what work is supposed to mean and achieve vary depending on the wider context. In Weimar Germany, for example, during the 1920s, public work-generation schemes intended to fight widespread unemployment used the same slogan of '*Arbeit macht frei*' that later was to become irrevocably linked with Nazi atrocities. From the point of view of some, the intention of the Weimar work schemes may have been to alleviate the misery of those suffering from structural economic factors beyond their control. For those who considered the unemployed as culpable loafers and criminal elements, they constituted a way of turning these people into morally less despicable citizens. Earlier usage of the phrase '*Arbeit macht frei*' during the late nineteenth century by authors such as the nationalist novelist and lexicographer Lorenz Diefenbach also accentuated the moral disciplining effect of work.[5] At the other end of the political spectrum, ant enthusiast, eugenic psychiatrist and one-time socialist Auguste Forel likened the 'free work' done by ants for the greater good of the insect colony to socialist collectivism, claiming, like Diefenbach, that '*le travail rend libre*'.[6]

The meaning of work is clearly subject to different interpretations that lend themselves to a range of ideological positions. The varied and wider social and political connotations and agendas that framed and influenced the perceptions of patient work in institutions, and the conditions under which it was performed, require as much attention as the medical ideas and regimes that are more commonly at the centre of histories of psychiatry.

Medical ideas

Activity or exercise has been a mainstay of a variety of medical paradigms. In the pre-modern period, they were, in the Graeco-Roman tradition, part of the six 'non-naturals', namely factors external to the body over which a person had some control. Motion or exercise (*motus*) was considered alongside rest and relaxation (*quies*), and together they figured alongside the other five constellations in Galen's pathology of the humours that required balancing out and use in moderation: atmosphere and environment; food (diet) and drink; sleep and wakefulness; retention and evacuation; and passions of the mind (emotions). Non-European traditions such as Ayurveda and Chinese medicine, too, identify activity as an integral part of their medical regimens. According to these medical systems well-designed activity has beneficial effects on both body and mind. Emphasis is on regulation of the body – and hence the mind – and on actions that facilitate its natural processes. Importantly, care has to be taken to avoid overexertion and strain. Therefore, in Ayurveda, exercise (*vyayama*) should avoid employing more than half the capacity of the individual and not consist of vigorous activities such as fast running. According to *Charaka Samhita* (*c*. 300–500 CE) 'death runs after one who runs'. Although Chinese Qigong exercises draw on various kinds of humdrum work activities, such as grinding the millstone, like Graeco-Roman and Ayurvedic medicine, it too emphasises moderation. Hard physical labour does not figure as part of a health-enhancing regime. In fact, in Ayurveda, for example, the facilitation of the capacity for work (*karma-smarthya*) constitutes one of the benefits of motion and exercise rather than a therapeutic aid in itself.

While the idea of activity, exercise and occupation as part of therapy is not confined to the modern period, the extent to which physical labour is supposed to be employed in medical regimens seems to have emerged only more recently. This may be linked to changes in the social and economic fabric of European societies that occurred from the mid-eighteenth century onwards. Some of these imbued work more generally with new connotations and accentuated particular meanings in the employment of activity as part of medical regimens. Foremost among these developments was the changing locus of the treatment of the mentally ill: To begin with, patients were confined in relatively small, mostly privately run madhouses, but, increasingly, from the mid-nineteenth century, they were housed in large-scale public lunatic asylums that provided for hundreds of inmates, in some cases even a couple of thousand. Institutionalisation on a progressively larger scale was expensive and an emphasis on motion or work rather than rest became a way of setting off the costs of public institutions during a period when the term 'industry' harboured its double meaning of 'processing of raw materials' and of 'industriousness'. Whole families, including women and children from the age of five or six, spent more time working than they had hitherto done in agricultural employment – in England between 1750 and 1800 annual working hours increased by at least one fifth.[7]

The idea of work as punishment also flourished, within the prison sector in particular, where inmates and those transported to penal colonies like Australia were forced to work. The ideal public institution, be it lunatic asylum or orphanage, was supposed to be, and frequently was, both a place of industriousness in the wider sense and, more specifically, an economically profitable place of industry, manufacture, or of otherwise usefully employed labour. We should not forget that in many countries the nineteenth century was not only the century of industrialisation and urbanisation but also the heyday of the workhouse, where inmates were forced to employ their labour power within a punitive context and to earn their keep. Work was an economic necessity and the workhouse was, as Jeremy Bentham put it, 'a mill to grind rogues honest, and idle men industrious'.[8] The workhouse also came to install, as Foucault suggested, a new 'ethical consciousness of labour', and turned it into a moral symbol that affirmed the value of work. Punishment, economic necessity and morals were intrinsically bound up. Attitudes of the elite towards work had evidently crystallised in Britain by the early and in Germany by the late nineteenth century as industrialisation took hold. Work was a moral duty and a source of individual improvement, both morally and materially. Values of thrift, toil and sobriety associated with the growing class of entrepreneurs derived, according to Max Weber, from a mindset he termed the 'Protestant work ethic'.

Within this context the meanings of 'motion', 'activity' and 'exercise' were no longer the same as in the Hippocratic or subsequent pre-modern medical traditions. Nineteenth-century and present-day social and medical understandings of work and of occupation as therapy are, from a historical perspective, very specific ways of conceptualising these terms. Currently, medical thinking chooses to focus on work as empowerment; on work satisfaction; on the aim of rehabilitation and reintegration; and on the dangers of 'bore-out' in the absence of meaningful and productive work (rather than of 'burn-out' in the face of overwork). Within institutional psychiatry, emphasis has shifted since the late eighteenth century. The aspects of punishment on the one hand and of self-improvement and economic and personal empowerment on the other were accentuated to a varying extent at different times, and both medical rationales and moral and economic considerations were appealed to by asylum superintendents and psychiatrists when they argued in favour of patient work.

During the eighteenth century patient work did not feature prominently within psychiatric institutions in Europe. It was employed by only some mad-doctors, such as Francis Willis who treated King George III in 1788. He set the monarch to work, alongside other men of distinction, on the farm and stables attached to Greatford Hall, near Bourne, Lincolnshire. Contemporary reports tell us that:

> As the unprepared traveller approached the town, he was astonished to find almost all the surrounding ploughmen, gardeners, threshers, thatchers and other labourers attired in black coats, white waistcoats, black silk breaches and stockings, and the head of each *'bien poudre, frise et arrange'*.
>
> These were the doctor's patients with dress, neatness of person, and exercise being a principle feature of his admirable treatment system where health and cheerfulness conjoined to aid recovery of every person attached to that most valuable asylum. (1796, French visitor)[9]

Willis's regime was based on the usual range of physical treatments such as blistering as well as on the carrot and the stick. Patients were told off for misdemeanours and symptomatic behaviour, fixed with the eye and put under physical restraint; when placid and symptom free they were allowed to engage in gentlemanly pursuits and polite conversation. More generally though, patient work was rarely used as part of asylum regimes.

With the emergence of 'moral treatment' around the turn to the nineteenth century, patient work became, as Andrew Scull put it, a 'major cornerstone' of treatment, with emphasis on the development of the patient's self-control, as distinct from control established by a therapist.[10] The York Retreat in Britain became the epitome of this kind of reformed regimen, along with Pinel's Salpêtrière. Historians have been divided on the role of work within moral treatment during the early nineteenth century. Foucault considered the Retreat's use of patient work as an attempt to impose 'a moral rule, a limitation of liberty, a submission to order, an engagement of responsibility' in order to 'disalienate' the mind.[11] Others believe that Foucault has overemphasised the repressive nature of occupation and moral therapy. While patient work might require subordination to routine and the acceptance of discipline, such habits were seen as important in preparing the convalescent patient for re-entry into the world outside the asylum.[12] On balance, it might be fair to suggest that work within the context of 'moral therapy' as practised at the Retreat aimed at social conformity through humane means.[13]

Moral therapy was a reform movement and for a while an inspirational ideal realised in but a few institutions in Britain, France and other Western and colonial countries around the world. Patients' experiences at the York

Retreat and establishments modelled on it were more salubrious than those persisting in old-style, unreformed institutions that made use of physical restraint and punishment. By the late nineteenth century, the principles of moral therapy were still widely celebrated, but the feasibility of implementing them in the large-scale public institutions that emerged all over Europe was restricted. Patient work, however, was more easily retained as a cornerstone of institutional management of the insane and an income spinner. Reference to patients' self-improvement through work was common in institutional reports and doctors' writings. The divide between rhetoric and practice and between favourable and even exquisite conditions for rich patients in private establishments and overcrowded and deteriorating circumstances for the poor in public asylums widened during the course of the nineteenth century and beginning of the twentieth century.

If we look at the available evidence on the wider context within which patient work was organised in the large public asylums of the late nineteenth and early twentieth centuries, we find that the emphasis came to be increasingly on institutional profit, intolerance to 'idleness' and work as the default setting rather than as a matter of patient choice. Reports of profiteering on the part of asylum staff, coercion of patients, and withdrawal of food and rewards such as cigarettes or outings as punishment for non-compliance were not uncommon for this period. The huge mental institutions of the late nineteenth and early twentieth centuries, were not only, as the anti-psychiatrist Thomas Szasz has suggested, places where madness was 'manufactured', but also became self-supporting if not lucrative manufactories or agricultural enterprises.[14]

The profit motive became in some countries entangled with eugenics during the first decades of the twentieth century. The *Gütersloh* model of Hermann Simon, for example, was for a while an inspiration not only for social psychiatrists in Europe and across the globe (for example Argentina and India) but also for those keen on ridding society of those who would or could not be productive.[15] His '*aktivere Krankenbehandlung*' or more active therapy entailed work being deployed in a planned and systematic way as a sheet anchor of psychiatric treatment. Those unable to work were labelled '*minderwertig*' (inferior) and considered as '*Ballastexistenzen*' (burdensome encumbrances) or '*soziale Parasiten*' (social parasites) who should undergo forced sterilisation or even be exterminated and hence '*erlöst*' (redeemed). Even if Simon's fully blown extermination regime was not adopted in other countries, his efficient, work-focused institutional design and the paradigm of work as social duty were well received.

Simon's and other late nineteenth- and early twentieth-century ideas on the role of work in the treatment of the insane were far removed from the classic, Graeco-Roman and other healing rationales that aimed at adjusting a patient's regimen of rest and motion in relation to his or her individual humour (or constitutional characteristics). Another major discontinuity with earlier and non-Western ideas during the modern period pertains to the emphasis on a person's social class or race rather than just their individual physical and mental condition. Willis may have got George III to engage in agricultural work, but the King laboured alongside gentlemen and other people of distinction. The emergence of large public institutions for the poor alongside private establishments for the rich during the nineteenth century occasioned a focus on what kind of work was suitable for what kind of social class. The work to be done by poor lunatics was very different from the active pursuits engaged in by gentlemen and ladies. In colonised countries, such as India, for example, racial considerations came into play, outweighing divisions of social class. Europeans of any social class were therefore exempted from physical work in mental hospital, instead being offered leisure activities for distraction and entertainment. Indians, in contrast, were expected to work and in some institutions their diet was cut if they did not comply. For Eurasians (people of mixed race), social class became again relevant, as those belonging to the higher classes were treated like Europeans and those of lower standing like Indians. It is particularly intriguing how race- and class-specific work therapy was justified. Medical and moral rationales were given, alongside economic considerations.

The poor in Europe and other races were seen to be used to physical work and hence there was a danger of alienating them from familiar pursuits if they were offered activities enjoyed by the higher classes and races. The rich in Europe and Europeans in the colonies would find physical work unseemly and therefore unsettling. Besides, their constitutions and moral sense were different from natives'. Class and racial differences were medicalised and environmental and hereditary factors that were seen to have a bearing on different social classes and races became criteria for the type of work, if any, that should be pursued in Europe and in the colonies. With the development of the discipline of anthropology during the late nineteenth and early twentieth century, considerations of 'culture' were linked up with medical and eugenic ideas, leading to the 'culturalisation' of race and the justification of varied work regimes in psychiatric institutions on those terms. The wider social, scientific and economic contexts impacted on how patient work was configured and rationalised, and how patients' experiences were framed.

It is from the early to mid-twentieth century onwards that patient work became increasingly viewed as an entitlement rather than a duty. Psychological paradigms were advanced by asylum reformers, which considered work as enabling, empowering and part of good physical and mental health. Periods of rest or leisure and work or activity had to be in balance and a new, professionally trained group of experts – occupational therapists – became responsible for this task. There remain debates on the cultural and social acceptability of particular types of work and activities for patients from different social and cultural backgrounds, but the link between work and coercion has been broken to such an extent that occupational therapists nowadays find it hard to consider that it had ever been part of their profession's history. Yet work, psychiatry and society are intrinsically bound up, and patients' experiences of work and activity in mental institutions have consequently been varied over time, being dependent not only on individual patients' predispositions and inclinations, but also on the wider social, institutional and medical contexts within which work is pursued.

Themes

The origins of work therapy have commonly been linked with the advent of moral therapy or moral management during the early nineteenth century. The first chapter, by Jane Freebody, investigates this link, identifying when patient work began to figure in English, French and Italian psychiatrists' publications on moral treatment. Freebody shows that while patient work was *de facto* employed in institutional regimes as part of the toolbox of asylum management from the later decades of the eighteenth century, it was not theorised as a central aspect of moral treatment in specialist publications until the early nineteenth century. This highlights the importance of considering both theories and practices in any historical account of a phenomenon such as work. Psychiatric textbooks and other publications may not always allow us to fathom what was actually happening on the ground. On the other hand, Freebody shows that in early psychiatrists' writings bodily exercise and mental distraction through activity *were* central aspects of moral treatment – albeit not necessarily in the shape of menial work. Moreover, they were almost exclusively conceptualised in relation to the humoral framework of the six non-naturals. In the late eighteenth-century treatises exercise remained invariably linked to the language and understandings of classic medicine, and no privileged role was attributed to menial labour in contrast to walks and active games. Later, in contrast, early nineteenth-century accounts increasingly tended to meld the previous, humoral conceptions with contemporary ideas about the moral and economic benefits of work.

The meaning of patient work within late eighteenth-century institutional contexts and its conceptual and tangible links with the prevalent medical, social and political ideas of its period varied from the way it was framed during the early nineteenth century. As medical theories gradually shook off the shell of humoral medicine, exercise, occupation and work became reconceptualised within new frames of medical theory and social conditions. Freebody maps this trend in relation to an emergent industrialising society struggling to contain the problem of the poor and the cyclically unemployed within a rapidly industrialising society (in the case of England); the post-revolutionary understandings of (aristocratic) idleness and productive labour (France); and a predominantly agricultural economy characterised by poverty and an acute rural-urban divide (Tuscany). Despite the very different social, economic and political circumstances in these states, the rise of moral therapy and of patient work occurred at a roughly similar time. This may be accounted for by the shared roots of humoral medicine and post-Enlightenment humanist thinking, which appear to have merged seamlessly with the ideas of moral treatment and the medical benefits of exercise in general and work in particular.

Freebody's account shows particularly well how specific ideas and practices travelled between institutions in France, Italy, Spain, England and Ireland, and across varied social and political cultures during the early period of patient work. The three chapters that follow focus on ideas and practices in institutions in northern America, which came to greatly influence European regimes of work therapy from the late nineteenth century onwards. Ben Harris highlights how ideas about, and practices of, patient work varied considerably at any particular period and over a range of private and public institutions in the United States. He traces the 'roller coaster ride in popularity/demonisation' (p. 56) of work regimens that were employed since the founding of asylums in the early nineteenth century. The nature of patient work changed concomitant on changing medical ideas, asylum management structures, and national ideology. Far from simply emulating ideas extant in the 'old country', American doctors developed their own, varied understandings and brands of what moral therapy and patient work ought to entail.

Harris deftly maps the waxing and waning of moral and psychological approaches and of patient work from the early days of therapeutic optimism to the rise of reductionist neurology in the 1880s, followed by 'a revival in the use of work therapy' at the start of the twentieth century – in New England in particular. The belief in the formation of good habits through regular work (which, as patients at Bethel, Maine, sang, while sawing wood, 'sets our spirits free!'), dovetailed with wider national sentiments of prosperity from natural resources and new technologies and with the corresponding belief that work could tap individuals' inner resources and restore good health. Alas, another wave of therapeutic pessimism in the wake of changes within the mind sciences, economic depression and the silting up of hospitals with chronic patients characterised institutional regimes from the 1920s onwards, with unpaid patient work coexisting alongside a variety of practices subsumed under the newly emerging specialism of occupational therapy (OT). The therapeutic value of patient work remained elusive well into the middle of twentieth century, when, as Harris points out, female patients, for example, 'may have worked as maids and janitors for much of their day with no therapeutic rationale, and then attended a brief OT class' (p. 71). The death knell of institutional care struck in the 1970s when the anti-psychiatry movement and the campaign against unpaid patient labour led a number of states to either close down institutions or therapeutic workshops.

As was the case in other countries, in the USA medical ideas and work practices travelled across national boundaries, some more so than others. Freudian psychotherapy and hypnosis were examples of the former, while, on account of Americans' sense of formal social equality during the nineteenth century, apprehension towards the socially segregative English system of separate institutions for the rich and the poor exemplified the latter. However, national sensitivities easily turned into prejudice and managerial, profit-orientated pragmatism, as the imposition of work regimes on immigrant paupers from Ireland attests. Harris points out that the Irish were considered a different race, 'accustomed to work' and beyond the reach of moral treatment. The economic value of Irish patient labour dominated over therapeutic considerations, in particular towards the late nineteenth century, when the profit motive was prominent more generally in the newly established hospitals for the chronic mentally ill. It is then that the observed lack of deference to authority on the part of American patients, in contrast to those from Britain, was remarked on by superintendents and the injunction against motivating incentives commonly used in European institutions (such as tobacco and beer) bemoaned. However, US practices and debates on patient work also echoed those in European countries, such as arts and crafts, Cabot's insistence on the therapeutic, socialising and intrinsically satisfying value of patients' work activities during the early decades of the twentieth century and the perceived gender-specific suitability of particular tasks (domestic chores for women; outside labour for men) during most of the nineteenth and twentieth centuries. The therapeutic and empowering effect on women who engaged in men's work (such as sawing wood), which was postulated and observed by Cabot and Gehring may, however, have stretched the sense of social and gender propriety of English middle and upper class observers.

James Moran explores the ways in which the 'cult of productivity' (p. 78) that characterised early to late nineteenth-century American society had a bearing on both civil trials in lunacy and on the organisation of patient life inside the New Jersey lunatic asylum. In his rich analysis of detailed case-studies he highlights how the capacity to work was seen by patients, families, doctors and court officials as central to good mental health. During court trials a person's willingness to perform productive work was a proof of a rational mind. Within psychiatric care settings, on the other hand, the connection between work and madness was framed in medicalised terms, with emphasis on the role of work in promoting rational behaviour through repetition of familiar tasks, stimulation of body and mind, and distraction from morbid thoughts.

Moran argues that the work–madness relationship assumed a central role in lunacy investigations and within the asylum respectively, but was configured in very different ways. Importantly, the link between work and mental status in the public and legal realms had been well established for centuries, while the idea of patient work inside an asylum was new to New Jersey, focusing on medical endeavours to rekindle rational thought and behaviour as well as on the financial and managerial benefits that could be derived. Within the asylum context, psychiatrists' promotion of patient work on account of the cost savings it entailed sat at times uneasily alongside their insistence that the labour of the insane was not real productive work. However, those who were admitted to the asylum, so Moran points out, 'were introduced to a very different world – one in which farm, garden and some domestic work may have been the most familiar element' (p. 95). Patients' involvement in various types of labour, it could be suggested, may have been more reassuring, and less alienating, than their experience of the other aspects of asylum life they were exposed to.

Like Moran's, Kathryn McKay's chapter provides a detailed analysis of work in a specific institution. She focuses on the Provincial Mental Hospital in British Columbia, Canada, during the late nineteenth and early twentieth centuries. Developments there differed considerably from those in the eastern provinces of Canada where colonial settlement had occurred nearly two centuries earlier. While by the late nineteenth century eastern provinces contained several well-established urban centres, British Columbia was still largely rural, relying on resource extraction and mobile groups of able bodied men, rather than agriculture and sedentary family units. The composition of the asylum population in the west therefore differed considerably from the social make-up of patients admitted to institutions of long standing in the eastern regions.

With regard to the establishment of health and welfare institutions, British Columbia may have lagged behind eastern provinces, but it shared with them a policy model that was very different from the one pursued in the neighbouring United States of America. There was an emphasis in the Canadian provinces on publicly funded rather than private provision, and on clear lines of financial and professional accountability for state employees. McKay notes that asylum staff and medical authorities in British Columbia were well aware of the need to economise and account for public funds as well as the contentiousness of patient work. This led superintendents to employ in their annual reports 'a number of strategies to address the tension between exploitation and therapy' lest they be accused of wrongdoings (p. 99). They had to tread a fine line between celebrating their managerial skills in saving public monies by making patients work for their keep, on the one hand, and establishing their own credentials as medical professionals skilled at implementing work as therapy, on the other. The annual reports were the means by which superintendents were able to account for and justify their practices.

McKay traces the shifts in the ways in which patient work was represented in the annual reports in line with changing governmental priorities. Given the relatively late emergence of publicly funded asylum provision in western Canada and persistent fiscal problems, patient work up to about 1900 was invariably presented as a 'most valuable means of medical treatment' (p. 105), yet predominantly framed in relation to monetary considerations and cost control. During the subsequent two decades, therapeutic concerns appear to have gained a higher profile alongside monetary matters and, what is more, the annual reports 'evolved from simple accounts of finances and patient statistics to a persuasive tool illustrating the modernity of the institution and, by extension, the province' (p. 106). Work as therapy was one of the ways in which staff at mental institutions could affirm that, despite allowances being made for local specifics (such as the prejudiced assignment of laundry duties to Chinese patients), their managerial and medical practices compared favourably with those pursued at the most progressive establishments in other provinces and in Europe. For an erstwhile frontier province known as 'the west beyond the west', the right balance between patient work as cost saver and medical treatment constituted an important way of affirming provincial pride and refuting potential contentions of backwardness.

Some aspects discussed by McKay, such as the role of well-organised patient work as a marker of modern hospital practice, and gendered and racially diversified work regimes, are echoed in the next two chapters on the two, very different, colonial contexts of the British West Indies and British India. While Jamaica, Guiana and Trinidad, like Canada, were settler colonies their economic rationale was based on the exploitation by a European minority of, first, imported African slave labour and, second, following emancipation in 1838, of *coolies* or unskilled labourers from South and South East Asia. British India, in contrast, while enabling European traders, merchants and industrialists to benefit from the wealth produced by indigenous labour, was never intended to become a region for wide-scale European settlement. Despite these differences, colonial policies and institutional practices in both the West and the East Indies drew heavily on British blueprints. With regard to the role of patient work, ideas and practices in both contexts followed closely those prevalent in the colonial mother-country during the nineteenth century, while at the same time dominant views of racial hierarchy and of different people's physical constitutions, mental characteristics and social milieus determined the ways particular activities were allocated to patients from varied backgrounds.

In the Caribbean, as Smith notes, the important role attributed to patient work in psychiatric regimes such as moral management fitted in well with colonial perceptions of the main role of colonised people. Given that 'the whole rationale for the existence of the Caribbean colonies was labour-intensive, large-scale production' of crops for European and American consumption, the resemblance to well-ordered plantations of the work and moral management regimes introduced into lunatic asylums from the late nineteenth century resonated with the broader colonial aims of the exploitation of cheap labour. However, superintendents also faced logistic limitations such as overcrowding (Jamaica, Guiana, Trinidad), shortage of material (Guiana) and lack of arable land (Trinidad) during the institutions' early decades. Belief in the curative role of work, however, was shared by superintendents, with Robert Grieve at Fort Canje, Guiana, in 1881 even attributing to labour 'a foremost place' in an asylum's 'pharmacopeia' (p. 149).

Smith also highlights the central role of the medical men who had been trained within the British public asylum system, were frequently charismatic and passionate about implementing European regimes of moral treatment and modern management to the colony, and increased institutional savings by rarely paying patients for their labours in cash or kind. On account of their previous experience in British institutions, superintendents would have been aware of contemporary controversies regarding the potential for exploitation of asylum inmates. From the point of view of doctors who found themselves within colonial contexts where the memories of pre-emancipation plantation labour were still vivid and work within asylums was elevated to a therapeutic in itself, unpaid patient work was not considered exploitative or a means of punishment but, as Robert Grieve put it, 'a privilege'.

Ernst's chapter highlights the shifts in the meaning of patient work. During the early nineteenth century, work tended to be firmly embedded in the rhetoric of 'moral therapy', with emphasis on kind and humane treatment of the insane. While still part of the wider framework of moral treatment, from the late nineteenth century, the prevention of 'idleness' was accentuated. In the early twentieth century, patient work became part of a medical paradigm that conceived of it as beneficial if not curative, alongside an array of other practices (such as hydrotherapy, sedation, tonics, and shock treatments). It was reconceptualised in the scientific terms of the period and, with the emergence of newly professionalised auxiliary medical disciplines, refashioned as 'occupational therapy'. The noted shifts largely echoed dominant psychiatric discourses prevalent in the West, but, as Ernst shows, the colonial context led to modifications in the ways in which particular work, as well as leisure, activities were employed highly selectively to fit the perceived needs and predispositions of different genders, races, castes and social classes. What is more, individual superintendents accentuated different aspects of patient work, employing it as therapy, to empower patients, as a means to combat idleness, to create institutional profit, and as forced labour. Patient work meant a number of different things and was implemented in varied ways.

The chapters by Akira Hashimoto and Osamu Nakamura consider another non-Western context. As in the West and East Indies, the trope of westernisation is at the centre of analysis. Japan did not suffer colonisation by any Western power, remaining an independent nation that began to industrialise and modernise rapidly in the wake of the emperor's restoration in 1868, achieving global military power. The opening up to external influences from the late nineteenth century encouraged the development of health and social welfare provision along Western lines. Hashimoto maps the prevalence of German influence in the conceptualisation and practice of patient work during the late nineteenth and early twentieth centuries and the impact of American ideas especially after the Second World War.

During the 1950s, the psychiatrist Kobayashi Hachiro developed a broader approach to OT, 'life therapy', which drew on the American habit training approach and included patient work as well as recreational activities. It became contested in due course, during the 1970s, when critics – in Japan as much as in Western countries – viewed patient work as exploitation of cheap labour. However, the American influence remained strong during the post-Second World War period, on account of the Allied occupation led by the Americans and the subsequent presence of British and American lecturers in training schools that delivered in English rather than Japanese curricula based on those devised for colleges in the United States.

Despite the prevalence of Western blueprints, modernisation has been closely entwined with Japanese nationalism. The lines between a narrow Japonism, critical challenges to unmitigated kow-towing to Western-centric discourses, and reflection on the cultural relevance of Western models of healthcare provision have been subject to debate in relation to psychological models that highlight the assumed cultural specificity of the Japanese character. The assumed specifics of the mental structure of the Japanese were focused on especially during the 1970s, when popular cultural theories and psychoanalytical ideas merged and dependence and immaturity were considered specifically Japanese traits. Around 2000, the ambition to move beyond Western blueprints led to the resurgence of these earlier ideas in the shape of an occupational therapy model (the *kawa* or river model) that has been portrayed as 'culturally relevant' to the Japanese context by its main proponent, Michael K. Iwama. However, as Hashimoto shows, and as was the case in earlier ethnopsychiatric paradigms, the *kawa* model, too, is based on the reification of Western-Orientalist ideas and cultural clichés such as collectivism and family orientation (in contrast to Western individualism and independence) and love of nature. Critics have argued that rather than freeing Japanese practices of OT from the predominance of Western paradigms that privilege individual autonomy and agency, culturalist models tend to reduce individuals to mere representatives of flawed role attributions such as 'Japanese', 'an Oriental' or 'a non-Westerner'. The issue of the relevance of therapeutic models developed in cultural contexts perceived to be different from those in which they are to be applied has been contentious in the wake of post-colonial and other critical thinking on the emergence of different kinds of modernity during the age of globalisation.

The impact of modernisation on the emergence of psychiatric services and patient work, and the role of wider religious practices and social concerns in this process, is also at the centre of Nakamura's chapter. He focuses on host family based care in the village of Iwakura near Kyoto. The practice began when pilgrims visiting the Daiunji-Temple for relief or cure of their mental afflictions were offered temporary or long-term accommodation by local guest-house keepers from the late eighteenth century onwards. The importance of temples, shrines and pilgrimage sites in mental healing and care provision has been documented for many places across the world. The expanding network of guest houses specialising in the reception of mental patients from the late nineteenth century in particular was likened to a Japanese version of the Gheel colony in Belgium. Hosts provided mainly for higher-class patients whose relatives were able to pay for their board, lodging and care by personal attendants and preferred the private and individualised arrangement to the more costly and potentially stigmatising admission into one of the private or public mental hospitals that began to emerge in Japan concomitant with modernisation. This system also relieved relatives of the responsibility of spending extended periods attending to their mentally ill family members at temples and shrines, as had previously been the case.

From the 1880s, doctors affiliated to the private mental hospital at Iwakura invariably emphasised the importance of patient work and leisure activities in the treatment of the mentally ill, framing existing institutional practices and the family host system extant in the village in reference to those prevalent in Germany and Belgium. Yet, the private host family arrangements were not consistently approved of by the provincial government on account of the lack of medical control and accountability, and patients' treatment within mental institutions was preferred. Notwithstanding these official preferences, guest houses continued to flourish, even after the Mental Custody Act of 1900, as existing institutions were unable to meet the demand for appropriate in-patient facilities. The scope for patient work within the family host setting was, however, very limited, as the paying, higher-class clientele did not necessarily consider it appropriate to engage in physical labour and domestic duties.

While the number of working patients remained low, Nakamura shows how the family host system contributed considerably to the local economy.

Local residents in an area with limited employment prospects and scarcity of profitable agricultural land were able to make a living from hosting the mentally ill. Once improvements in the local infrastructure enabled villagers to find paid work further afield and facilities for the institutionalisation of the mentally ill were extended rapidly during the post-Second World War period, the family care system declined. Attempts in the 1970s on the part of staff at the new mental hospital at Iwakura to introduce an open medical care system failed on account of local residents' resistance. Changes in the wider economic context and emphasis on institutionalisation of the mentally ill led to the decline of the 'Japanese Gheel'.

In contrast to Japan, family host care was considered mostly inappropriate within the context of two of the principalities of Wallachia and Moldavia, as the chapter by Valentin-Veron Toma shows. Medical doctors considered the local population in rural areas disinclined or unsuitable to act as hosts and carers for the mentally ill on account of their economic and educational backwardness, and prevalent prejudice and stigmatisation. Notwithstanding the introduction of land reforms and a democratic constitution during the 1860s and after the Second World War, some of the regions discussed by Toma were subject to feudal conditions based on the exploitation of the peasantry. Social unrest was rife in the principalities of Moldavia and Wallachia until 1878, when the new Kingdom of Romania was formed, while Transylvania was under Austro-Hungarian rule from 1867 until 1918, becoming part of Greater Romania in 1920. Notwithstanding the high level of political, social and economic instability in the region from which Romania emerged as a Soviet Union-ruled state between 1946 and 1950, institutional psychiatry was funded by charities and developed along western European lines in the former principalities up to the Second World War. The latter attests to the ambition of a local medical elite to seek out modern knowledge in neighbouring nations, in particular Austria, Germany, Switzerland, France, Belgium, Scotland and England.

As Toma shows, Romanian psychiatrists were highly qualified and knowledgeable about the organisation of patient work in Europe and America. They frequently visited the asylums considered most advanced at the time and reflected on the suitability for the varied Romanian contexts of the different models of psychiatry and patient work mooted abroad. Earlier French influences (in Sutzu's asylum at Bucharest, for example) were followed by reliance on mainly German, Belgian and American blueprints until a narrowly Pavlovian psychiatry emerged for a while after the Second World War. Psychiatrists like Sutzu, who ran the asylum at Bucharest from 1867, discussed the scope and limitations of the various organisational frameworks mooted in Europe, within which mentally ill people in Romania could be cared for and engaged in work activities. First among these was confinement in a lunatic asylum, with patients being involved in domestic and workshop activities. Second, was the German open door or agricultural colony system, in which farm work was done on land within or adjoining an asylum. Both of these options were implemented in the principalities, with the latter being considered by some (Sutzu and Obriega in Bucharest, Wallachia, and Braescua in Iasi, Moldavia) the most suitable for an agriculture-based region such as Romania. The third model, the British cottage or pavilion system, was championed by Mileticiu in Craiova (Wallachia). It allowed a high degree of segregation of patients and engagement in a range of workshop, garden and other activities. The fourth model, a modified version of the Belgian family care system was realised only at Sibiu in Transylvania. Here economic development and educational standards were considered high enough to allow for its implementation in the form of an agricultural colony that made use of family care under asylum doctors' medical supervision (under Szabo from 1872) and, subsequently (under Kalman from 1911) in conjunction with the open door system.

The institutional developments and work regimes prevalent in the different regions in Romania during the late nineteenth and early twentieth centuries, showcase particularly well the plurality of models for the cost-effective and therapeutically efficient organisation of patient work in psychiatry that were available at the time. As in other countries, from the 1930s the concept of 'science-based' work regimes emerged, which implied that patients' activities in knitting, rug making, basket weaving workshops were monitored regularly, and changed and adapted to individual patients' capabilities and needs. This practice, a version of Simon's 'more active work therapy', was referred to as 'scientific ergotherapy' in Romania and used for chronic and convalescent patients, alongside the 'old' standard regimes that involved domestic and agricultural work and small production workshops.

The chapters on patient work in German mental hospitals focus on two very different regions: the northern port city state of Hamburg and southern, rural Württemberg. Müller traces the unfolding of psychiatric provision in the oldest institution in Württemberg, Zwiefalten, from its early conversion from a Benedictine monastery in 1812 to the tragic impact of Nazism on the fate of patients. Work figured highly at Zwiefalten, in various configurations. During most of the nineteenth century patients performed domestic chores and from 1838 some were also employed outside the institution, contributing their labour to the local economy by assisting in the construction of roads and buildings and as journeymen to local craftspeople. By the 1870s, about two thirds of patients worked and agricultural activities were extended. Unlike in Romania, where wages were saved up until patients' discharge from the institutions, at Zwiefalten inmates received a small salary from 1816, which was paid out on a weekly basis to allow the purchase of small luxuries and additional food items. Superintendents stressed the voluntary nature of patient work, noting that the freedom to choose to engage in work constituted 'one of the main differences between an asylum and a forced labour facility' (p. 225). However, Müller alerts us to the fact that patients lost privileges and rewards if they declined to work. He notes that the 'boundaries between well-intentioned and therapeutically meaningful occupation and economic exploitation' may have been fluid (p. 225).

In contrast to rural Romania, where family care was considered unsuitable, in rural Zwiefalten the system was implemented in 1896. It was proposed by a nearby resident, the widow of the eminent psychiatrist Wilhelm Griesinger, and evidence suggests that it was well liked by patients, not least because restricted food provision in the hospital led to severe malnutrition and starvation among in-patients during the First World War and during the subsequent years of economic crisis. Although family care was considerably cheaper than in-patient services, even if hospital staff was required to monitor the arrangement during weekly visits as was the case at Zwiefalten, only about 3 to 4 per cent of patients were boarded out to local families who seem to have welcomed the presence of an extra worker in their midst. In contrast, a larger number of patients benefitted from the establishment of agricultural colonies in 1897, which allowed them a greater degree of independence than work within the asylum itself.

In relation to staff and food shortages, which led to the decline of work and leisure activities and the rise of mortality rates and illnesses, Müller raises again the uncomfortable question as to what extent the therapeutic role of work would still have figured prominently under these circumstances. No less distressing is the fact that 500 patients from Zwiefalten were killed during the 1930s and 1940s. These were mainly people considered as incurable and chronic cases. The inability to work was central for selection for gassing at Grafeneck under the central euthanasia programme, T4, or by lethal injection as part of decentralised euthanasia, euphemistically referred to as 'mercy killing'.

Monika Ankele's chapter highlights the central role attributed to the ability to work within and outside mental institutions. Ankele shows that earlier nineteenth-century medical conceptions of patient work that focused on diversion from unwholesome thoughts, relaxation and tiring out of inmates continued alongside an increased awareness of the economic usefulness of and psychological satisfaction gained through work, while the ambition to reintegrate inmates whenever possible into the labour market and life outside the institution gained prominence in the early twentieth century. She notes that the 'aims of work therapy resonated strongly with social and political mores that lay beyond the realm of the merely medical' (p. 243). Work and employment were central to the vision and identity of the Weimar Republic as a modern democracy and successful economy. As Ankele shows, both staff and patients at the Langenhorn asylum and agricultural colony near Hamburg were acutely aware of the wider social conditions during a period characterised by civil war-like episodes, hyperinflation, poverty and unemployment. She stresses that the meanings of patient work and of work outside institutions differed from those extant during the nineteenth century. They changed during the Weimar period in accordance with developments in the labour market and measures such as the introduction of accident insurance and welfare benefit schemes. Patients' perceptions of work inside Langenhorn, their willingness to submit to work therapy and their hopes and fears about rehabilitation were informed by what was happening in society outside the walls of the institution.

The permeability of the boundaries between work inside and outside the walls of the institution are a major focus of this chapter. Ankele explores this aspect through the lens of patients' varied understandings of their roles as inmates; their attitudes towards work therapy; and their prospects on discharge. Notwithstanding the fact that many of the patients at Langenhorn were considered as chronically ill (though able to work), inmates considered their confinement as a stage in their working life rather than as a permanent solution. Some even complained that while handicraft, agricultural and domestic work may have been beneficial for the institution's self-sufficiency, these outdated activities did not qualify them for employment in a modern, urbanised society. Others requested to be put into workshops in which they could make sensible use of and further hone their existing skills in order to increase their employability on discharge. On the other hand, there were also patients who were willing to work but did not wish to leave the institution, for fear that they would be unable to find employment outside and become a burden on their families. Unemployment had soared to record levels between 1928 and 1932 and Hamburg as a port city had been badly hit by the world economic crisis. In other cases, even patients employed in skilled work (such as in bookbinding) at Langenhorn felt that extended institutionalisation and separation from the outside world had made them unable to compete on the labour market. Ankele's evidence from the patients' case files shows the wide variety of patients' views.

There were also instances when patients felt demotivated once they realised that their chances of getting a job outside were slim. Ankele notes that staff understood patients' realistic concerns and worries, encouraging them to remove themselves from the institution gradually as part of an open door policy that made it possible to stay at Langenhorn while adjustment to working outside occurred. On the basis of evidence from Hamburg, Ankele suggests that the enduring trope in the history of psychiatry of the asylum as a place where inmates were kept against their will does not encapsulate what was happening at Langenhorn, where, as in Ireland during the famine years, mental institutions offered a refuge and shelter in a period of economic hardship.

Sonja Hinsch's contribution complements Ankele's and other chapters. It highlights that ideas on work prevalent in society at large and the application of work regimes within penal and other institutions are highly relevant for any comprehensive assessment of meanings and practices of patient work within mental hospitals. Hinsch examines how different kinds of work and nonwork were conceptualised during the interwar period in Austria, focusing in particular on those sent to forced labour facilities (*Zwangsarbeitsanstalten*). About 210 men and women were confined in these institutions in the mid-1930s. Under Austrian prison, workhouse and forced labour laws, conviction for vagrancy, begging or prostitution led to imprisonment. But those considered amenable to moral improvement and likely to develop an industrious attitude, were sent to forced labour facilities. Hinsch explores the criteria employed in definitions of industriousness and of socially and legally acceptable work and non-work. She shows that the criteria were multifaceted, including legal, moral and medical judgements. The multiply determined meanings of work and non-work contributed to the blurring of the boundaries in particular between illness and immorality, madness and badness.

Detainees in the forced labour facilities were seen to have failed to lead a morally and socially compliant life with engagement in a steady and socially and legally acceptable occupation. Not every kind of activity that guaranteed a living (such as prostitution) exempted a person from incarceration. On the other hand, the presumed disinclination or unwillingness to work, referred to as 'work shyness', was differentiated from the fate of those unable to find employment during a period of economic crisis. Depending on the type of activity and a person's perceived proclivity, non-work could be construed as morally and legally acceptable or as reprehensible. There was room for interpretation, as had been the case also in regard to the Vagrancy Act of 1885, which had not clearly stipulated the difference between begging due to necessity and begging on account of perceived work shyness.

Given this wider context, the implementation of patient work in mental hospitals can be expected to have engendered a variety of mixed feelings and complex attitudes among patients and staff even if it occurred within medical contexts – as Ankele has shown for Langenhorn. However, in contrast to mental hospitals, work in the forced labour facilities was designed to be backbreaking and challenging, with explicit emphasis on punishment rather than therapy. Resistance to the work regime or under-performance were invariably punished and inmates risked their lives if they tried to escape. Last, but not least, the criteria for discharge were related to proof of industriousness and improvement of attitudes and manners rather than relief from mental symptoms.

Sarah Chaney's chapter continues the theme of how wider social, political and economic concerns impacted on the meanings of occupation and on the perception of refusal to work or 'malingering'. Hers is the first of five chapters that focus on the meanings and development of patient work in Britain. As Hinsch shows for Austria and Ankele for Germany in the early twentieth century, Chaney notes for Britain also an increased focus on the rehabilitative dimension of patient work from the 1870s to the beginning of the First World War. Asylums aimed at turning patients into 'useful members of society' – both during their confinement within and, following discharge of those considered cured, outside the institutions' perimeters. Wider economic concerns drove the understanding of a person's usefulness. However, this understanding was still imbued with moral concerns and beliefs in the curative role of occupation. During a period characterised by debates on racial degeneration, mental deficiency and mental hygiene on both sides of the Atlantic, usefulness was seen to signify not only the capacity to earn a living but also entailed engagement in acts that were not considered morally or physically degraded. Within this wider context, those who refused to engage in useful activity were viewed with apprehension.

Chaney maps the shift from earlier understandings of malingering as moral failure to fulfil one's military or civil duty in society towards a predominantly economic meaning. This went along with psychological views of individual functioning that established links between behaviour and internal mental state, and between outer appearance and moral and psychological inclinations. The expansion of health insurance systems such as the Workmen's Compensation Acts of 1897 and 1906 (equivalent to the earlier German Sickness Bill 1883 and Accident Bill 1884), further accentuated the importance of medical experts acting as assessors for insurance companies differentiating between a person's physical or mental inability to engage in work and wilful or motiveless malingering.

While these wider changes framed the meanings of work both in society at large and inside mental institutions, there were also significant differences in the perception of patients' occupations. Any kind of occupation, be it leisure pursuits or work such as engagement in domestic chores, workshop activities and outdoor labour, were considered favourable to physical and mental health if not a means to recovery or even cure. Notwithstanding the emphasis in asylums on occupation or activity as part of the medical regimen of cure and care, the model of 'usefulness' could still be employed in relation to acute and curable as well as incurable or chronic patients. This was exacerbated under conditions of financial constraints that adversely affected many, severely overcrowded county lunatic asylums during the late nineteenth and early twentieth centuries.

Oonagh Walsh's chapter on work in the Connaught District Lunatic Asylum in Ballinasloe, County Galway, during the late nineteenth century further highlights the importance of the wider socioeconomic and political context in relation to medical practice and the status of patient work. The situation in the early Free State of Ireland was very different from England and Wales, marred by economic stagnation, little industrialisation, high levels of un- and underemployment, and long periods of starvation. Asylum inmates shared a homogenous background, with two thirds being made up of agricultural labourers and domestic servants. There was a scarcity of skilled and semi-skilled patients who could perform any more complex tasks than manual labour on the institution's farm. Although medical staff at the time recognised the therapeutic benefits of meaningful, non-monotonous activity, and considered inmates' ability and willingness to engage in steady work as a means of assessing their mental state and readiness for discharge, in practice occupations for male patients in particular were highly restricted. Female inpatients fared better in terms of variety of activities available to them, as they were engaged in a multitude of domestic chores for which they were considered suitable on account of their former lives as domestic servants or homemakers. Those among them who were diagnosed as suffering from 'puerperal mania' were also exempted from work duties, as medical staff were sympathetic towards their plight. These women were malnourished and exhausted and hence allowed to rest and eat before their discharge back into the community. Superintendents in Ireland were clearly well aware of the basic needs of over-worked and under-fed pregnant women and mothers.

Notwithstanding the importance attributed to patient work in terms of the therapeutic value of distracting patients from morbid introspection and exhausting the maniacally inclined as well as its substantial contribution to the maintenance of the institution, it did not generate any sizeable profit. The main income was derived from the few private patients' fees. As Walsh shows, it would have been difficult for the institution to market any produce or products during a period of economic stagnation, characterised by oversupply of cheap labour. With the majority of the population teetering on the verge of starvation throughout the nineteenth century, the English 'open-door system' and employment of patients in the surrounding area, which was implemented so successfully at the Zwiefalten Asylum in rural Germany, for example, was neither viable nor welcome in the Irish context. In fact, the establishment of the Connaught District Lunatic Asylum had been hailed on account of the expected boost to the local economy in the form of staff wages, tenders and rental of farm lands. It was hoped, as a local newspaper had put it in 1830, that it would 'transform this backward and remote district, bring a humane refuge for the mentally distressed, as well as the not inconsiderable benefit of substantial economic investment' (p. 307).

Walsh notes the resistance of the population to the institution's efforts to minimise costs and make the asylum self-sufficient. What they wanted was employment opportunities for the sane outside, not for the insane inside who had the benefit of food and shelter. Life was dire and people were at breaking point, as is attested by heart-rending petitions that Walsh has unearthed: 'The use of inmates denies men the opportunity to fend for their families, and greatly speeds the departure of those who are forced to seek employment on foreign shores' (p. 307). Inmates were clearly not the only ones who were yearning for the benefits of useful occupation at the most basic level. Protests against patient work and pressure to employ local labour and use locally made goods rather than relying on asylum produce sharpened from the 1880s, with the upsurge of the Catholic nationalist movement and the Irish Revival's attempts to replace English imports with local products. This indicates that an assessment of patient work needs to extend its glance and look not only from the inside out but also from the outside in.

John Hall's account of the development of OT within the wider context of patient work and occupation after the First World War returns our gaze to the more palatable grounds of governmental policies and the formation of professional bodies that provided the administrative frameworks within which a new profession emerged in England and Wales. While patient work in the main continued on similar lines as before within publicly funded mental hospitals, activities in private and charitable, or registered, hospitals became increasingly subject to guidance by specialist occupational therapists who had studied for a professional qualification in training colleges established during the 1930s and early 1940s.

Several themes emerge with regard to the rise of OT as a profession in its own right rather than a multitude of approaches to the organisation of patient work and activities supervised by staff from varied backgrounds and vocations. First, Hall notes the progressive shift from hospital-based work and activity regimes aimed at the occupation of patients with tasks thought to be beneficial to them alongside other therapeutic interventions towards activities that might facilitate social and economic rehabilitation. New approaches to the ways in which psychiatric in-patient facilities could be organised, such as therapeutic communities and sheltered workshops, were part of this process. Second, Hall notes the development of OT alongside other forms of patient activity that became professionalised during the same period, namely IT (focused on tasks and structures similar to those prevalent on the labour market outside institutions) and creative therapies (favouring engagement in art, music, and drama). Third, he identifies the reception of Continental and in particular American ideas and practices by those concerned with the establishment of professional training colleges in Britain, like Dr Elizabeth Casson at Dorset House, Bristol, and Dr Thomas Tennent at the Maudsley Hospital, London. Fourth, Hall's chapter highlights the tension and potential conflict between the formal authority of medical doctors and the increasingly perceived need for collaboration within multidisciplinary teams of experts from different professional backgrounds (psychiatry, nursing, OT, IT, creative therapies).

Last, but not least, the establishment of a peculiarly British brand of OT, which, in contrast to practices in other European countries, privileged arts and crafts, or pastimes and hobbies, rather than manual labour to the extent that students from arts colleges provided teaching input in the OT training colleges (Dorset House, Maudsley Hospital) is focused on. These kinds of activities were well suited to fee-paying patients from the higher social classes and attracted trainees who were in the 1920s referred to as 'well-educated, intelligent, refined type[s] of girl[s]' (p. 319). Given this class-specific trend, economic and financial considerations come less to the fore in Hall's account of the professionalisation of OT than might have been the case if work regimes in the hospitals dedicated to the reception of the poor had been at the centre of analysis. This highlights not only the pluralities of meaning in the conceptions of work and therapy, but also the issue that hospital practices and patients' experiences of work in a wide range of contexts cannot be mapped adequately and comprehensively through an assessment of the concerns and aims of one particular professionalised group. This is not to say that the rise of OT itself was not also, as Jennifer Laws has shown, subject to multiple experiences and meanings, continued contestation of what constituted therapeutic work and meaningful activity, and characterised by paradigm shifts that did not necessarily follow a linear trajectory.[16]

Following on chronologically from Hall's chapter, Vicky Long looks at the development of IT from the 1950s onwards. IT developed later than but alongside OT, further accentuating within the British context the divide between work, on the one hand, and leisure activities such as arts and crafts on the other. Long shows how patient work that was designed to resemble activities in factory environments lost its therapeutic function. She concludes: 'industrial therapy focused on work, at the expense of therapy'. There were also other problems. While the aim of rehabilitating long-stay patients in particular into the wider community and the labour market may have been achievable at a period of labour shortages during the decades following the Second World War, it became increasingly unrealistic from the mid-1970s when high unemployment and the deinstitutionalisation of the mentally ill occurred in Britain. Between 1957 and 1967 the number of industrial units attached to hospitals rose from 21 to 100, leaving only twenty-two psychiatric institutions without such provision. With the closure of mental hospitals in the 1970s, emphasis came to be on extra-mural, community-based provision. However, the focus on factory activities was no longer viable at a time when a shift in the economy from manufacture to the service sector occurred, resulting in IT becoming increasingly a means of occupying chronic long-stay patients in the few remaining hospitals. Once the full effect of the rundown of institutions changed the social demographic of in-patients, with mainly elderly patients remaining, the acquisition of workplace skills was no longer indicated, while newly admitted acute patients did not spend long enough in the hospital to make IT units viable. The emerging community-based day centres increasingly tended to focus on recreational as opposed to work-orientated activities.

Long's chapter highlights a number of themes that have been to the fore also in other chapters. The issue as to whether certain activities and the monotony of factory-style industrial labour for example constitute therapeutically valuable occupations meaningful for patients is one. It raises the question of whether potentially alienating work activities could be justified in therapeutic terms as helpful in the dis-alienation of patients' minds. As in Hall's chapter and those that focused on the German and Austrian contexts during the early twentieth century, the increased emphasis on patient work as a means of rehabilitation and on the dictates of the labour market contrasts with the nineteenth-century weight given to the benefits of work and leisure for in-patients as well as the finances of the institutions.

By the mid-1980s only a quarter of attendees at government-funded Employment Centres managed to secure employment in the free market, and the question was raised whether psychiatry ought no longer be involved in occupational matters, not least because sheltered workshops, Remploy activities and the like were more expensive to run than the cost engendered by unemployment benefits. Therapeutic considerations and concerns about whether life on unemployment benefits was good for people's mental health were less prominent in debates, while insistence on the principles of social inclusion have led to the withdrawal of government subsidies from the only remaining facilities that had enabled unemployed or unemployable mentally ill and disabled people to earn a living. Like everyone else, the mentally ill and disabled are expected to integrate into society and the labour market and share the social and mental costs concomitant to unemployment. As in earlier periods, the mentally ill themselves have rarely had a say in the matter of how they could lead a meaningful social and working life – inside or outside institutions.

Jennifer Laws' chapter challenges us to consider how patients' voices can be gleaned even from evidence that is not primarily concerned with the patient's view. In her elegant and methodologically sophisticated analysis of two case scenarios from the early nineteenth and early twenty-first century respectively, she puts emphasis on the *petits recits* or smaller, localised narratives that are embedded in the grand narratives of occupation as therapy, distraction, empowerment, improvement, punishment and as path to rehabilitation and employability. She identifies the recurring tensions between a perspective that couples work with rationality and reason (accentuated most vividly in Freud's contention that work connects an individual to reality, rationality and reason, and in Foucault's reading of the York Retreat as a place that exemplifies an episteme of governance) and an approach that appreciates the personal and affective encounters and the relationality inherent in humans' connectedness to work. Her analysis therefore moves beyond medical rationales of therapy, moral discourses of improvement, the intensifying economic rationalisation within therapeutic practice, and the statistics that chart the percentage of patients engaged in work inside and outside of institutions and their employability in the labour market. Laws explores the unquantifiable and elusive, yet deeply felt, friendships and kindly or hostile relationships that emerge alongside the formalised and increasingly standardised therapeutic encounter or 'alliance' between patient worker and staff member which defy quantification and rationalisation of their 'success' or 'failure' by means of audit trails and output statistics.

Laws' chapter rounds off the edited volume in more ways than one. It shows that regardless of the many changes that have occurred in the organisation of patient work and leisure activities, from the time of the Tukes' moral therapy to present-day therapeutic work and rehabilitation projects, and notwithstanding the varied models of patient work employed in different localities, we can identify in all of these scenarios traces of patients and their staff achieving what Marx called their 'species being'; moments when humans realise their humanity through their working relationships.

Notes

1 The few currently available case studies include: Jennifer Laws, 'Crackpots and basket-cases: A history of therapeutic work and occupation', *History of the Human Sciences*, 24 (2011), 65–81; Heli Leppaelae, 'Duty to entitlement: Work and citizenship in the Finnish post-war disability policy, early 1940s to 1970', *Social History of Medicine*, 27:1 (2013), 144–64; Urs Germann, 'Labour, silence and order: visualising modern psychiatry – strategies for legitimising Swiss asylum psychiatry in the context of occupational therapy in the interwar period', *Medizin, Gesellschaft und Geschichte*, 26 (2006), 283–310; Martina Huber and Thomas Müller, 'Patientenarbeit in Zwiefalten. Institutionelle Arbeitsformen des ausgehenden 19. Jahrhunderts zwischen therapeutischem Anspruch und Oekonomischem Interesse', in Thomas Müller, Bernd Reichelt and Uta Kanis-Seyfried (eds), *Nach dem Tollhaus. Zur Geschichte der ersten Königlich-Württembergischen Staatsirrenanstalt Zwiefalten* (Zwiefalten: Verlag Psychiatrie und Geschichte, 2012), pp. 71–84; Geoffrey Reaume, 'Patients at work: Insane asylum inmates' labour in Ontario, 1841–1900', in James Moran and David Wright (eds), *Mental Health in Canadian Society: Historical Perspectives* (Montreal: McGill Queen's University Press, 2006).

2 Vicky Long, 'Rethinking post-war mental health care: Industrial therapy and the chronic mental patient in Britain', *Social History of Medicine*, 26:4 (2013), 738–58.
3 Occupational health has recently become a well-established field: Vicky Long, *The Rise and Fall of the Healthy Factory: The Politics of Industrial Health in Britain, 1914–60* (Basingstoke: Palgrave Macmillan, 2011); Arthur McIvor and Ronnie Johnston, *Lethal Work* (London: Tuckwell, 2000); Arthur McIvor, *Working Lives: Work in Britain since 1945* (Basingstoke: Palgrave Macmillan, 2013); Roger Cooter and Bill Luckin (eds), *Accidents in History: Injuries, Fatalities and Social Relations* (Amsterdam: Rodopi, 1997); Janet Greenlees, '"The dangers attending these conditions are evident": Public health and the working environment of Lancashire textile communities, c. 1870–1939', *Social History of Medicine*, 26 (2013), 672–94; Barbara Harrison, *'Not Only the Dangerous Trades': Women's Work and Health in Britain, 1880–1914* (London: Taylor & Francis, 1996); Paul Weindling (ed.), *The Social History of Occupational Health* (London: Croom Helm, 1985); Carolyn Malone, *Women's Bodies and the Dangerous Trades in England, 1880–1914* (Woodbridge: Boydell, 2003); Joseph Melling, 'An inspector calls: Perspectives on the history of occupational diseases and accident compensation in the United Kingdom', *Medical History*, 49 (2005), 102–6; Steve Sturdy, 'The industrial body', in Roger Cooter and John Pickstone (eds), *Medicine in the Twentieth Century* (Amsterdam: Harwood, 2000), 217–24; S. Thompson, *Unemployment, Poverty and Health in Interwar South Wales* (Cardiff: University of Wales Press, 2006).
4 'Loving you is driving me crazy/People say that you were born lazy/'Cause you say that work is a four-letter word …/… .'
5 See Lorenz Diefenbach's work *Arbeit macht frei: Erzaehlungen* (Bremen: Kuethmann, 1873).
6 See Auguste Forel, *Les fourmis de la Suisse* (1874; La Chaux-de-Fonds: Imprimerie coopérative, 2nd edn, *1920)*; L. Daston and F. Vidal (eds), *The Moral Authority of Nature* (Chicago, IL: University Press, 2004); B. Kuechenhoff, 'The psychiatrist August Forel and his attitude to eugenics', *History of Psychiatry*, 19 (2008), 215–23.
7 Hans-Joachim Voth, 'Time and work in eighteenth-century London', *Journal of Economic History*, 58:1 (1998), 29–58, 33.
8 Roy Porter, *English Society in the Eighteenth Century* (Harmondsworth: Penguin, 1991), p. 131.
9 'Détails sur l'établissement du docteur Willis, pour le guérison des aliénés', *Bibliothèque Britannique*, Littérature (Geneve: Bibliotheque Britannique, 1806), pp. 759–73, quoted in W. L. Parry-Jones, *The Trade in Lunacy* (London: Routledge & Kegan Paul, 1972), pp. 183–4.
10 Andrew Scull, *The Most Solitary of Afflictions: Madness and Society in Britain, 1700–1900* (New Haven, CT: Yale University Press, 1993), p. 102.
11 *Ibid.*, p. 248.
12 Anne Digby, 'Moral treatment at the Retreat, 1796–1846', in W. F. Bynum *et al.* (eds), *The Anatomy of Madness: Volume II* (London: Routledge, 1988), pp. 52–72, 68.

13 Fiona Godlee, 'Aspects of non-conformity: Quakers and the lunatic fringe', in W. F. Bynum *et al.* (eds), *The Anatomy of Madness: Volume II* (London: Routledge, 1988), pp. 75–6.
14 Thomas Szasz, *The Manufacture of Madness* (London: Harper & Row, 1970).
15 Yolanda Eraso, '"A Burden to the State". The reception of the German "Active Therapy" in an Argentinian colony-asylum', in Waltraud Ernst and Thomas Müller (eds), *Transnational Psychiatries. Social and Cultural Histories of Psychiatry in Comparative Perspective, c. 1800–2000* (Newcastle: Cambridge Scholars Publishing, 2010), pp. 51–79.
16 Laws, 'Crackpots and basket-cases'.

1

The role of work in late eighteenth- and early nineteenth-century treatises on moral treatment in France, Tuscany and Britain

Jane Freebody

This chapter will assess whether British, French and Tuscan authors writing about the moral treatment of insanity in the late eighteenth and early nineteenth centuries advocated work as an essential aspect of this new method of treatment.[1] It will be argued that work was not considered an integral part of moral treatment throughout the period 1750–1840. The sources comprise sixteen contemporary publications focusing on the treatment of insanity, selected on the basis of their advocacy of moral treatment (rather than traditional methods), many of which have not hitherto been analysed with regard to patient work. Some of the publications, such as those of Samuel Tuke and Philippe Pinel, are famous, while others, such as those of Vincenzo Chiarugi and William Hallaran, are less well known. The texts published prior to 1813 were selected on the basis of their being the first known writings to include recommendations for moral treatment. More attention is given in this chapter to those that include references to work rather than advocacy of moral treatment more generally. Although Chiarugi does not mention work in his *Treatise*, the topic does arise in the hospital regulations for which he was believed to be responsible. The later texts were selected on the basis of their emphasis on the concept of work as a key element of moral therapy, following its introduction by authors Pinel, Hallaran and Tuke. The textual analysis is restricted to those aspects of the treatment that relate to recommendations for patient work, occupation and exercise. Most of the texts were written by physicians, although some were penned by non-medical proprietors of madhouses. The texts were meant for different purposes – as a practical guide to treatment, advertising a private madhouse, providing a reference book for other physicians, making a political statement or celebrating a relative's achievements – but they all offer an insight into the way moral treatment for insanity was perceived differently both regionally and over time. What the texts do not communicate is what was actually happening inside institutions for the insane, including those linked to some of the authors; such information can be found in monographs concerning individual institutions and is not the focus of this chapter.

The emergence of moral treatment and patient work

Historians of medicine have debated at length the emergence of moral treatment, but relatively little about the role of patient work within that framework. William Tuke and Philippe Pinel are the most well-known early proponents of moral treatment and both recommended patient work. But whether they were the originators of moral treatment is a contested area. Roy Porter traced the origins of moral treatment in England to the mid-eighteenth century. He believed that William Battie's insistence that 'management did much more than medicine'[2] and the methods outlined in his *Treatise on Insanity* (1758) set the standard for what became known as moral therapy in the nineteenth century. In his 1981 article, 'Was there a moral therapy in eighteenth-century psychiatry?' Porter claimed that, following Battie, eighteenth-century writers recommended 'occupational therapy', including some form of work for men, as an aspect of moral treatment.[3] The sources indicate, however, that work was not incorporated into moral treatment *theory* prior to the publication of works by William Hallaran and Samuel Tuke in 1810 and 1813 respectively.

Andrew Scull has argued that Porter was overstating the case in his insistence that 'both in rhetoric and in reality, "moral" forms of therapy were well tried and tested long before the close of the eighteenth century'.[4] Scull did not support William Bynum's claim that 'the pre-history of the concept of moral therapy appears quite meagre', nor the traditional view that Tuke's introduction of moral treatment at the Retreat at York represented a complete rupture with the past.[5] He disagreed with Porter's assessment of the level of continuity between eighteenth-century practices and the 'Utopian programmes of the nineteenth-century lunacy reformers', who advocated elaborate work schemes for their patients.[6] Leonard Smith agrees with Scull, claiming that 'the elevation of work to become a rationalised central element of therapy and rehabilitation in public lunatic asylums' did not occur until the early 1820s.[7] For Scull, the Tukes' emphasis on the development of the patient's self-control, as distinct from control established by a therapist, represented a distinct departure from the earlier methods of moral management. Work was a 'major cornerstone' of this new form of moral treatment, helping patients to restrain themselves.[8]

The role of work at the York Retreat has been evaluated in very different ways. Michel Foucault found the work regime at the Retreat repressive, referring to its 'constraining power', through which the patient was returned to 'the order of God's commandments', submitting 'his liberty to the laws that are those of both morality and reality'.[9] He accused the Retreat of using work to impose 'a moral rule, a limitation of liberty, a submission to order, an engagement of responsibility' in order to 'disalienate' the mind.[10] Anne Digby believed that Foucault overemphasised the repressive nature of employment at the Retreat. While the work might require subordination to routine, the acceptance of discipline or maintaining concentration were seen as important in preparing the convalescent patient for re-entry into the world outside the asylum.[11]

Focusing on developments in France, Jan Goldstein has pointed out that Philippe Pinel (1745–1826) never claimed sole responsibility for developing the moral treatment.[12] Dora Weiner draws attention to Pinel's awareness of the moral treatment methods practised in certain Spanish hospitals, which included work regimes for patients, praising these at length in his *Traité* of 1800.[13] Although no treatise appears to have been written by the early Spanish practitioners of moral treatment, reports by French travellers on the impressive treatment received by lunatics in Spain drew attention to their methods. At the Hospital General de Nuestra Senora de Gracia in Zaragoza, for example, records from the 1760s show that patients worked on the hospital farm, in the bakery and in the kitchens; others helped with cleaning the wards and with transporting patients unable to walk unaided. The work was not to be too arduous and the patients were visited by a physician twice daily.[14] Goldstein notes that Pinel also paid homage to a number of lay individuals of various nationalities, including Poussin, his superintendent at Bicêtre Hospital, whose daily care for the insane allowed him to glean much valuable experience.[15] Karen Grange referred to Pinel's admiration for the 'enlightened care in England' and his desire to follow the English lead, citing Pinel's article, 'Observations on the moral regime' of 1789, in which Pinel discussed the English methods, such as those of Dr Francis Willis.[16] Despite these influences, Pinel maintained that he was the first to explicate the 'moral treatment' fully and develop the technique scientifically.[17] Weiner claimed that Pinel's *Memoir* of 1794, which included a recommendation for patient work and was incorporated into his *Traité* in 1800, represented the 'earliest formulation of important new concepts and attitudes'.[18] Pinel is seen by psychiatrist Alexander Walk as a contradictory figure, on the one hand, adopting the coercive practices of Willis while, on the other, displaying great compassion for the insane with innovative humanitarian methods.[19] Pinel's use of coercion, however, was a last resort. If a patient ignored or took advantage of kindly treatment, the latter would have to be abandoned temporarily in favour of restraint. Pinel was clear that such measures should never involve corporal punishment and were not to be executed out of animosity or anger. Pinel believed that those who worked with the insane should exude a natural authority which could be deployed in circumstances requiring coercion, and it was this quality that he admired in Willis and Haslam. Pinel's attitude to coercive measures, which featured in his much earlier writing on insanity, coupled with his advocacy of therapeutic work, could be regarded as a crossover between moral management and moral therapy, according to Scull's definitions.

In contrast to the number of publications on moral treatment in England and France, works in English on the history of Italian psychiatry are limited; even in Italian, there are surprisingly few. Furthermore, according to Patrisia Guarnieri, those that exist tend to be written from a nationalistic and Whiggish perspective.[20] Most authors cite Antonio Maria Valsalva (1666–1723), Joseph Daquin (both the Italians and the French claimed Daquin as their own) and Vincenzo Chiarugi as the Italian precursors to Philippe Pinel. Although Valsalva, most famous for his work on the ear, is recognised as one of the first physicians to address and implement humanitarian treatment for the insane, Chiarugi does not mention him.[21] In fact, as Italian-American psychiatrist George Mora points out, Chiarugi made no reference to previous attempts to treat the insane humanely, nor did he cite the English literature alluded to by Pinel, save a brief mention of Battie.[22] Pinel was disparaging of Chiarugi's traditional approach, claiming in the introduction to his 1800 *Traité*, that 'it was Chiarugi's lot to follow the beaten track ... to return again to the old scholastic order of causes, diagnosis, prognosis and symptoms'.[23] Certainly Chiarugi, like many of the early English and French authors whose work is examined below, appeared to remain greatly influenced by the ancients, indicated by repeated references to the 'six non-naturals' and the centuries-old concept of 'regimen'.

The six non-naturals and attitudes towards exercise

The six non-naturals comprised air, food and drink, exercise and rest, sleep and waking, repletion and evacuation and the passions and emotions. These had to be carefully regulated in order to maintain a balance between the four bodily humours. Health would thus be maintained in a well person and restored in a sick person.[24] The non-naturals featured in the work of many influential seventeenth-century physicians, including Hermann Boerhaave (1668–1738) and Thomas Sydenham (1624–89). Their influence is reflected in the early texts on moral treatment, which stress the importance of routine, diet and the patient's surroundings, as well as exercise and amusements. Exercise is a recurrent, and frequently unexplained, aspect of the moral treatment texts. Moderate exercise was an important aspect of the six non-naturals and was discussed by a number of early modern writers. The Italian physician Hieronymus Mercurialis (1530–1606), whose work *De Arte Gymnastica* (1569) remained the standard text on physical exercise for centuries, argued that sport aided the body's metabolism and detailed a variety of exercises including running, jumping, wrestling, boxing, riding, ball games and dancing. Francis Bacon (1560–1626) suggested moderate exercise to protect the body against disease, but warned that overexertion could be detrimental to health.[25]

Joseph Addison, writing in the *Spectator* in 1711, extolled the benefits of exercise for 'the faculties of the mind' and advocated an hour's daily exercise. He noted that while both country life and industrious physical labour involved exercise, those engaged in studious or sedentary occupations were liable to neglect exercise and to suffer ill health, such as melancholia, as a result.[26] George Cheyne (1671–1743), in his *Essay on Health and Long Life* (1724), recommended exercise as part of a daily regimen for a healthy mind and body, noting the particular benefits of billiards and cricket for rheumatism, tennis for feeble arms and bell-ringing or pumping for a bad back. His book was extremely popular, running into eight editions.[27] Cheyne's theories were brought to the masses by preacher John Wesley (1703–91), whose *Primitive Physick* (1744) ran to twenty-three editions by the time of his death. Wesley aimed to make available to the public a simple guide to remaining healthy; he advocated daily exercise, such as walking or riding, in the open air.[28] The writing of Samuel Johnson (1709–84) indicated that swimming, dancing, riding, boxing, climbing, cricket and skating were all regular sources of exercise for the upper-class mid-eighteenth-century English male. Johnson remarked that exercise promoted health and a sense of wellbeing and that a lack of it led to mental and physical malaise.[29]

In France, Enlightenment philosopher Jean-Jacques Rousseau (1712–78) argued that manual labour and bodily exercise strengthened the constitution; in his book *Émile* (1762) he observed that men who exercised both their minds and their bodies lived longer.[30] The *Encyclopédie* (1751–72), edited by Denis Diderot and Jean d'Alembert, highlighted the health benefits of such sports as bowling, croquet, billiards and tennis. Other articles in the *Encyclopédie* advocated regular exercise as a means of promoting good health, through stimulation of the movement of the humours, ensuring good circulation and digestion.[31] The Revolutionary medical reformer, Pièrre-Jean-Georges Cabanis (1757–1808), while taking a more scientific approach, also regarded physical fitness as fundamental to health.[32]

The health benefits of regular, physical exercise for both the mind and the body were well recognised by the mid-eighteenth century in the context of both humoral and scientific medicine. However, while Addison's article, for example, suggests an awareness of certain occupations exercising the body, and of the need for those in sedentary professions to exercise during their leisure time, there is no suggestion that the term 'exercise' could mean 'work'. The authors of the texts on moral treatment, when recommending exercise for their patients, tended not to specify the type of exercise. But it would appear that exercise usually meant some form of sport or physical activity, such as walking or riding, rather than work.

English publications on moral treatment 1758–1810

William Battie (1703–76) was the first English writer to advocate 'management' of the insane, in preference to medicine, in his *Treatise on Insanity* (1758). Battie only eschewed medical methods of treatment when injudiciously applied, however, and much of his treatise refers to the appropriate administration of medicines and physical interventions, such as vomits or cathartics. Battie claimed that 'madness … like most other morbid cases, rejects all *general* methods' (italic in the original).[33] His adherence to medical and physical interventions, together with his readiness to inflict 'bodily pain' to 'divert the mind from its delirious attention', indicates considerable continuity with more traditional methods of treatment.[34] Battie suggested 'bodily exercise' as a remedy for idleness, even if a patient 'who has long indulged in idleness' was unwilling to 'put his body in motion'. While he was not specific about what constituted voluntary bodily exercise, Battie maintained that involuntary 'bodily exercise' could be stimulated through the use of 'vomits, rough cathartics, errhines, or any other irritating medicines', which would incorporate 'a great deal of exercise into a small portion of time, and that without the consent of the patient, or even the trouble of contradicting his lazy intentions'.[35] This suggests external control of the patient's behaviour, rather than the encouragement of self-control, and is coercive in tone. Battie did not mention work (therapeutic or otherwise) although observers noted in 1789 and 1799, and again in 1815 (subsequent, it must be noted, to Battie's retirement from St Luke's in 1764), that patients were engaged in occupations at St Luke's Asylum; some assisted with household tasks and others in building maintenance.[36] The motivation for such activities appeared to have been a mixture of economy and engaging the patients' attention, rather than actual therapy.[37]

William Perfect's (1731–1809) earliest work, *Methods of Cure in Some Particular Cases of Insanity*, appeared in a total of seven editions between 1778 and 1809, under a variety of titles. Constructed around a series of case histories, the first edition advocated a blend of medical treatment and management based on 'gentle methods' and 'temperance and moderation'. There was no mention of work, although Perfect described one patient who became insane after retiring from work and city life. While the man 'languishe[d] for want of employment' Perfect's proposed treatment plan of a light diet, bleeding and gentle purging, did not involve any alternative occupation.[38] His observations came tantalisingly close to recognising the importance of work to an individual's wellbeing, but Perfect did not actually recommend it as a remedy.

Benjamin Faulkner (? –1799), who was not medically qualified, ran a private madhouse at Little Chelsea in London. Faulkner wrote in 1790 that medicine could only offer partial relief and advocated treating the insane person as 'a rational creature' by 'presenting objects of amusement, directing the attention, and humouring the imagination', but not by working.[39] Both lay and medical proprietors of private madhouses, such as Faulkner and Perfect, advertised their premises on the basis of mild treatment in order to attract patients; the prospect of effective moral treatment methods were more attractive to patients' relatives than harsh, traditional regimes.[40] Upper-class patients, who could afford private madhouse fees, would have been unaccustomed to work, which may explain its absence from Faulkner's and Perfect's recommendations.

William Pargeter (1760–1810) aimed to gain control over the patient, as he revealed in his very practical account of insanity first published in 1792. His technique involved catching and holding the patient's gaze and establishing a rapport. Pargeter recounted his first meeting with one female patient: 'I went suddenly into the room, and had her eye in a moment'.[41] This technique, known as 'catching the eye', was associated with Dr Francis Willis, the physician and clergyman who successfully attended George III during his episodes of madness in 1788 and 1789. (Willis wrote neither treatise nor memoir, so his theories are not included in this chapter, but he was known for his harsh treatment of the King, which included forcing the latter to work in the fields.) Pargeter's methods did not extend to coercion, however. He emphasised his belief that 'brutish violence' was unnecessary and that beatings were ineffective, claiming that 'if maniacs are not to be subdued by *management*, or by the operation of fear, or both – *beating* will never effect it' (italic in original).[42] Pargeter declared that 'the government of maniacs is an art' and recommended that the physician 'employ every moment of his time by mildness or menaces, as circumstances direct, to gain ascendancy over them and to obtain their favour and prepossession'.[43] Pargeter's case histories mentioned the efficacy of proper diet, exercise (unspecified) and amusements, reminiscent of the classical regimen, but he did not mention work.

Based on his experiences as assistant physician (1789–90), and then honorary physician (from 1790), to the Manchester Infirmary's lunatic hospital, John Ferriar (1761–1815) advocated moral treatment in his *Medical Histories and Reflections* of 1795. He recommended 'a system of mildness and conciliation' when dealing with the insane, which, although it might not cure a madman, might at least 'soften the destiny of the sufferer'.[44] He sought to instil self-restraint through promoting discipline without terror or pain. He used solitary confinement and deprivation of light or food as punishment, and a system of rewards, including privileges (such as the use of a special room for convalescents) or demonstrations of confidence, to boost self-esteem.

Ferriar believed the patient must 'minister to himself' to affect a cure.[45] His methods were close in tenor to those of the Tukes, in their attempt to foster self-control by rewarding good behaviour rather than through inducing fear. Ferriar's writing predated the opening of the Retreat by one year, but he did not mention patient work. A large garden was available to certain patients at the Manchester Infirmary from 1783, however, although this could have been simply for exercise and a change of air.[46]

John Haslam (1764–1844) also recommended that the superintendent exert his authority over patients, having 'first learned management of himself'.[47] Haslam's 1798 work was based on his treatment of several hundreds of patients at Bethlem Hospital, and was referred to by both Pinel and Tuke. Although discoveries by the 1815–16 Select Committee investigation into madhouses revealed the dubiousness of Haslam's support for moral treatment,[48] in this early work Haslam stressed the need for 'gentleness of manner and kindness of treatment'.[49] Alongside the usual range of medical treatments, physical restraint (regularly deployed at Bethlem) should be used where necessary. Haslam maintained that instilling 'regular habits' would help madmen control their behaviour and insisted that lunatics should be 'made to rise, take exercise, and food at stated times', which would not only contribute to their health, but make them more manageable.[50] He advocated 'occupying the mind [of madmen] on different subjects' to prevent them from dwelling on erroneous ideas and opinions,[51] but Haslam did not suggest work as a diversion until much later. However, the records at Bethlem Hospital reveal that patients were being rewarded in money and alcohol for a variety of tasks at the end of the eighteenth century, such as assisting the cook, capturing escapees and needlework.[52] Such revelations are at odds with the Committee of the House of Commons' report of Bethlem in 1815 as a place of idleness and dissipation, although the work carried out by patients may have been due to understaffing rather than therapeutic considerations.[53]

The methods of Joseph Mason Cox (1763–1818) elucidated in his *Practical Observations on Insanity* (1804, 1811) sought to achieve external control of the patient. Cox's book, considered by Daniel Hack Tuke (1827–95) to be 'the best medical treatise of the day on insanity', discussed the therapeutic technique of 'swinging', using a rotary device designed by Cox, to whirl the patient around, inducing vertigo, vomiting and, eventually, unconsciousness.[54] Cox described the treatment as 'both a moral and medical mean', since its 'valuable properties' were 'not confined to the body' and acted on the mind as a powerful deterrent: 'Compliance was frequently procured by a threat of employing it [the swing]'.[55] Cox found the swing 'an excellent mode of secure confinement, and of harmless punishment'.[56] Cox readily admitted that his device invoked 'the passion of fear'.[57] While his methodology suggests coercion, in other passages Cox stressed his preference for gentle techniques, claiming that 'Maniacs of almost every description, are sensible to kindness and tenderness, and, in general, are to be managed and controlled with more facility by these than by harsher means'. Cox maintained that securing 'either fear or confidence' could be effective, although he preferred the latter. Deception of the patients by medical staff or attendants, however, was unacceptable.[58]

Thomas Arnold (1742–1816) published a three-volume work on insanity, the third volume of which focused on treatment (1809). He claimed that it was written on the basis of experiences gleaned during his forty years of running a private madhouse.[59] He advocated gaining the patients' 'esteem and confidence' in order to ensure their 'obedience to orders' and 'submission to due control'. Arnold believed that 'gaining Authority over them [the lunatics] is absolutely necessary', but on no account should any 'severe coercion, or painful chastisement' be deployed. Arnold's *Observations on the Management of the Insane* was probably produced to promote his Belle Grove madhouse and to counter criticism of his management of the Leicester Asylum.[60] Nonetheless, Arnold was clear that his humane management methods were not merely an end in themselves, but the most effective means of achieving a cure.[61] Arnold's treatise recommended regular exercise (the type was not specified) and 'various amusements and recreations of the mind and body'; he did not suggest patient work.[62]

A pattern emerges (although not entirely consistently) whereby the earlier English publications tended to focus on external control of the patient while publications produced at the end of the eighteenth century, such as that of Ferriar, as Scull observed, began to put more emphasis on establishing internal control, a concept later developed by the Tukes.[63] While some authors, such as John Haslam, did not mention patient work, records at their establishments suggest that work may have been going on, but not necessarily pursued for therapeutic aims. These aims might have been to render the patients more manageable, to assist with the smooth running of the establishment, to save money, or as a form of distraction. Such rationales might explain why no specific recommendations for work were made within the context of guidelines for moral treatment. Furthermore, work may have been considered less of a social duty in the closing decades of the eighteenth century, when the full impact of the industrial revolution was yet to be felt in Britain, than would be the case from the late 1810s, by which time modern working practices had become more widespread.

Early French authors, 1791–1801

The earliest French writer to advocate moral treatment methods, and deeply critical of contemporary care of the insane, was Joseph Daquin (1732–1815), whose work *Philosophie de la Folie* was first published in 1791. A revised edition, published in 1804, was dedicated to Pinel, although this was never acknowledged by Pinel.[64] Daquin's work was based on his experience as chief physician to the hospital at Chambéry, which had a special area reserved for the insane. Daquin expressed his humanitarian sentiments and the humane methods he preferred, and was sceptical about the efficacy of medicine. In line with the six non-naturals, he maintained that 'diet, exercise, roaming at liberty and above all, gentle words and kind treatment' were the most effective means of cure.[65] He disagreed with keeping the insane locked in their cells, and advocated that they should be allowed to wander in the gardens between meals, supervised by attendants, where the wonderments of nature could distract them.[66] Daquin did not mention work.

Philippe Pinel advocated a mix of both internal and external control of his patients. In his *Traité* of 1800 Pinel quoted at length John Haslam's views on 'gaining ascendancy' over the insane patient, which he regarded as essential in certain cases of 'periodical maniacs' and convalescents. He remarked that governing madmen of extreme irascibility and sensitivity required their superintendent to possess a rare combination of physical and 'moral' qualities, including firmness, an authoritative manner and physical strength. He should never threaten, but always deliver punishment swiftly if disobeyed. However, 'stupidity, ignorance and unprincipled behaviour ... may occasionally excite fear but will always inspire contempt'.[67] No acts of violence towards the patient, nor corporal punishment of any kind, were sanctioned by Pinel, not simply because of their cruelty, but because they exacerbated the patients' condition.[68]

Pinel first mentioned work in his *Memoir* of 1794, considerably earlier than any of the British authors. Here, in a lecture, he lamented the 'idleness of the inmates [of Bicêtre], and the lack of some manual labour to provide useful distraction from their sombre thoughts'.[69] In his *Traité*, Pinel praised the work practices adopted in the Zaragoza asylum in Spain:

> Mechanical work was not the sole objective: the institution's founders utilised the satisfaction gained through working the land, and the pleasure man derives from growing his own food and providing for his own needs, as a sort of counterweight to mental aberration.[70]

The patients worked hard in the fields all day, fulfilling a variety of functions according to the season, and returned to the hospital happy, calm and ready for sleep. 'Prolonged experience at this hospital [Zaragoza] has demonstrated this to be the most effective and reliable means of restoring reason; aristocrats who reject mechanical work, regarding it with disdain and arrogance, simply perpetuate their condition'.[71]

Pinel observed that children's natural vices – disobedience and idleness – disappeared during play, when they became active, focused and keen to obey the rules. He regarded those convalescing from insanity in the same light; they were undisciplined and reluctant to take exercise, after such a long period of inactivity. When given recreational activities or some sort of work, however, they were distracted from their wayward thoughts, their circulation was stimulated and they were later able to enjoy a tranquil sleep. When appropriate work (such as that provided by certain Paris merchants) was found for Pinel's patients at Bicêtre, they immediately became calm, responsive and lucid. Pinel expressed his desire that land could be found near the hospital so that his patients could grow their own produce and thus accelerate their recovery.[72]

Pinel maintained that all asylums for the insane should provide employment for their patients; even the furious should have some kind of physical occupation. In fact, physical work, rigorously executed, was, in Pinel's opinion, the only way to maintain health, good spirits and order. Idleness exacerbated madmen's symptoms, while physical work fixed their attention on something satisfying and helped them to maintain self-control (which Pinel described as *la police intérieure*).[73] Pinel's strong endorsement of work indicates his adoption of post-Revolutionary attitudes towards work and what it meant to be a useful citizen.

Tuscan publication, 1793–94

Chiarugi's three-volume work, *On Insanity* (1793–94), advocated inculcating fear in the maniac which Chiarugi believed was necessary 'for the safety of the attendants and which has a beneficial, sedative effect'. In order to win the patient's respect, 'the behaviour of the attendants, and of the doctor too, should be authoritative and impressive, but at the same time sympathetic'. Although he claimed that beating was forbidden at his institution, the Bonifazio Hospital, Chiarugi recommended 'whipping at the waist' for some unruly inmates. He suggested another way of inculcating fear in a maniac, namely submersion in water, 'until he starts showing signs of asphyxia'.[74] In another section, on treatment for 'inertia' or 'languor', Chiarugi recommended a 'light flogging on the back, arms and thighs' with 'bunches of nettles' to cause painful sensations lasting several hours.[75] These remedies were based on humoral ideas about the assumed benefit of counter-irritation and physical shock. Chiarugi did not appear concerned about inflicting pain, or at least discomfort, to bring about desired behaviour.

Chiarugi recommended travel for melancholic patients since it not only stimulated the mind and distracted the patient from fixed ideas, but 'The unusual physical movements are of great help for the body'.[76] He pointed out that the benefits of 'pleasant walks, long travels, merry company [for] insane persons' had been observed 'by Celsus, Hoffmann and many others',[77] and remarked that 'exercise of the body and of the spirit' would be useful in the treatment of inertia, although excessive exercise could be harmful. It was up to the physician to gauge the appropriate degree of both 'the time and the intensity of the exercise' and to apply 'the same reasoning' to 'exercise of the mind', although there was less danger of overstimulation to the mind than there was of over-exercise to the muscles.[78] As the disease subsided, the patient should be kept away from the factors which caused his condition, avoiding stress and adopting regular habits, which maintained a balance between the 'six non-natural things'. Care should be taken to 'keep the mind distracted, and relieved through moderate physical exercise, and, in line with the teaching of Celsus, through a yearly journey'.[79]

Chiarugi's advocacy of exercise appears greatly influenced by the classics, and less so by more recent scientific ideas on the health benefits of exercise.[80] His treatise does not mention exercise in the context of work. However, the regulations for the Hospital Bonifazio, which are believed to have been written by Chiarugi in 1788, or at least overseen by him, suggest that some work was carried out by inmates. Patients were not expected to do any work without the permission of the physician, but the latter might recommend it from time to time. If patients did engage in activities such as weaving, repairing shoes or sewing, they were to be paid accordingly, their money kept in a safe by the hospital administration, and given to them on discharge.[81] Reference to work in the Regulations suggests a recognition of the value of work as a distraction, or as a financial necessity for some patients. It is curious that Chiarugi did not mention the therapeutic value of such work in his treatise. He may, however, have considered it superfluous to emphasise something so obvious to those familiar with humoral medicine.

Later British publications, 1810–20

The first Irish and English works to specifically advocate patient work were those of William Saunders Hallaran, appearing in 1810 and of Samuel Tuke, published in 1813. William Hallaran (1765–1825), who was medically trained in Edinburgh, founded Ireland's Cork Lunatic Asylum in 1791 and wrote the first Irish textbook on insanity.[82] The institution at Cork was singled out by an (unnamed) Irish lunacy reformer as the best managed asylum he had not only ever seen, but ever heard of, 'realising all the advantages of Took's [sic] Asylum at York'.[83] Hallaran's 1810 text featured a whole section on patient work, the first of its kind, predating Samuel Tuke's *Description*.

Hallaran claimed that the advantages to be gained from regular bodily exercise could only be bettered by 'the union of corporeal action, with the regular employment of the mind'.[84] Hallaran lamented the fact that so many physically healthy lunatics 'for want of some suitable occupation' were 'obliged to loiter away the day in listless apathy', condemned to 'unavoidable sloth'.[85] He noted that some lunatics with appropriate experience 'from previous habits of industry in the handicraft line' could assist with house maintenance and repairs. This was encouraged, not merely to 'benefit the house' but 'with a view of affording some interruption to the *taedium vitae*' so common in institutions for the insane. Hallaran observed that the patients employed in moderate labour were happily oblivious of 'their real or imagined grievances'.[86] He monitored his patients' progress carefully to ascertain 'the practicability of employing the mind, by any species of bodily exertion' once they were in a convalescent state. This proved more difficult in the case of female patients, who were less inclined to accept 'more active employments out of doors', although once engaged in household duties, these rarely failed to 'accelerate the prospect of recovery'.[87]

It was important to ascertain the character of the patient 'by which means a suitable occupation' could be devised.[88] Hallaran described how one patient, who had hitherto shown no signs of recovery, was discovered painting pictures on the walls of his apartment. When furnished with the 'necessary apparatus for painting' the man began creating portraits of the attendants, demonstrating considerable skill. After leaving the asylum fully cured, the patient pursued a successful career in London painting miniatures.[89] Hallaran concluded that in addition to being indisputably beneficial for convalescents, a 'systematic arrangement of daily labour' was also appropriate for incurable maniacs who were capable of physical exertion. It would enable them to 'acquire the habit of rendering themselves useful to society', by diminishing the cost of their maintenance at the same time as allowing them some respite 'from the horrors of a hopeless malady'.[90]

Hallaran recognised the difficulties involved in putting this plan into action, but believed that its effectiveness made the extra effort required to enforce discipline worthwhile. He commented that of the 642 patients consigned to his care over the previous ten years, only fifty were incapable of 'devoting from six to eight hours daily to the ordinary duties of husbandry and horticulture'.[91] Here was a clear and unambiguous endorsement of the value of work and activity, published some three years before that of Samuel Tuke. The York Retreat opened in 1796, fourteen years before Hallaran's book was published, but the Cork Asylum had been established by Hallaran in 1791. While the Irish lunacy reformers appeared to be suggesting that the Cork Asylum incorporated the Retreat's methods, rather than vice versa, it may well be that Hallaran's methods were adopted by the Tukes. While Hallaran paid tribute to Cox (whose swing he adapted) and Haslam in his book, he made no mention of the Tukes. Furthermore, Samuel Tuke's phrasing of remarks relating to employment combined with bodily action bears a marked resemblance to Hallaran's text, suggesting that Hallaran's writing could have influenced that of Tuke.

Samuel Tuke's (1784–1857) *Description of the Retreat Near York* (1813) was written as a celebration of his grandfather William Tuke's (1732–1822) achievement, and although he aimed for 'candour and sobriety of representation' despite his 'partiality', he may have been overly laudatory.[92] Early experimentation led the Tukes to abandon 'drugs and medicaments' in favour of a 'moral regimen' designed to assist the patient 'to control himself'.[93] While Tuke acknowledged that 'the principle of fear' could be efficacious, he maintained that 'desire of self-esteem' acted 'still more powerfully' and encouraged madmen to 'struggle to conceal and overcome their morbid propensities'.[94] It would appear, however, that in the early days the Tukes used fear and methods of gaining authority over patients rather more than is suggested by Samuel Tuke's *Description*. The Swiss physician De La Rive, writing in the *Bibliotheca Britannica* in 1798, noted that, 'At first they [the patients] must be subjected; afterwards encouraged, taught to work, and this work rendered agreeable to them by attractive means'.[95] The word 'subjected' suggests that some form of intimidation was deployed, although Samuel Tuke, who quoted from De La Rive in an Appendix to his *Description*, was anxious to point out that such practices were no longer carried out.[96]

Samuel Tuke, like Pinel, regarded treating the insane rather like rearing children. He spoke of restraining them from certain activities and encouraging others.[97] Chiarugi also recommended that those in charge of maniacs should assume 'the role of a parent who restrains his children'.[98] Tuke remarked that 'As indolence has a natural tendency to weaken the mind, and to induce ennui and discontent, every kind of rational and innocent employment is encouraged'.[99] He advocated 'bodily exercise, walks, conversation, reading and other innocent recreations', activities which would 'fix the attention on objects opposite to their [the madmen's] illusions'.[100] But 'of all the modes by which the patients may be induced to restrain themselves, regular employment is perhaps the most generally efficacious', particularly employment 'accompanied by considerable bodily action'.[101] Tuke discussed the improvement in the mental health of a former gardener who was given work in the Retreat's garden,[102] and described how female patients were employed in sewing, knitting or other domestic affairs. The attendant should gauge the most appropriate employment for the patient in his care, aiming to indulge his wishes unless 'the employment he desires obviously tends to foster his disease'.[103]

In John Haslam's later work, *Moral Management of the Insane*, published in 1817, two years after the damning report on Bethlem by the House of Commons Select Committee, he emphasised the importance of occupation and amusements, including work. This publication may have been produced as a riposte to the accusations of patient idleness contained in the Committee's report, or in recognition of the popularity of the Retreat's methods. 'Whatever may be recommended as the mode of occupation ... labour or rational employment, and a varied union of both, will probably be found most advantageous', claimed Haslam.[104] He maintained that 'the secret of employment consists in discovering something which may rationally occupy the mind ... . And not an occupation which would induce idle habits, or tend to confirm his [the patient's] disillusion'.[105] Haslam stressed the importance of correctly judging when occupation should be introduced, since premature introduction could be detrimental to recovery. Such reflections on occupation, however, ran alongside a recommendation for manacles, rather than strait waistcoats, as a means of restraint and thus of external control.[106]

The assessment of publications on moral treatment from 1750–1815 shows that patient work did not figure prominently in British, French and Italian publications until the turn of the nineteenth century. As far as is known, work was not advocated in written form by Spanish authors recommending moral treatment, but it was definitely practised at Zaragoza. It would also seem that work was not considered an essential aspect of treatment by Chiarugi; it was, however, *de facto* part of the institutional regime and referred to in the hospital regulations. Pinel, Hallaran and Tuke were the earliest authors to regard work as an integral element of treatment. They recognised the benefits of exercise, but suggested that the value of exercise was greatly enhanced when combined with some sort of physical work. The latter was supposed to be tiring, satisfying and distracting. Work that did not involve physical exertion, such as sewing, was still considered beneficial as a distraction and a means of improving concentration and self-discipline. Late eighteenth-century English theories of moral treatment emphasised the principle of control through fear, but this was gradually being diluted and would eventually be supplanted by a recognition of the efficacy of self-control and desire for self-esteem. Although in the early stages, intimidation was also used as a means of control at the Retreat, the Tukes saw work as an effective means of instilling self-control, discipline and concentration. William Tuke, a successful businessman and a Quaker imbued with the Protestant work ethic, understood the value of such habits. Hallaran also suggested an economic motive, enabling even incurable patients to become useful members of society by contributing to the cost of their care. Pinel recognised the efficacy of both intimidation and efforts to instil self-control through work and other means, deploying both as the situation required, while Chiarugi paid less attention to attempts at establishing self-control and did not recommend work in his writings. While Hallaran and Tuke recommended that appropriate work was found for patients, the tasks themselves were relatively unsophisticated. The authors mentioned above devoted far less space to discussing the types of work, or the specifics of organisation, than authors writing a decade or two later.

English publications on patient work, 1820–40

It was only in the 1820s, when industrialisation and modernisation of the economy accelerated after the French Wars, and concerns about poverty and the unemployed escalated, that English recommendations for work practices in asylums became considerably more sophisticated. A much greater proportion of monographs on insanity written between 1820 and 1840 were devoted to discussion of the therapeutic benefits of work practices and how to organise them. For example, George Man Burrows (1771–1846), who had greater faith in medical than moral treatment to provide a permanent cure for insanity, still advocated a blend of both in his 1828 work and observed that 'inactivity debilitates the powers of body and mind'.[107] He recommended exercise, occupations and amusement, to which he attributed equal importance as 'auxiliaries to the powers of medicine'.[108] Burrows advised that 'each should be suited as much as possible to the rank and tastes of the patient' since 'a man of refined education would find exercise and occupation in digging, but no diversion of his morbid ideas'.[109] All public asylums should have a garden or land available for horticultural or agricultural work. Burrows commented that asylums located in manufacturing areas had the advantage that 'the majority of lunatics may be made to follow their several callings', which illustrates a direct link between new working practices and patient work. 'Such occupations not only tend to the amelioration of the patients' state', explained Burrows, 'but to diminish the expense of keeping them'.[110] At Wakefield, he reported, the patients manufactured the materials for their clothing and the surplus was sold.[111] He remarked that 'most lunatics are disinclined to work' but 'kind entreaties' or the promise of rewards encouraged them.[112] Burrows' concern for economic issues reflects the contemporary debate about the 'social question' in England and antagonism regarding the cost of maintaining the poor.

Sir William Charles Ellis (1780–1839) took the theme of occupation to a new level. Ellis, although raised in the Church of England, became a Methodist and was greatly influenced by the methods deployed at the York Retreat. He recommended patient work when his candidature was being considered for the role of superintendent to the new West Riding Asylum. According to Len Smith, his commitment to promote schemes of work, illustrated by his declaration that 'nothing is found so efficacious as employment', influenced his selection by the authorities, and he was appointed to the role in 1817.[113] He remained there until 1831, when he was invited to supervise another new asylum, at Hanwell in London.

At both institutions he introduced a comprehensive work programme for almost all physically capable patients, making significant cost savings.[114] 'In all institutions for paupers, workshops should be provided in which the patients may perform different branches of mechanical labour to which they have previously been accustomed', Ellis maintained in his 1838 treatise. Where this was impractical, the patient could be taught a new skill. Ellis recounted that at the Hanwell Asylum, 'there are no less than six shoemakers now at work, who never did anything of the kind before their admission'. Other patients were taught twine spinning and rope making.[115] Female patients, organised by a 'workwoman', helped in the kitchen and storerooms, were employed in the gardens or engaged in sewing and mending. Women capable of fine needlework were occupied making 'useful and fancy articles' for sale at a bazaar organised by the workwoman. Ellis reported that this activity was highly beneficial, generating great enthusiasm among the patients and a profit for the asylum, which was used to purchase an organ.[116] He claimed that around eighty-eight patients were regularly employed in the gardens at Wakefield.[117]

It is evident from Ellis' account that work was not only seen to be most efficacious but had also become a sophisticated operation, carefully geared to the patient's needs and previous occupation, and a means of instilling regular work habits. Ellis was writing his work at a time when debates concerning the Old Poor Law were at their peak; the work was published after the New Poor Law, with its emphasis on productivity and self-sufficiency, had come into effect in 1834.

French publications, 1820–40

Étienne-Jean Georget (1795–1828), a favoured pupil of Esquirol who wrote his treatise, *De La Folie* in 1820, before his master penned his own, held that work, which taxed the body more than the mind, was helpful in restoring physical fitness and diverted the attention away from fixed ideas. However, he made the point that work was more appropriate for the labouring classes than the higher classes, claiming that 'a great lady would not want to exercise her fingers, nor would a gentleman, used to doing nothing, want to tire his body'.[118] Gender was not made much of in the texts, but the allocation of appropriate work was emphasised, appropriate to the patient's sex, class and previous occupation. Georget noted that at the Salpêtrière, women benefited from knitting and making garments and every effort was made to find work for the men in line with their previous livelihood. Those who could not, or would not, work, however, were allowed to go for walks – even the furious. The rich could travel.[119] Here is a specific recognition of the different therapeutic requirements of upper and lower classes, which could reflect a renewed tolerance of the aristocracy (not shared by the Revolutionary Pinel) following the Restoration of 1815.

Jean-Étienne Dominique Esquirol (1772–1840), Georget's teacher and Pinel's dedicated disciple, published his treatise, *Mental Maladies*, in 1838. He recommended 'corporeal exercises, riding on horseback, the game of tennis, fencing, swimming and travelling' especially in cases of melancholy and epilepsy.[120] He claimed that 'exercise, in whatever manner it may be taken, is, without contradiction, one of our greatest resources, in combating lypemania'.[121] He advocated diversions such as travelling, taking charge of a garden, carriage driving or the 'practice of some profession'.[122] Attention should also be paid to the mind as well as the body, with the provision of appropriate stimulation for the imagination. In cases of mania, furious patients should be allowed out into the open air 'to surrender themselves to all their susceptibility of motion' and thus exhaust themselves.[123]

Esquirol commented upon Pinel's enthusiasm for occupying patients in cultivating the earth and supported his recommendation that every asylum should have a farm connected to it where patients could work. He observed that at the Salpêtrière hospital, the best results derived from the women engaged in manual labour. The women sewed, knitted, performed household chores or tended the garden. The rich, however, chose to substitute this 'precious resource' with 'walks, music, readings, [and] assemblages'.[124] Esquirol remarked that, 'the habit of idleness among the wealthy counterbalances all the other advantages which this class enjoy for obtaining a cure'.[125] He remarked that at the Hospital for the Insane at Zaragoza, the rich patients failed to recover, while the poor, who worked, were cured.[126] In his section on 'Melancholy', he noted that 'corporeal labour ... is the best check upon the passions, which it moderates'.[127] Esquirol suggested that 'an idle and inactive life' or the transition from an active to an indolent one, could bring on 'moroseness and mental torpor'.[128] Excessive study could have the same effect, particularly if it encroached on time which should have been spent resting or exercising. Musicians, poets, actors and 'merchants who are engaged in hazardous speculations' were also susceptible to melancholy, since their professions 'exalt the imagination and passions' and disrupt a balanced regimen.[129] Esquirol's emphasis on maintaining a balanced regimen, and taking care not to overexert the mind or body, still sounds very traditional and wedded to the classics. While English authors had developed more sophisticated recommendations for patient work by this time, neither Esquirol nor his immediate followers advanced their theories very far beyond those of Pinel.

Conclusion

It would be too simplistic to conclude that advocacy of patient work as an essential part of moral treatment corresponded directly to levels of industrialisation or to political circumstances. However, there is arguably a link between the introduction of recommendations for specific types of work activities, as opposed to mere physical exercise, and the recognition that self-control and self-discipline were effective means of improving insane patients' behaviour, and bringing it in line with what was considered appropriate for the time. The earlier recommendations for moral treatment were focused on controlling patients through the ascendancy of the physician, rather than by summoning their *police intérieure*. The problem with external control, as Scull noted, was that 'it could force outward conformity, but never the ... internalisation of moral standards'.[130] Some authors, such as Pinel, recommended a blend of both approaches.

In France, where the political situation had a greater influence than industrialisation on attitudes towards work, the Revolutionary emphasis on productivity and becoming a useful citizen can be clearly detected in Pinel's advocacy of work for insane patients, although Pinel also recognised the efficacy of measured intimidation. After 1820, the impact of industrialisation and social issues were much more evident in England. This is the stage at which, in England, recommendations for patient work became more sophisticated, coinciding with debates regarding the Poor Law and the costs of maintaining those unable to work. The level of sophistication in terms of the organisation of patient work was not mirrored in France at this time, which could be linked to the slower, less dramatic pace of industrial growth. The later French authors recognised the reluctance of the upper classes to co-operate in menial work, which was considered to be to their detriment.

In England, early nineteenth-century work practices required a flexible and efficient workforce; those who could not work needed to be 'remoulded', either in the workhouse or the asylum, and, if possible, returned to society to make their economic contribution. Tuscany, within the context of a united Italy, would have to wait until the 1880s for industrial growth to take off. What is more, Chiarugi, as Pinel commented, was more traditional in his recommendations for treatment, adhering closely to the classical concept of regimen. In Ireland, the dire economic situation may have compelled Hallaran to recommend ways in which his patients could not only contribute to the cost of their care, but also give themselves the best chance of securing employment outside the asylum.

In conclusion, patient work was not mooted as an integral part of moral treatment in Britain, France and Tuscany before the nineteenth century, although it was carried out in a number of asylums. Work was introduced at different times depending on: first, whether the author emphasised external or internal methods of controlling patient behaviour; second, the prevailing political, socio-industrial or economic circumstances; and, third, the extent to which the author relied on classical teaching with regard to exercise and occupation, rather than absorbing or promulgating emerging views on moral treatment.

Notes

1 Following Scull, I have used the phrase 'moral treatment' to include 'moral management' (largely based on control of the patient by the practitioner) and what became known as 'moral therapy' (based on the encouragement of *self*-control). For the purposes of this chapter, Britain comprises England and Ireland, but not Scotland. Scottish authors do not feature in this account.
2 William Battie, *A Treatise on Madness* (London: J. Whitson and B. White, 1758), p. 68.
3 Roy Porter, 'Was there a moral therapy in eighteenth-century psychiatry?' *Lychnos* (1981–82), 19.
4 Andrew Scull, *The Insanity of Place, The Places of Insanity – Essays on the History of Psychiatry* (London and New York: Routledge, 2006), p. 45.
5 William F. Bynum, 'Rationales for therapy in British Psychiatry, 1780–1835', *Medical History*, 18 (1974), 319.
6 Scull, *Insanity of Place*, p. 45.
7 Leonard Smith, *Lunatic Hospitals in Georgian England, 1750–1830* (London and New York: Routledge, 2007), p. 156.
8 Andrew Scull, *The Most Solitary of Afflictions: Madness and Society in Britain, 1700–1900* (New Haven, CT: Yale University Press, 1993), p. 102.
9 Michel Foucault, *Madness and Civilisation: A History of Insanity in the Age of Reason*, trans. Richard Howard (New York: Random House, 1965), pp. 247–8.
10 *Ibid.*, p. 248.
11 Anne Digby, 'Moral Treatment at the Retreat, 1796–1846', in W. F. Bynum *et al.* (eds), *The Anatomy of Madness: Essays in the History of Psychiatry, Volume II, Institutions and Society* (London and New York: Tavistock, 1985), p. 68.
12 Jan Goldstein, *Console and Classify; The French Psychiatric Profession in the Nineteenth Century* (Chicago and London: University of Chicago Press, 2001), p. 65.
13 Dora B. Weiner, 'The Madman in the Light of Reason. Enlightenment Psychiatry, Part I', in Edwin R. Wallace and John Gach (eds), *The History of Psychiatry and Medical Psychology: With an Epilogue on Psychiatry and the Mind–Body Relation* (New York: Springer, 2008), pp. 258–61.
14 Asuncion Fernandez-Doctor, 'Psychiatric Care in Zaragoza', *History of Psychiatry*, 15 (1993), 391.
15 Goldstein, *Console and Classify*, p. 72.
16 Kathleen M. Grange, 'Pinel or Chiarugi?', *Medical History*, 4 (1963), 375.
17 Goldstein, *Console and Classify*, pp. 65–6.
18 Dora B. Weiner, 'Philippe Pinel's "Memoir on Madness" of December 11, 1794: A fundamental text of modern psychiatry', *The American Journal of Psychiatry*, 6 (1992), 728.
19 Alexander Walk, 'Some aspects of the 'moral treatment' of the insane up to 1854', *The Journal of Mental Science*, 421 (1954), 820.
20 Patrisia Guarnieri, 'The history of psychiatry in Italy: A century of studies', in Mark S. Micale and Roy Porter (eds), *Discovering the History of Psychiatry* (Oxford: Oxford University Press, 1994), p. 249.

21 Steven H. Yale, 'Antonio Maria Valsalva (1666–1723)', *Clinical Medicine and Research*, 3 (2003), 35.
22 George Mora, 'Introduction', in Vincenzo Chiarugi, *On Insanity and Its Classification*, trans. George Mora (1793–94; Canton, MA: Watson Publishing International, 1987), p. cviii.
23 Ibid., p. cix.
24 Stanley W. Jackson, 'Introduction', in *Observations on Maniacal Disorder* by William Pargeter, ed. Stanley W. Jackson (Abingdon and New York: Routledge 1989), p. xxx.
25 Neil Carter, *Medicine, Sport and the Body – A Historical Perspective* (eBook: Bloomsbury, 2012).
26 Robert Batchelor, 'Thinking about the gym: Greek ideals, Newtonian bodies and exercise in eighteenth-century Britain', *Journal for Eighteenth Century Studies*, 2 (2012), 189.
27 Ibid., p. 186.
28 Samuel J. Rogal, 'Pills for the poor: John Wesley's primitive physick', *Yale Journal of Biology and Medicine*, 51 (1978), 86.
29 Julia Allen, *Swimming with Dr Johnson and Mrs Thrale: Sport, Health and Exercise in Eighteenth-Century England* (Cambridge: Lutterworth Press, 2012), pp. 10–12.
30 Carter, *Medicine, Sport and the Body*.
31 James H. Overfield, *Sports and Physical Exercise in Diderot's Encyclopédie* (University of Vermont, 1996), http://library.la84.org/SportsLibrary/NASSH_Proceedings/NP1996/NP1996g.pdf (accessed 23 July 2014).
32 George Lachmann Mosse, *The Image of Man: The Creation of Modern Masculinity* (Oxford: Oxford University Press, 1996), pp. 61–2.
33 Battie, *Treatise on Madness*, p. 93.
34 Ibid., p. 85.
35 Ibid., pp. 86–7.
36 Smith, *Lunatic Hospitals*, p. 156.
37 Ibid., p. 156.
38 William Perfect, *Select Cases in the Different Species of Insanity, Lunacy or Madness* (London: W. Gillman, 1787), p. 43.
39 Benjamen Faulkner, 'Observations on the general and improper treatment of insanity' [1790], in Richard Hunter and Ida MacAlpine, *Three Hundred Years of Psychiatry 1535–1860: A History Presented in Selected English Texts* (Oxford: Oxford University Press, 1963), p. 525.
40 Charlotte Mackenzie, *Psychiatry for the Rich – A History of Ticehurst Private Asylum, 1792–1917* (Abingdon and New York: Routledge, 1992), p. 26.
41 William Pargeter, *Observations on Maniacal Disorders* (Reading: Smart and Cowslade, 1792), p. 59.
42 Ibid., p. 130.
43 Ibid., p. 49.
44 John Ferriar, *Medical Histories and Reflections, Volume II* (London: T. Cadell, 1795), pp. 187–8.

45 *Ibid.*, p. 188.
46 Smith, *Lunatic Hospitals*, p. 155.
47 John Haslam, *Observations on Insanity* (London: F. & C. Rivington, 1798), p. 122.
48 Jonathan Andrews, 'Haslam, John (1764–1844)', *Oxford Dictionary of National Biography* (Oxford: Oxford University Press, 2004), www.oxforddnb.com/view/article/12548 (accessed 2 April 2014).
49 Haslam, *Observations*, p. 128.
50 *Ibid.*, pp. 129, 132.
51 *Ibid.*, p. 130.
52 Jonathan Andrews *et al.*, *The History of Bethlem* (London: Routledge, 1997), p. 213.
53 *Ibid.*, p. 213.
54 Hunter and MacAlpine, *Three Hundred Years*, p. 596.
55 Joseph Mason Cox, *Practical Observations on Insanity* (Philadelphia, PA: Thomas Dobson, 1811), pp. 152, 182.
56 *Ibid.*, p. 154.
57 *Ibid.*, p. 155.
58 *Ibid.*, p. 56.
59 Smith, *Lunatic Hospitals*, p. 154.
60 Peter K. Carpenter, 'Thomas Arnold: A provincial psychiatrist in Georgian England', *Medical History*, 33 (1989), 209.
61 Smith, *Lunatic Hospitals*, p. 156.
62 Thomas Arnold, *Observations on the Management of the Insane* (London: Phillips, 1809), pp. 10–13.
63 Andrew T. Scull, 'Moral treatment reconsidered: Some sociological comments on an episode in the history of British psychiatry', *Psychological Medicine*, 9 (1979), 421, 425.
64 Evelyn Woods and Eric Carlson, 'The psychiatry of Philippe Pinel', *Bulletin of the History of Medicine*, 35 (1961), 18.
65 Joseph Daquin, *La Philosophie de la Folie*, ed. Claude Quétel (Paris: Frénésie, 1987), p. 78 (trans. author).
66 *Ibid.*, pp. 92–3.
67 Philippe Pinel, *Traité medico-philosophique sur l'aliéntation mental, ou la manie* (Paris: Chez Richard, Caille et Ravier, 1800), pp. 194–5 (trans. author).
68 *Ibid.*, p. 195.
69 Philippe Pinel, 'Memoir on madness', cited in its entirety in Weiner, 'Philippe Pinel's "Memoir on Madness"', p. 732.
70 Pinel, *Traité*, pp. 225–6.
71 *Ibid.*, p. 226.
72 *Ibid.*, pp. 198–9.
73 *Ibid.*, pp. 224–5.
74 Vincenzo Chiarugi, *On Insanity and Its Classification*, trans. George Mora (1793–94; Canton, MA: Watson Publishing International, 1987), par. 176, pp. 691–4.
75 *Ibid.*, par. 100, p. 367.

76 *Ibid.*, par. 137, p. 516.
77 *Ibid.*, par. 103, p. 379.
78 *Ibid.*, par. 103, p. 378.
79 *Ibid.*, par. 187, p. 737.
80 Mosse, *Image of Man*, pp. 61–2 (in relation to Cabanis).
81 Mora, 'Introduction', pp. lvii–lix.
82 Brendan D. Kelly, 'Mental health law in Ireland, 1821–1902: Building the asylums', *The Medico-Legal Journal*, 1 (2008), 19; Brendan D. Kelly, 'Dr William Saunders Hallaran and psychiatric practice in nineteenth-century Ireland', *Irish Journal of Medical Science*, 177 (2008), 79–84.
83 Hunter and MacAlpine, *Three Hundred Years*, p. 649.
84 W. S. Hallaran, *An Enquiry Into the Causes Producing the Extraordinary Addition to the Number of the Insane* (Cork: Edwards and Savage, 1810), p. 101.
85 *Ibid.*, p. 101.
86 *Ibid.*, pp. 102–3.
87 *Ibid.*, p. 104.
88 *Ibid.*, p. 104.
89 *Ibid.*, pp. 104–5.
90 *Ibid.*, p. 106.
91 *Ibid.*, p. 106.
92 Samuel Tuke, *A Description of The Retreat, An Institution Near York* (1813; Charleston, SC: BiblioLife, LLC, 2009), p. xii.
93 *Ibid.*, pp. 133, 139.
94 *Ibid.*, p. 157.
95 Walk, 'Aspects', p. 817.
96 *Ibid.*, p. 817; Tuke, *Description*, p. 223.
97 Tuke, *Description*, p. 150.
98 Chiarugi, *On Insanity*, par. 173, p. 681.
99 Tuke, *Description*, p. 180.
100 *Ibid.*, pp. 152, 162.
101 *Ibid.*, p. 156.
102 This case is discussed by Jennifer Laws in Chapter 17.
103 Tuke, *Description*, p. 181.
104 Walk, 'Aspects', p. 823.
105 *Ibid.*, p. 823.
106 *Ibid.*, p. 823.
107 George Man Burrows, *Commentaries on the Causes, Forms, Symptoms, and Treatment, Moral and Medical, of Insanity* (London: Thomas and George Underwood, 1828), p. 704.
108 *Ibid.*, p. 706.
109 *Ibid.*, pp. 705–6.
110 *Ibid.*, p. 706.
111 *Ibid.*, p. 706.
112 *Ibid.*, p. 707.

113 Leonard D. Smith, '*Cure, Comfort and Safe Custody*', *Public Lunatic Asylums in Early Nineteenth-Century England* (London: Leicester University Press, 1999), p. 229.
114 *Ibid.*, pp. 231–2.
115 W. C. Ellis, *A Treatise on the Nature, Symptoms, Causes and Treatment of Insanity* (London: Samuel Holdsworth, 1838), p. 283.
116 *Ibid.*, pp. 299–300.
117 *Ibid.*, p. 304.
118 Étienne-Jean Georget, *De la Folie* (1820). Textes choisis et presentés par J. Postel (Toulouse: Edouard Privat, 1972), p. 144 (trans. author).
119 *Ibid.*, p. 145.
120 Jean-Étienne Dominique Esquirol, *Mental Maladies, A Treatise on Insanity* [1838], trans. E. K. Hunt (Philadelphia, PA: Lea and Blanchard, 1845), pp. 83, 168.
121 *Ibid.*, p. 227. Esquirol coined the term lypemania, to be used instead of melancholia.
122 *Ibid.*, p. 227.
123 *Ibid.*, p. 398.
124 *Ibid.*, p. 83.
125 *Ibid.*, p. 83.
126 *Ibid.*, p. 83.
127 *Ibid.*, p. 212.
128 *Ibid.*, p. 212.
129 *Ibid.*, p. 212.
130 Scull, 'Moral treatment reconsidered', p. 425.

2

Therapeutic work and mental illness in America, c. 1830–1970

Ben Harris

This chapter looks at patient labour in the United States from the birth of the asylum to the start of its demise in the 1960s. The focus is on the Northeastern states, where separate psychiatric hospitals originated in the 1840s and multiplied over the next half century. The story told here comes from histories of individual hospitals and histories of psychiatry, supplemented by the medical and popular literature on mental illness, and accounts written by former patients. These show patient labour playing a central role in the creation of asylums, their change from curative to custodial institutions and finally their dissolution.

One of the most compelling accounts by a patient is the 1946 novel *The Snake Pit* by Mary Jane Ward, based on her own hospitalisation at New York's Rockland State Hospital. Her protagonist, Virginia Cunningham, shared Ward's red hair, career as a writer and sharp sense of humour. Relevant to this chapter, Virginia was chronically sceptical about the therapeutic jargon of her hospital, where patients sat around doing simple embroidery that was deemed 'occupational therapy' or 'OT'. In response to the hospital's jargon Virginia:

> [I]nvented a private therapy. Thinking therapy she called it, T. T. All Right T. T. Lady, she would say to herself and then she would have her class in thinking … It seemed queer to her that the hospital had no interest in teaching its patients to think. [Its] goal was to Keep Them Quiet. Let people think and at once they are drawing up petitions and demanding Rights. There simply were not enough nurses to handle thinkers.[1]

Although patients produced little of value in OT in *The Snake Pit*, much of their days was devoted to free labour to help keep the hospital running. On the wards, patients mopped and scrubbed and did other janitorial tasks. Healthier patients worked in the hospital kitchen and when Virginia improved she served on a crew that cleaned the outbuildings where some of the staff lived. This labour was not called OT, but gave patients some diversion and allowed the staff to notice the patients' ability (or lack thereof) to follow instructions and act purposefully.

As Virginia came to realise in *The Snake Pit*, by the middle of the twentieth century most of the work performed by psychiatric patients had little if any claim to the status of therapy. A hundred years earlier, however, work by patients was often part of a therapeutic regimen. While this did not survive the death of therapeutic optimism in the late nineteenth century, the start of the twentieth century saw a revival in the use of and faith in work therapy. It centred in New England, where clergy, psychologists and physicians briefly collaborated in developing a pre-Freudian therapy as an alternative to the reductionist neurology of the 1880s. This did not last, as Freudians came to dominate psychiatric thought and the optimism of the 1910s was replaced by another wave of therapeutic pessimism. These internal trends in the mind sciences were accompanied by economic depression and the silting up of hospitals with chronic patients as quickly as they could be built. The results were the conditions so starkly conveyed in *The Snake Pit*, in which Virginia Cunningham cures herself when confronted by squalid conditions and a lack of real therapy.

Because the history of work therapy spans centuries and involves millions of patients, a full catalogue of its roller-coaster ride in popularity/demonisation is beyond the limits of this chapter. It would require a retelling of the entire history of psychiatry and allied fields, in which disputes over money, labour, patients' rights and therapeutic authority were a constant feature.[2] Instead, I look at key individuals, ideas and events in the development of patient work. My emphasis is on the relation of patient work to changes in therapeutic ideas, psychological theory, institutional realities and national ideology. As often happens in medicine, motives do not match outcomes and even small changes in practice could be overdetermined – as forces internal to a field interacted with political trends, changes in patient demographics and public attitudes.

Moral therapy and the birth of the asylum

The concept of therapeutic labour accompanied the birth of the asylum in America. Before the asylum could be created, madness had to be seen as a medical condition. Consistent with the Enlightenment view of man as existing in a rational universe, eighteenth-century medicine began to see madness as something other than caused by the supernatural. Still, the mad were often equated with brute animals and treated as such. To restore sanity, physicians devised 'heroic' methods to create dramatic bodily changes – such as gross changes in blood circulation – the most famous being Benjamin Rush's device to increase blood flow by whirling the patient and another to bind the patient's head and limbs to reduce the flow of blood to the brain.

More relevant to the birth of the asylum were *psychological* methods designed to restore the patient to his or her previously rational self. These included diversions from unhealthy thoughts or habits, and the use of fear, guilt and argument to steer the patient toward reason. As Nancy Tomes explains in her history of the Pennsylvania Hospital for the Insane, a variety of forces combined to create a more 'domestic' – and psychological – approach to mental illness in the 1830s. These included a changed view of human nature, the wealth brought on by the Industrial Revolution, and a more egalitarian view of social relations.[3]

This changed approach to mental illness first appeared on a separate ward created for lunatics at the Pennsylvania Hospital, before the Pennsylvania Hospital for the Insane was opened in 1841. Its inhabitants included the wealthy, justifying an environment and staffing appropriate to their social rank. They had games, personal musical instruments and a shared pianoforte, and staff who would converse, walk with patients and interact in a manner 'to awaken their minds'. The patients, in turn, seemed less fearsome.

> Playing on the harpsichord or working at their crafts, they hardly recalled the wild beasts of [Benjamin] Rush's generation ... The image of the furious, fierce, and dangerous madman so prominent in early hospital folklore gradually gave way to a more romantic vision of the insane as victims of human passion and frailty.[4]

Although some might attribute this change in therapeutic philosophy to the influence of Philippe Pinel and William Tuke, the physicians and Quaker overseers of the Pennsylvania Hospital appear to have changed their approach to madness independently of overseas examples. In Tomes' account, asylum directors in Italy, France, England and the United States had a shared problem of how to handle the insane. What they all discovered was the superiority of a 'sympathetic milieu' to heroic medical treatments and to confining the mad in individual cells in alms houses. The result was a new view of the physician and his relation to his patients and the hospital in which they lived.

In both the United States and abroad, the treatment of patients by a psychological milieu became known as 'moral therapy'.[5] As the director of McLean Hospital explained in 1841, its key components were 'separation, direction, classification, and occupation'.[6] That is, patients were first separated from the family and home situation that was blamed for their illness. They were then directed toward healthy thoughts and behaviour by their new environment, which included buildings, furnishings, and the asylum staff. Finally, they were occupied by diversions and work.

'Occupations and amusements' for the patients

Initially, this system was understood to operate in an implicit comparison to the religious conversion of the Second Great Awakening – a postmillennialist revival movement of the late eighteenth and early nineteenth centuries.[7] The patient would be saved from his illness through guilt over his degraded state, incentives for better self-control, and by emulation of the healthy – those closer to salvation. Later, the concepts of phrenology provided a more scientific version of how moral therapy worked. More specifically, its 'occupations and amusements [were] designed to stimulate the patients' latent reason and capacity for self-control'.[8]

Whatever the theoretical rationale, the key to moral therapy was the asylum superintendent. As exemplified by Thomas Kirkbride (1809–83) of the Pennsylvania Hospital for the Insane, this physician lived in the hospital and supervised every detail of asylum life. With the patient population capped at 250, he could supervise the staff, deal with crises and come to know each patient and customise the mix of the therapeutic measures he or she received. Initially this was how moral treatment seemed to work so well. Later, it was its undoing as large numbers of patients, housed in separate quarters could not be given the individual attention and treatment necessary for success.

At its best, however, this system of moral therapy was both effective and widely admired, as seen in this report of Charles Dickens's 1842 visit to the Boston Lunatic Asylum:

> Every patient in this asylum sits down to dinner every day with a knife and fork; and in the midst of them sits the [superintendent]. At every meal, moral influence alone restrains the more violent among them from cutting the throats of the rest; but the effect of that influence [is] a hundred times more efficacious than all the strait-waistcoats, fetters, and handcuffs that ignorance, prejudice and cruelty have manufactured since the creation of the world.[9]

When Kirkbride was at the height of his influence during the 1850s and 1860s, his hospital was a model for both lay reformers and his peers at other hospitals. What set it apart from later asylums was its mixture of social classes, with non-indigent families providing the funds that supported an individualised approach by staff. Most relevant to this chapter were the customised programmes of work or physical activity for each patient. They differed by gender and social class, with working-class patients employed in the garden and workshop (males), or kitchen (females). Wealthy patients, in turn, received their exercise in carriage rides and diversion in needlework. All these activities were part of a hospital-wide programme to occupy and divert the patients, which included calisthenics, lantern slide lectures and patient-created poetry and religious sermons.

In Dickens's account, the benefits of both work and amusement were clear:

> In the labour department, every patient is as freely trusted with the tools of his trade as if he were a sane man. In the garden, and on the farm, they work with spades, rakes and hoes. For amusement they walk, run, fish, paint, read, and ride out [in carriages] to take the air ... They have among themselves a sewing society to make clothes for the poor, which holds meetings, passes resolutions, never comes to fisticuffs or bowie-knives, as sane assemblies have been known to do elsewhere ... The irritability, which would otherwise be expended on their own flesh, clothes and furniture, is dissipated in these pursuits. They are cheerful, tranquil, and healthy.[10]

Patient interactions, orchestrated by the staff, were part of the therapeutic milieu. Two processes that authors cited as curative were emulation and ambition. In a process described a hundred years later in *The Snake Pit*, patients who lacked motivation were shown worse-off patients to inspire self-control and improvement. They were also supervised by patients doing better, to be a positive social influence rather than a money-saving device. In Kirkbride's scheme this worked because patients lived in a single building, allowing the best behaved to live closer to the centre core of rooms – where the paternalistic superintendent and his family lived.

Soon, political and economic pressures motivated younger physicians to call for alternatives to Kirkbride's system of moral treatment in one elaborately arranged hospital. A major factor was the increasing number of patients needing treatment, many of whom were chronic and failed to satisfy the optimistic assumptions of Kirkbride and his supporters. The Boston asylum visited by Dickens, for example, was soon overwhelmed by a mass of immigrant paupers and abandoned all pretences of therapy. Part of the problem was the number of patients and part was their ethnicity. In the northeast, a surge in Irish immigration meant that most of the asylum poor were of that nationality, which was considered a different race and part of 'the cast-off humanity of Europe'.[11] The Irish were considered more subject to insanity, either because of their poverty or poor heredity. They were also less likely to benefit from moral treatment. As prominent alienists explained, it was often impossible to establish the trust and easy communication with Irish patients that were required by this type of therapy.[12] They could, however, be put to work.

Dissident alienists argued in favour of emulating European experiments with alternative styles of housing. These included small, private asylums for the recovering wealthy and farm colonies of indigent patients who worked and lived apart from hospitals. As American physician Pliny Earle (1809–92) complained, 'We are looking too much toward comfort and too little toward labor; we are running after luxury, and away from work.'[13] In the view of reformers like Dorothea Dix (1802–87), changes in hospital design were needed that took advantage of 'the providential fit between the value of work in moral therapy and the capability of asylums [for the poor] to self-finance'.[14]

In 1862, psychiatrist and statistician Edward Jarvis (1803–84) offered an unsentimental, social psychological rationale for work-oriented hospitals for the chronically insane poor in Massachusetts, who were 'almost all natives of Ireland [and] accustomed to work':

> [I]f they work in the almshouses, they will do so at the hospitals; and if they work readily on the ward, they doubtless will be induced to work as readily in the shops … Let employment be established as the general habit, and idleness the exception, then the law of custom and sympathy would operate, powerfully on the few who would otherwise be induced to do nothing. Let the fields and the shops be the populous places, and they will be the popular ones. Then the wards will be lonely and wearisome to those who have life sufficient for action, and the self-control enough to direct their powers to any purpose.[1]

Defenders of the Kirkbride plan countered that the English system of poor farms and wealthy 'homes' violated Americans' sense of social equality. As Nancy Tomes explains, the traditionalists believed that 'separate facilities for the chronic insane implied acceptance of a stratified society with a permanent pauper class, a development that few Americans of Kirkbride's generation wished to accept'.[16] Those who knew political realities explained that colonies for chronic patients would be funded at the level of almshouses, reversing a hundred years of effort at bringing the insane out of prisons and poorhouses.

New hospitals for the chronic mentally ill

In an attempt to serve chronic patients but avoid the decent into the squalor seen in county institutions, the state of New York built Willard Asylum in 1869. Promoting itself as both fiscally prudent and humanitarian, it boasted twice as many staff as county-run poorhouses, which it hoped to afford by making money from patient work. Thus work was a defining characteristic of this type of asylum from the start, rather than a hidden scheme to subvert its founders' ideals.

In the years preceding Willard's creation, its design was vigorously debated in the National Association of Asylum Superintendents, showing the divergent ethical and therapeutic visions within the field. As both sides of the debate realised, this was a turning point in the care of the mentally ill, with consequences that took a hundred years to fully develop. The advocates for an exclusively chronic population explained that the existing hospital in Utica had a standard procedure of returning unimproved patients to their county of origin, where they were confined to almshouses. In both Massachusetts and New York, state-wide investigations produced reports condemning the conditions in which the non-hospitalised mentally ill were held.

As the New York legislature proclaimed in 1866, 'many have become, and others are fast becoming incurable from inefficient care and treatment. The time has arrived when legislative provision for them should be made', particularly because at least a quarter of these patients 'are capable of some labor [that] might be made productive in the maintenance' of an asylum.[17] Countering the argument that an asylum for chronics would be historically regressive, physician George Cook (1824–76) explained that the current conditions were medieval in the dirty cells where the untreatable were housed by county authorities.

Work also played a role in the debate on the question of whether acute patients should be included in an asylum such as Willard. Advocates of a mixed population suggested that some acute patients would help keep hospital conditions from receding from the public's consciousness. Advocates of a purely chronic hospital countered that 'having under care large numbers of recent cases [means that] the labor of patients is of little comparative value'.[18] Here one sees the economic value of work deemed more important than its therapeutic potential. To the advocates of Willard Asylum, both value and patient benefit could be achieved with a stable, non-excitable population. As the superintendent of Utica Asylum promised, 'with a good farm connected to [chronic] asylums, and the judicious arrangement and management of shops, one-half of the incurable insane of our country would perform sufficient labor to support themselves, and would be the happier and more healthy for the exercise.'[19]

Once built, Willard Asylum demonstrated the benefits and perils of a hospital founded to be less expensive than a regular asylum, more humanitarian than a poor house (in theory) but essentially non-therapeutic. In her study of the Willard and Utica asylums, Ellen Dwyer notes that the daily routine for the patients and attendants changed little from the asylums' opening until 1890.[20] They woke at 5:30 a.m. and began a rigid schedule of activities that was supposed to teach discipline. Patients took care of their less competent comrades, ate meals, washed dishes, cleaned the wards, and those who were able worked on the farm, in the wards, or in the asylum's workshops. Some cottages housed patients based on their work assignments, so that gardeners lived with gardeners, farm workers with farm workers, and so forth.

Patients were bribed or coerced into work, which was mostly unskilled and repetitive, particularly for women – who worked in the laundry or mended clothing (figure 2.1). Men helped build roads and buildings within the asylum (figure 2.2). They also built the roadbed for a privately owned railroad that brought coal and freight to the asylum and may have carried patients to off-site jobs as labourers.[21]

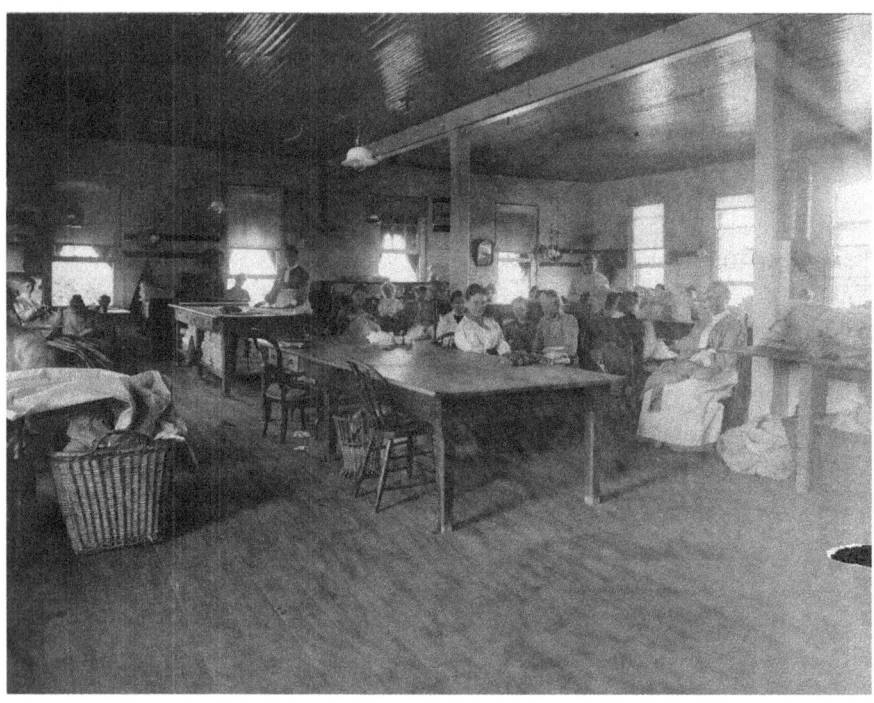

2.1 Sewing room, Willard Asylum, *c.* 1890.

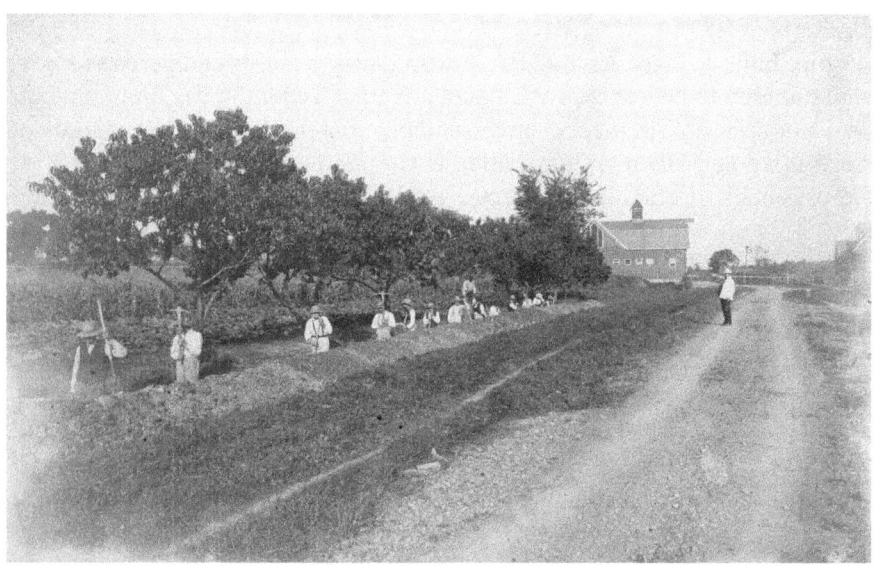

2.2 Men working outside, Willard Asylum, *c.* 1890.

Asylum superintendents complained that American patients were more difficult to motivate to work compared to those in England. This they attributed to the lack of deference to authority by American labourers and the significantly better conditions that English patients encountered compared with life in poorhouses. The psychiatrist and forensic scientist Isaac Ray (1807–81) also noted that English superintendents motivated their patients with rations of tobacco and beer, a practice not permitted in America.[22]

As Dwyer notes, the superintendent revived the rhetoric of moral treatment to justify the heavy reliance on work programmes. But, unlike Thomas Kirkbride, the medical staff was unlikely ever to meet most patients, relying on poorly trained attendants for information and interventions. Illustrating the asylum's lack of interest in work as rehabilitation or social reintegration, one patient lost his permission to leave the hospital grounds when it was discovered that he rented himself out to local farmers as a hand.[23] Apparently, he was talented enough to earn their admiration – but not earn a place in a less restrictive alternative to the asylum. And, despite the promise of the asylum superintendent, a large percentage of the patients did not participate in work programmes.

After the creation of Willard Asylum in 1869, other states built hospitals that housed patients in less expensive, smaller buildings and emphasised patient work to reduce costs. The most notable were the Eastern Illinois Hospital at Kankakee and the sixteen county hospitals built in Wisconsin on farmland, where patients worked and lived closer to their families. At the same time, more traditional hospitals were built and older ones were expanded.[24]

By the late 1880s, the creation of hospitals designed to house large numbers of poor patients 'inevitably returned to almshouse standards of care'.[25] The smaller, cheaply built buildings deteriorated at asylums like Willard, and overcrowding produced large hospitals that expanded to house more than 1,000 souls. As Nancy Tomes explains:

> [T]he developments Kirkbride had most feared – the abandonment of moral treatment, a purely clinical approach to patients, huge custodial hospitals, and a sharply class-differentiated system of mental health care – all came to pass in the late nineteenth century. What might be styled a 'cult of pessimism' thoroughly supplanted the old cult of curability.[26]

The eclipse of moral therapy

In the last two decades of the nineteenth century, the era of moral therapy ended in America. This happened as the spirit of the Kirkbride-style hospital was replaced by the custodial ethos of asylum bureaucracies, depriving moral therapy of its institutional home.[27] It also ended under an onslaught of criticism by neurologists practising the new, 'scientific' psychiatry. To them, the laboratory, dissection theatre and autopsy table were where one learned about the nature of insanity and its milder relatives, neurasthenia and hysteria.

One measure of this shift were the papers read at the annual meeting of hospital psychiatrists. By the early 1880s, their focus had shifted from managing hospitals to the diseases of the patients. And the discussion of disease 'reflected a new interest in pathology, physiology, and pharmacology, and a willingness to experiment with surgical and endocrinological treatments of insanity. All these approaches had relatively little in common with mid-nineteenth-century moral therapeutics.'[28]

By today's standards, the flaw in the new psychiatry was its extreme somaticism, which created a backlash that would revive moral therapy under a different guise in the 1910s. But in the 1880s, the list of embargoed concepts were not just spiritual and moral ones. Also rejected were mental processes, cognitions and beliefs, not to mention anything subliminal or unconscious. While skilful neurologists like S. Weir Mitchell (1829–1914) *used* psychology to understand and cure their private patients, the writings of Mitchell and his colleagues were generally anti-psychological.[29]

In Nathan Hale's history of psychotherapy, the intransigent somaticism of late-nineteenth-century neurology is exemplified by the reaction of neurologists to a paper by their senior colleague George Beard (1839–83). The author of *American Nervousness*, Beard was a model of scientific rectitude and biological enthusiasm. No friend of metaphysical or spiritual concepts, in 1874 he attended a seance in Vermont in disguise to gather evidence exposing two brothers who made their living as mediums.[30] Relevant to psychiatric problems, Beard believed in a biological energy that obeyed the laws of thermodynamics and fuelled the human organism and its systems. Neurasthenia, he believed, was caused by nervous depletion.

Two years after exposing the spiritualists, Beard read a paper to fellow neurologists, 'The influence of the mind in the causation and cure of disease'. In it he cautioned that mental factors could either neutralise or aid other therapies, and needed study. To his surprise, the response to his paper was furiously negative. One senior neurologist said Beard's ideas would lead the field 'back to monkery – give up our instruments, give up our medicines and enter a convent'.[31] James Jackson Putnam (1846–1918), who would later embrace psychotherapy and Freudianism, asserted in 1876 that no disease had ever been cured by a therapist's psychological influence, and that the study of emotion was inherently unscientific.[32] In such an atmosphere, the personal influence that was the basis of moral therapy was no more welcome than the practices of Christian Science or Theosophy.

From rest cure to work cure

Less than two decades later, dissenters from this anti-psychological consensus surfaced in New England, the home of transcendentalism, Swedenborgianism, Christian Science and a number of mind cure sects. By the 1890s a group of neurologists, psychologists and psychiatrists centred in Boston was openly promoting psychological healing, which included therapeutic work. To Harvard-affiliated neurologist Morton Prince (1854–1929), *psychotherapy* could create proper habits in patients and would prevent nervous breakdowns in times of stress. The process was two-fold and used the psychology of suggestion. 'The attitude of the physician,' Prince wrote, 'should be largely that of the trainer to the athlete. He is to teach the patient to help himself.'[33] This would occur by autosuggestion, inculcating new habits of the sort described by William James. For bad thoughts or habits that were resistant, the physician himself would use direct suggestion and personal influence.

James Jackson Putnam was another Harvard neurology professor who converted to psychotherapy. He spoke in 1899 of a wave of research 'sweeping us toward a better knowledge of the secrets of the mental life in health and disease'.[34] A third colleague was Richard Cabot (1868–1939), a young physician who became head of out-patient medicine at Massachusetts General Hospital in 1898 and founded the profession of medical social work. It was Cabot who first explained to the public in 1908 the nature of 'psychotherapy' in a new periodical with that title. In his view, psychotherapy was simultaneously 'mental, moral [and] spiritual'.[35]

Most relevant to this chapter, Cabot became the leading advocate of the work cure for neurosis in North America. Before explaining the work cure's benefits, Cabot described its relation to the 'rest cure', popularised by S. Weir Mitchell as treatment for the nervous depletion described by Charles Beard. Writing in *Psychotherapy*, Cabot cited William James (1842–1910) and New Thought maven Annie Payson Call (1853–1940) on the need to re-educate patients in the exercise of their will. As they explained in their 'gospel of relaxation', fatigue is caused not by excess exertion but frantic misdirection of the patient's energy. Thus, rest must be accompanied by changing the beliefs ('the old adhesions of the mind') that caused the frenzy and misapplication of the will to useless or harmful ends.[36]

Comparing the neurotic to someone with a sprained ankle, Cabot explained that re-education through work was equivalent to bodily exercise under the doctor's supervision. 'Many neurasthenics were born tired and have been getting more tired the more they rest,' he explained. 'Nothing will ever rest them but work, just as nothing cures the weak sprained ankle except exercise, painful though that is.'[37] Switching metaphors, he said the neurotic was like a prodigal son who has run up debts and seeks his father's help. A wise father, Cabot explains, will demand a reformed life just as the psychotherapist will demand new behaviour and new beliefs from his patient:

> The essential point is to change his heart, to reform his habits, to help him to find out how he can live in the future so as to run up no huge bills ... It is true that the neurasthenic is constantly fatigued and that the slightest exertion of mind or body increases his fatigue, but this is ... not because he has done so much work, but because his mental and moral machinery revolves with so much internal friction of part upon part.[38]

Having established that a rest cure could only be a first step in recovery, Cabot explained how work could be therapeutic. First, it must not be drudgery – tasks that are repetitive with little value. More positively, it should be part of a well-organised programme, 'moving on with a steady current into which the patient can put himself'.[39] Second, it should produce something that seems worthwhile, possibly benefitting others. Third, its performance should be social, providing contact with other people engaged in work and showing positive attitudes.

Cabot's theory of how this would be therapeutic was a mixture of Transcendentalism, Jamesian habit training, social psychology and cognitive restructuring (short-circuiting obsessions and teaching positive expectations). Following James, Cabot explained that work provides routine, which acts like a 'heavy fly wheel [to] carry us beyond the dead-points and moody states' that everyone experiences.[40] It also engages the worker and makes him 'forget the anarchical fancies or dispiriting languors of the morning'.[41] The *social psychology* of work routine comes from others' counting upon us to turn up at a certain time, which serves as a motive that 'makes it easier for us to work, and makes us so far the happier'.[42] The cognitive benefit came from all the morbid decision making that was avoided when one had scheduled tasks to perform each morning and afternoon.

For women, getting out of the house to work would provide a break from domestic worries and a 'fresh mental surface' to replace the grooves of daily worry and obsessing. In one example, Cabot told of a widow who was urgently needed to run her late husband's business. She threw herself into the job and found 'the healing power of work in her misfortune'. Sounding a feminist note, Cabot quoted the woman's exclamation, 'How much more natural a man's life is than a woman's' when one needs distraction and a sense of usefulness.[43] In other words, upper-middle-class men have schedules, goals and daily accomplishments, while 'women's work is never done'. Although the audience for Cabot's articles in *Psychotherapy* was upper middle class, the work therapy that he advocated became adopted in public hospitals and used to treat all social classes.

The larger shift in thinking that Cabot advocated was seeing humans' nervous systems not like storage batteries, becoming depleted and needing time to recharge. Instead, 'we run [like] a trolley responding to currents of energy supplied from without, by our fellow men, by nature, and by God.' Nervous disorders, in this metaphor, resulted from the person becoming disconnected from the overhead source of power. 'To get an invalid to work is as essential as to get a trolley car onto a trolley wire. It is not the whole cure but it is a *sine qua non* for cure.'[44] As Jackson Lears explains in *Rebirth of a Nation*, this change from a negative to a positive model of the nervous system was part of a broader, sociocultural transformation. By 1909, economists and politicians had proclaimed 'that the US had passed from an "era of scarcity" to an "era of abundance"'.[45] Just as the nation prospered from natural resources and new technologies, individuals could draw strength from their inner resources, which were refreshed by higher powers and human fellowship. Useful work would tap those resources and restore good health and spiritual abundance.

Work cures in practice, 1890–1920

Given the clinical success and cultural resonance of the work cure, it is not surprising that numerous practitioners emerged in the early 1900s, even before Cabot endorsed the practice and provided a scientific rationale. Missing from histories of OT is perhaps the most successful work-cure practice in the nation. It was an idiosyncratic, one-man operation in rural Maine by former Cleveland surgeon, John G. Gehring (1857–1932). In the late 1880s, Gehring suffered a mental breakdown during an operation, quit medicine and travelled for his health. He settled in Bethel Maine and treated his emotional problems by taking up horticulture and the raising of chickens and vegetables.[46] In the 1890s he learned suggestion and hypnosis, first from a Portland, Maine, physician and then in Europe where he visited leading practitioners like Hippolyte Bernheim.

In 1897 Gehring began to treat neurotics and soon had a patient list that read like a who's who of professors, politicians, artists, businessmen and club women. He restored the health of so many Harvard professors that Bethel became known as the 'Cambridge of the North' and Gehring was called 'the Wizard of the Androscoggin' (referring to the nearby river). Housed in Gehring's home and a nearby inn, his patients chopped and sawed wood, worked in the garden, and took daily plunges in an outdoor pool. They met regularly with Gehring, took meals together and performed theatricals after dinner. Gehring designed all the activities to teach good habits, impart hope, foster spiritual uplift and inhibit negative thoughts. This earned Gehring the loyalty of his patients, ecstatic press coverage and a novella based on his life, *The Master of the Inn*.[47]

Gehring's philosophy included a variant of William James' theory of habit training. To Gehring, 'training, not teaching is required from birth' because behaviours learned through *training* are activated through an indirect, subconscious network, producing habits that become automatic.[48] The relevant habits were physical activities that were incompatible with anxiety, depression and phobias. Gradually, the amount of healthier behaviour was increased, and it was assumed that thoughts would follow along – as William James learned when healing himself. Gehring's idea of the dynamics of his work cure was expressed in a letter to James Jackson Putnam in 1908:

> I find sometimes that to put these ideas [about the patient's strengths and weaknesses] straight to the patient – from the shoulder – helps them greatly. But a patient has to have a certain caliber before this is likely to do good. I have certain patients here now for whom I would like to prescribe the wash-line, every Monday morning, and then the week's ironing & the daily dish-washing the rest of the week! I know it would save them.[49]

In other words, hard work stiffens the mental backbone and cures illness, because it was hard to believe that one was a hopeless invalid when one was doing chores, sawing wood or performing other healthy behaviour. Such work also required patients to inhibit their negative thoughts and persevere despite fatigue or distraction. As Gehring explained it in his book, *Hope of the Variant*, emotions are secondary to the Jamesian 'muscular settings' that one can acquire in work. For one quiet shy man, Gehring prescribed going out into the woods and practising college yells as loud as possible, throwing his hat into the air for emphasis.[50]

The benefits of work were expressed in a song that was improvised at a reunion organised by grateful patients in 1916. To the tune of *Johnny Harvard* they sang:

> We try to saw so very fast, and yet the wood it will not last
> And summer time will soon be past …
> For our clothes or the pose naught care we,
> 'Tis sawing wood that sets our spirits free![51]

As suggested by that song, work also occurred in a landscape and social environment that was as curative as the activities themselves. In that environment there were also leisure activities from sleigh rides to tennis matches, which complemented the physical labour that most dramatically showed patients' improvement.

The positive social psychology of Gehring's work cure was captured by a letter home from Austin Riggs, a general physician who was treated by Gehring and then founded his own psychotherapeutic retreat in Stockbridge, Massachusetts:

American therapeutic work and mental illness

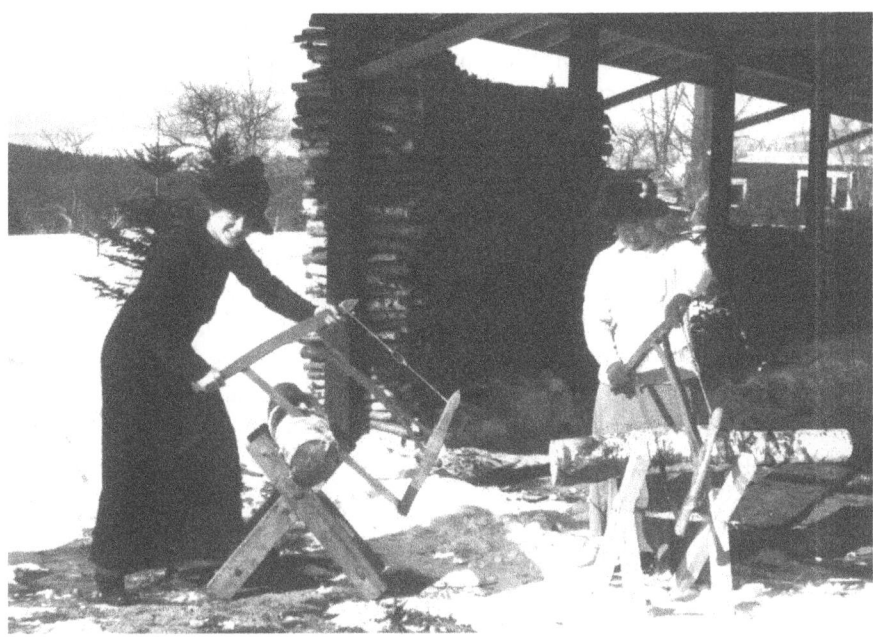

2.3 Women sawing, John Gehring's Asylum, Bethel, Maine, c. 1910.

I had another wonderful talk with Dr. Gehring last night ... I'd better stay a day or two longer, and I shall do it. I am enjoying dear Aunt Bess [a patient of Gehring's] and also my charming Mrs. Warner very deeply. I sat on the woodpile yesterday and laughed at Aunt Bess while she sawed some huge logs. My this is a funny place! I'm fine as a fiddle, It is snowing a little today.[52]

As expressed by Riggs – and seen in figure 2.3 – women engaged in outdoor, manual labour that one might expect to be reserved for men. Freed from the gendered work assignments of public asylums, these private patients found women's labour to be a source of amusement and a contribution to group solidarity and positive thinking.

Another therapy practice that was founded before Cabot endorsed the work cure was the creation of a general physician operating out of a former mansion, in this case in Marblehead, Massachusetts. The doctor was Herbert Hall (1870–1923), who like Gehring had convalesced from a serious illness and was inspired to put patients to work. Compared with Gehring, Hall emphasised crafts, not just outdoor chores. In 1904 Hall created a pottery, weaving and carpentry workshop to treat hysteria, neurasthenia and neurosis.[53] Employing trained artists and craftsmen as supervisors, Hall emphasised the value of patients' work, which he said gave them pride and connected them with the larger world of commerce. When well done, crafts were morally strengthening and helped patients cast off despondency. Consistent with the English Arts and Crafts Movement, Hall also believed that handicrafts connected patients with 'the history of the race' and provided the happiness that comes from 'being able to get into ready contact with the minds of others'.[54]

In 1910 Hall described his success in treating 100 patients (nine out of ten of whom were women), and in 1915 he co-authored a book that tried to integrate his results with work programmes at large psychiatric hospitals.[55] Until recently, he complained, patient work 'has been desultory'. Now, there was a 'new science of work which will not be satisfied with the demand of household service from those who are most able'.[56] Productive work was curative, he explained, and cited a hospital shoe shop that employed a 'long row of happy boys hammering out a cobbler's chorus'.[57]

He also praised hospitals that used patient work to construct roads and buildings, and to farm:

> Every stroke of the shovel and hoe that does not overtax the strength is clear gain to the patient, and to the commonwealth. The idle farm and the idle patient seem existing for each other. The time has come when economy and therapeutics both demand the raising of crops, road-making, the grading and draining of land.[58]

He also touted Danvers State Hospital's programme for patients' making soap from fat left over from food preparation. It saved $1,400 per year and 'the men who do this work enjoy it and take great pride in their product' the physician in charge wrote to Hall.[59] What seems unclear is the essential difference between a patient who might be satisfied mopping the floor and one who found release in digging a trench or hoeing weeds out of a field of vegetables. And one might blame Hall's lack of psychological training to his endorsement of a hospital official's claim that soap making was ennobling for all the patients who participated.

Therapeutic work after 1920

In the 1920s, therapeutic work in psychiatric hospitals was reshaped by the creation of new specialties and theoretical changes in the profession of psychiatry. The result was the division of work therapy into various forms, including OT, vocational training, and rehabilitation, in addition to the unpaid patient labour that asylums relied upon from the 1880s onward – and that was of questionable therapeutic value. OT comprised a variety of practices, united only by their being supervised by people calling themselves occupational therapists. Theoretically eclectic, OT drew some of its authority from Herbert Hall's arts and crafts workshop, and its reforming spirit from the settlement house and mental hygiene movements.[60] In its infancy some of its leaders looked to Adolf Meyer's (1866–1950) ideas of personal adjustment for theoretical grounding. As Jennifer Laws notes, the sheltered workshops that became the hallmark of OT compromised the therapeutic principles of both Hall and Cabot, who wanted patient work to be more artistically viable and connected to the world of extramural labour.[61]

OT professionals distinguished what they did from rehabilitation, which was given to injured soldiers, and downplayed the vocational benefits of their activities. From an outsider's viewpoint, however, such distinctions seem elusive. When done conscientiously, OT was something that took place in dedicated spaces within hospitals and clinics, required significant staff, and was based on general principles of diverting patient thinking and training new habits.[62] Photos from the early history of OT show crafts and activities that would be difficult to teach to the severely mentally ill, and that would require a huge staff to offer to even a moderate percentage of patients at most state hospitals.[63] Thus it seems as if most patient work took place on wards, asylum farms and in shops that were run by foremen rather than OT nurses and attendants. As described in *The Snake Pit*, mid-twentieth-century patients may have worked as maids and janitors for much of their day with no therapeutic rationale, and then attended a brief OT class.

If post-First World War in-patients or out-patients were lucky enough to have an individual psychotherapist, however, work therapy might have been part of the treatment. In 1923, for example, the author Olive Higgins Prouty (1882–1974) suffered a breakdown and travelled from Worcester, Massachusetts, up to Stockbridge to be treated by Austen Riggs (1876–1940), the physician who had been taught the work cure by John Gehring in Bethel, Maine. As Prouty later wrote, Riggs:

> [W]asted no time searching for the cause of my slipping into such a slough but offered me tools to help pull myself out. He prescribed a daily schedule of activities, announcing I would be required to study the nervous system and presented me with a textbook on which I would be questioned by one of his assistants. I studied the lessons assigned, worked in the shop, walked, exercised, rested, played, mixed. His methods worked. No cure could have been more permanent.[64]

After reading her novel *Stella Dallas*, Riggs told Prouty that she should maintain her writing career after leaving his asylum. 'When you leave here,' he said, 'I want you to hire a room outside your home and work there on your writing three or four hours daily, five days a week.' When she replied, 'What about my children?' he responded, 'That New England conscience of yours! You mustn't let it lead *you*. You must get on to the right end of the leash and lead *it*.'[65] Grateful for the therapy that helped her recover, Prouty included a sympathetic psychiatrist in her novel *Now Voyager*, which became a successful Hollywood film. She also paid for the out-patient therapy of Sylvia Plath (1932–63), who attended Smith College on a scholarship provided by Prouty.[66]

In the novel *The Snake Pit*, Virginia Cunningham's psychiatrist provided *her* with a typewriter when she was well enough for a private room, so that her recovery could include the resumption of her career as a writer. The head nurse, however, did not understand how writing could be therapeutic and interfered with the planned work cure. In the film version of this story, Virginia's recovery was more the result of Freudian psychotherapy than of a combination of will power and the shock of seeing the worst-off patients – as happened in the novel.

The insertion of a psychoanalytic cure into *The Snake Pit* reflected the dominance of Freudianism in hospital psychiatry by the middle of the twentieth century.[67] That dominance ended psychiatric support for work therapy as a programme of retraining habit and suppressing symptoms. To Freudians, such modifications of behaviour were short sighted and ethically suspicious. Instead, patients' work at crafts or art was valued for revealing unconscious feelings and helping resolve them.[68] In elite hospitals that could afford the creation of a therapeutic milieu, the milieu was of psychoanalytic design, not the nineteenth-century sort that obeyed the principles of moral therapy. Instead of suggestion, auto-suggestion and therapeutic work, patients were offered the opportunity to express their unconscious conflicts in a safe, permissive environment (as described, for example, by Joanne Greenberg).[69]

For most patients, however, there was no milieu therapy. Instead, those well enough to work spent their hospital lives performing unpaid labour. One could argue that this was better than sitting idle in a ward dayroom. Often, however, success at a hospital job interfered with psychiatric assessment and movement toward discharge. A poignant example is the life of Lawrence Marek (1878–1968), as told in *The Lives They Left Behind*, a history of Willard state hospital from a patient-centric perspective.[70] Marek was admitted to Willard in 1918 as a socially avoidant paranoid schizophrenic with a bad temper and broken English. Assigned to work in the hospital cemetery, he showed a talent as a gravedigger. Devoted to his job and the isolation it provided, he dug graves and supervised the graveyard for 50 years – until his death in 1968. Although his symptoms seemed to have disappeared after a few decades, he was judged to be better served by his career in the hospital than anything that could be arranged outside. One wonders about the validity of this judgement, since there were few, if any, programmes to successfully move such a patient into the non-hospital world.

By the time of Lawrence Marek's death, patient work had come under attack by the movement to restore the civil rights of patients in psychiatric hospitals. In the early 1960s, activist lawyers began to argue that patients committed to a hospital had a right to treatment that would improve their condition or cure them. Otherwise, it was argued, their confinement violated the due process guarantees of the US Constitution. Within a decade, the Federal courts handed down rulings (e.g., *Wyatt* v. *Stickney*) that established minimum standards for hospital staffing, housing, and therapy that most states failed to meet. Instead, they discharged patients to nursing homes and other community facilities.[71]

A related legal campaign was mounted against unpaid patient labour, whether or not the purpose was therapeutic. This coincided with psychiatrists' accounts of the exploitative nature of patient work, which they called 'institutional peonage' and without which hospitals could not survive.[72] The legal attack on unpaid patient work succeeded in the case of *Souder* v. *Brennan*, a class action lawsuit in which a judge ruled that patient workers were state hospital employees, covered by labour laws such as the Federal minimum wage. This included patients participating in OT workshops that produced goods.[73] As they did in response to the right to treatment rulings, most states chose to either empty their hospitals or close down all therapeutic workshops. Critics of the patient rights movement have accused its lawyers of having deinstitutionalisation as their real goal, a charge refuted by at least one activist who argued that patient work was therapeutic but also worthy of payment.[74]

As mentioned at the start of this essay, patient work has played an important role in most major changes in the institutional treatment of the mentally ill in the United States. It was present at the birth of the asylum, as a key feature of both theory and practice. In the late nineteenth century, its change to non-therapeutic drudgery corresponded with the ascendance of custodial pessimism and the warehousing of the chronically ill poor. Its revival at the start of the twentieth century was engineered by an optimistic alliance of psychotherapists, clergy and physicians, reflecting the national mood of expansionism and financial promise. Soon, however, both Freudians and harried hospital bureaucrats put an end to the idea that work would help individuals overcome their symptoms and redirect their inner resources. And when the asylums were dismantled in the 1970s and 1980s, the politics of patient work helped move the process along. Few participants in these events could trace patient work as a thread that connected most major therapeutic changes, but hindsight allows us to see it as such.

Acknowledgement

The author thanks Ellen Dwyer for her comments on an earlier draft of this work.

Notes

1. Mary Jane Ward, *The Snake Pit* (New York: Random House, 1946), pp. 238–9.
2. Gerald N. Grob, *The Mad Among Us: A History of the Care of America's Mentally Ill* (New York: Free Press, 1994).
3. Nancy Tomes, *The Art of Asylum-Keeping: Thomas Story Kirkbride and the Origins of American Psychiatry* (Philadelphia, PA: University of Pennsylvania Press, 1994).
4. Tomes, *The Art of Asylum-Keeping*, p. 31.
5. Eric T. Carlson and Norman Dain, 'The psychotherapy that was moral treatment', *American Journal of Psychiatry*, 117 (1960), 519–24; Roy Porter, 'Was there a moral therapy in eighteenth-century psychiatry?' *Lychnos* (1981–82), 12–26.
6. Grob, *The Mad Among Us*, p. 66.
7. Ibid.
8. Tomes, *The Art of Asylum-Keeping*, p. 5.
9. Charles Dickens, *American Notes for General Circulation* (1842; Harmondsworth: Penguin, 2004), p. 56.
10. *Ibid.*, p. 56.
11. Gerald N. Grob, *Mental Institutions in America: Social Policy to 1875* (New York: Free Press, 1972), p. 240.
12. Gerald N. Grob, 'Introduction' to *Insanity and Idiocy in Massachusetts* (Cambridge, MA: Harvard University Press, 1971).
13. Tomes, *The Art of Asylum-Keeping*, p. 287.
14. *Ibid.*, p. 295.
15. 'Annual meeting of the Association of Medical Superintendents of American Institutions for the Insane', *American Journal of Insanity*, 19 (1862), 22–86, 54–6.
16. Tomes, *The Art of Asylum-Keeping*, p. 289.
17. George Cook, 'Provision for the insane poor in the State of New York', *American Journal of Insanity*, 23 (1866), 45–75, 47.
18. *Ibid.*, p. 66.
19. *Ibid.*, p. 65. County authorities believed this promise to be unrealistic and were proven right.
20. Ellen Dwyer, *Homes for the Mad: Life Inside Two Nineteenth-Century Asylums* (New Brunswick, NJ: Rutgers University Press, 1987).
21. Linda S. Stuhler, *1886 Hayt's Corner's, Ovid & Willard Rail-Road* (2011), http://inmatesofwillard.com/2013/01/09/1886-hayts-corners-ovid-willard-rail-road/ (last accessed 6 February 2015).
22. 'Annual meeting of the Association of Medical Superintendents' (1862), p. 59.
23. Dwyer, *Homes for the Mad*, p. 17.
24. Gerald N. Grob, *Mental Illness and American Society, 1875–1940* (Princeton, NJ: Princeton University Press, 1983).
25. Tomes, *The Art of Asylum-Keeping*, p. 309.
26. *Ibid.*, p. 314.
27. *Ibid.*, p. 7.
28. Grob, *Mental Illness and American Society*, p. 70.

29 David G. Schuster, *Neurasthenic Nation: America's Search for Health, Happiness, and Comfort, 1869–1920* (New Brunswick, NJ: Rutgers University Press, 2011).
30 Eric Caplan, *Mind Games: American Culture and the Birth of Psychotherapy* (Berkeley, CA: University of California Press, 1998).
31 Nathan G. Hale Jr, *Freud and the Americans: The Beginnings of Psychoanalysis in the United States, 1876–1917* (New York: Oxford University Press, 1971), p. 66.
32 *Ibid.*, p. 66. George Prochnik, *Putnam Camp: Sigmund Freud, James Jackson Putnam, and the Purpose of American Psychology* (New York: Other Press, 2006).
33 Morton Prince, 'The educational treatment of neurasthenia and certain hysterical states', *Boston Medical and Surgical Journal*, 139 (1898), 332–7, 335.
34 James Jackson Putnam, 'Not the disease only, but also the man', *Boston Medical and Surgical Journal*, 141 (1899), 53–7, 53.
35 Richard C. Cabot, 'The American type of psychotherapy', *Psychotherapy*, 1:1 (1908), 5–13, 7.
36 Richard C. Cabot, 'The use and abuse of rest in the treatment of disease', *Psychotherapy*, 2:2 (1909), 23–33.
37 *Ibid.*, p. 31.
38 *Ibid.*, p. 31.
39 Richard C. Cabot, 'Work cure', *Psychotherapy*, 3:1 (1909), 24–9, 28.
40 Richard C. Cabot, 'Work cure II', *Psychotherapy*, 3:2 (1909), 20–7, 22.
41 *Ibid.*, p. 23.
42 *Ibid.*, p. 22.
43 Cabot, 'Work cure', p. 27.
44 *Ibid.*, p. 29.
45 T. J. Jackson Lears, *Rebirth of a Nation: The Making of Modern America, 1877–1920* (New York: HarperCollins, 2009), p. 247.
46 Lawrence S. Kubie, *The Riggs Story: The Development of the Austen Riggs Centre for the Study and Treatment of the Neuroses* (New York: Hoeber, 1960).
47 William D. Andrews, 'Dr John G. Gehring and his Bethel clinic: Pragmatic therapy and therapeutic tourism', *Maine History*, 43 (2008), 189–216.
48 John G. Gehring, *The Hope of the Variant* (New York: Scribner's, 1924), p. 60.
49 Countway Library, Harvard University, Cambridge, MA, James Jackson Putnam Papers, letter from J. G. Gehring, Bethel, Maine, to James Jackson Putnam, 14 January 1908, p. 1.
50 Gehring, *The Hope of the Variant*, p. 133.
51 Western Reserve Historical Society, Cleveland, OH, William Bingham II Papers, container 1, folder 6, The Bethel League, second reunion dinner programme, 18 September 1915, p. 4.
52 Kubie, *The Riggs Story*, p. 16.
53 Herbert J. Hall, 'The systematic use of work as a remedy in neurasthenia and allied conditions', *Boston Medical and Surgical Journal*, 152:2 (1905), 30–2.
54 Herbert J. Hall and Mertice M. Buck, *The Work of our Hands: A Study of Occupations for Invalids* (New York: Moffat, Yard, 1915), p. 93.
55 Herbert J. Hall, 'Work cure: A report of five years' experience at an institution devoted to the therapeutic application of manual work', *Journal of the American*

Medical Association, 54:1 (1910), 12–14; Hall and Buck, *The Work of Our Hands*, pp. 166–79.
56 Hall and Buck, *The Work of Our Hands*, p. 13.
57 *Ibid.*, p. 15.
58 *Ibid.*, p. 18.
59 *Ibid.*, p. 25.
60 At Chicago's Hull House, modelled after London's Toynbee Hall, Jane Addams and colleagues tried to lessen the alienation of women industrial workers by teaching them arts and crafts. Eleanor Clarke Slagle, a pioneer of OT, applied the philosophy of Hull House to psychiatric patients at the Phipps Clinic in Baltimore and then returned to Chicago to teach OT to young, middle-class women, who would then work in hospitals and clinics. Virginia A. M. Quiroga, *Occupational Therapy: The First 30 Years 1900 to 1930* (Bethesda, MD: The American Occupational Therapy Association, 1995).
61 Jennifer Laws, 'Crackpots and basket-cases: A history of therapeutic work and occupation', *History of the Human Sciences*, 24 (2011), 65–81, 71.
62 Susan Hall Anthony, 'Dr. Herbert J. Hall: Originator of honest work for occupational therapy 1904–1923, part II', *Occupational Therapy in Health Care*, 19:3 (2005), 21–32.
63 Quiroga, *Occupational Therapy*, p. 265.
64 Olive Higgins Prouty, *Pencil Shavings: Memoirs* (Cambridge, MA: Riverside Press, 1961), p. 180.
65 *Ibid.*, p. 181.
66 Judith Mayne, 'Afterword' to *Now, Voyager* (New York: Feminist Press, 2004), p. 269.
67 Fishbein has argued that the Freudian plot was anti-feminist propaganda designed to put women back into the home in the post-Second World War era. Leslie Fishbein, '*The Snake Pit* (1948): The sexist nature of sanity', *American Quarterly*, 30 (1978), 641–65.
68 Laws, 'Crackpots and basket-cases', p. 74.
69 Joanne Greenberg (writing as Hannah Green), *I Never Promised You a Rose Garden* (New York: Holt, Rinehart & Winston, 1964), p. 251.
70 Peter Stastny and Darby Penney, *The Lives They Left Behind: Suitcases from a State Hospital Attic* (New York: Bellevue Literary Press, 2008).
71 Gerald N. Grob, 'The paradox of deinstitutionalisation', *Society* (July–August 1995), 51–9.
72 F. Lewis Bartlett, 'Institutional peonage: Our exploitation of mental patients', *Atlantic Monthly* (July 1964), 116–19; James Arscott Raleigh Bickford, 'Economic value of the psychiatric in-patient' *Lancet*, 281 (1963), 714–15.
73 Michael L. Perlin, 'The right to voluntary, compensated, therapeutic work as part of the right to treatment, a new theory in the aftermath of *Souder*', *Seaton Hall Law Review*, 7 (1976), 298–339.
74 *Ibid.* Treatment Advocacy Centre, '*Souder* v. *Brennan*, in historic case digests' (undated), www.treatmentadvocacycentre.org/legal-resources/historic-case-digests/345 (accessed 2 June 2014).

3

Travails of madness: New Jersey, 1800–70

James Moran

By the mid-twentieth century, the questions prompted by our considerations of psychiatric patient work in institutional settings had formed a familiar subject in the broader history of the asylum. Ellen Dwyer, Nancy Tomes, Steven Cherry, Patricia D'Antonio, James Moran (and others) have all noted that patient work formed an essential part of the broader therapeutic system of moral therapy in asylum settings.[1] Partly grounded in much earlier humoral considerations of the mind/body relationship, physicians thought that the physical stimulation of work increased blood flow, thereby stimulating brain activity. Patient work in an asylum setting was also designed to divert mad minds from irrational thought. Though the models varied among institutions, and from one period to the next, myriad forms of physical labour, and less strenuous asylum activities such as walking the asylum grounds and lawn bowling, were seen as essential components to the highly regulated moral therapy milieus of asylum life.

However, as Geoffrey Reaume notes in his forceful critique of the relationship between patient work and asylum development, there were always two aspects to the phenomenon of patient work at the asylum. In 'Patients at work: Insane asylum inmates' labour in Ontario, 1841–1900', Reaume argues that over the course of the nineteenth century the reality of asylum patient work had strayed mightily from its original therapeutic rationale.[2] For Reaume, 'moral "therapy", when stripped of its therapeutic veneer, was in reality a public works programme run on "free" labour of people confined in insane asylums'.[3] Indeed, Reaume traces a massive increase in the percentages of asylum patients working at Ontario asylums between 1841 and 1900, and an ever-increasing array of work duties, including washing, knitting and sewing, domestic work, digging ditches, gardening, farming, masonry, manufacturing, carpentry and asylum nursing. Like other historians of asylum development, Reaume also points out the contradictions of psychiatrists' promotion of the savings reaped by patients' work, on the one hand, and their downplaying of the extent to which the labour of the insane constituted real productive work, on the other hand.

This historical dynamic of asylum patient work that became commonplace in Europe and North America, and the contradictions within it pointed out by Reaume, can be partially explained by bringing into consideration Andrew Scull's pioneering revisionist studies of English asylum development. Scull grounds the very rationale of the asylum in the anxieties of an emerging middle class about unproductive labour – the mass casualties of capitalist production whose unemployment rankled the busy middling sorts who were ever mindful of the powers of productive labour. The cult of productivity was, in turn, partly grounded in Protestant ideals that linked religious piety to work. Scull notes:

> The establishment of a market economy and, more particularly, the emergence of a market in labour, provided the initial incentive to distinguish far more carefully than hitherto between different categories of deviance [including madness]. If nothing else, under these conditions, stress had to be laid for the first time on the importance of distinguishing the able-bodied from the non-able bodied poor.[4]

Drawing on Karl Marx and Max Weber, Scull notes that a pillar of capitalism 'was the existence of a large mass of wage labourers who were not merely "free" to dispose of their labour power in the open market, but who were actually forced to do so'.[5] Under these circumstances the contradictions that Reaume and others have found between the therapeutic rationales of asylum work as therapeutic, and asylum work as exploitative, are accounted for. Work as a rehabilitative strategy in the public asylum for psychiatric patients was synonymous with the mid-nineteenth-century middle-class ideal of productivity. Psychiatrists may have conveniently altered their accounts of the productivity of patient work depending on their audience, but productivity and rehabilitation remained on one side of the ledger – idleness and mental illness were on the other.

If moral therapy was the central therapeutic model for early-to-mid nineteenth-century asylum care, and asylum work a central pillar of moral therapy, how did this compare with ideas and understandings about the relationship between work and madness outside the walls of the institution?[6] This chapter offers a preliminary consideration of this subject through the evaluation of civil trials in lunacy in New Jersey. Evidence from trials in lunacy suggests that people in farm and town settings in New Jersey understood the capacity to work effectively as central to good mental health. Conversely, various states of madness were marked according to witnesses in these trials by a person's relative lack of work acumen. This strong relationship between work and madness was partially built into the civil law of lunacy itself. It also made sense in a society that regarded success in work as essential to success in the social organisation of the family and the community. And, as with other farm and town contexts of capitalism in nineteenth-century North America, effective and productive work was very likely to be seen as proof of a rational mind.

After articulating the ways in which participants in New Jersey lunacy trials made the links between work and madness, this chapter briefly explores how New Jersey's first lunatic asylum superintendent, John Buttolph, understood the value of patient labour within his institution. Buttolph vigorously downplayed the likelihood that the domestic context could provide any hope of recovery for the insane. Like many other self-respecting psychiatric professionals in charge of institutions newly established in the United States, Buttolph compared asylum care favourably against the perils of managing madness at home and in the community. Like others, he was justifying himself professionally, while drumming up business for the new state institution. For Buttolph (and other asylum superintendents) part of the effectiveness of asylum care was the use of patient work, which was meant to be both therapeutic and practically useful. While in both the institutional context of the asylum and the local contexts of family and community in New Jersey it is clear that work was closely connected to mental health and to varying states of madness, the work/madness relationship operated very differently in each setting.

The civil trial process

Civil trials in lunacy formed part of a body of law that I call lunacy investigation law, which placed individuals on trial to see whether or not they were *non compos mentis*. The trials were primarily concerned with individuals who may have lost their ability to govern themselves and their property. The origin of this legal process dates back to fourteenth-century England. Over a 500-year period, lunacy investigation law developed into a powerful mechanism in the determination of, and response to, madness in England. It was also successfully transplanted across the Atlantic into colonial settings like New Jersey where it thrived well beyond the colonial period until at least the late nineteenth century.[7]

Much like in England, New Jersey trials in lunacy normally involved a jury of twelve property-owning, respectable men, a judge, and witnesses who were usually family members, neighbours and local authorities. In New Jersey, if the burden of evidence convinced the jury and judge that the individual on trial was insane, a verdict of *non compos mentis* was issued and two committees were created through the orphans court – one to take care of the person deemed to be insane, and the other to take responsibility for his or her property. There was provision in the lunacy investigation law for individuals to overthrow the decision of *non compos mentis* through *supercedas* – in effect a retrial which could determine that the individual was once more fit to govern him- or herself and his or her property. In New Jersey, the trials were open to the public and usually held in the taverns of local towns.

As an inheritance of English civil law, lunacy investigation law developed in colonial New Jersey and grew in significance from the American War of Independence until the late nineteenth century. The roots of this law therefore preceded the establishment of lunatic asylums in New Jersey. The law itself also developed in tandem with the development of the New Jersey State Lunatic Asylum, which was established in 1848, and with other mental institutions – some private, some public – in neighbouring states starting in the early nineteenth century. The documents relating to lunacy trials in New Jersey offer a unique opportunity to examine how witnesses – neighbours, friends and relatives of those on trial for insanity – and legal officials understood the relationships of madness, work and rehabilitation. As the asylum became an increasingly important response to madness in New Jersey after mid-century, it is possible to evaluate how those ideas about work and madness that were generated around lunacy investigation law compared with the ideas about work as therapy that formed part of psychiatric care in an asylum setting.[8]

The relationship between work and mental state was built into the very structure of lunacy investigation law. In all trials the point of the exercise was to determine if the person was in a fit mental state to govern his or her property and person. In New Jersey's version of the law, the property in question could range from large holdings (farms and businesses) to a few chattels. By comparison, in England, trials in lunacy were, on the whole, the prerogative of the wealthy. Regardless of the value of the property at stake, it was the owner's mental capacity to maintain it responsibly that was at issue. Responsible maintenance of property revolved around effective work, whether it was productive farming, wise business transactions or profitable investment. As we shall see, the point at which a lunacy trial was considered necessary was very often the point at which the work habits of individuals in New Jersey became suspect. This ineffectiveness at work could be accompanied by other displays of unusual behaviour, but a range of odd behaviour was tolerated, especially in pre-asylum New Jersey, as long as the individual was mentally responsible in the management of his or her property.

As the chief legal mechanism for determining the mental status of individuals considered as insane, the law of lunacy investigation was primarily concerned with male property holders. The majority of legal investigations that were held during the eighteenth and nineteenth centuries in New Jersey focused on the mental status of men. While there were some very notable exceptions in which women's mental states were examined, and a handful of cases in which verdicts of *non compos mentis* among women were challenged, most of these do not shed much light on the relationship between female labour and madness in New Jersey communities. Nevertheless, some trials that focused on women highlight both the differences in work tasks of rural New Jersey residents and the importance of work in relationship to mental health that obtained to women as well as men.

Wasting property

Some of the more obvious connections between work and madness highlighted in New Jersey lunacy trials involved concerns about the 'wasting' of property. For example, in 1826 John Barron's brother and father petitioned that John had for several months:

> [W]asted a considerable part of his property by buying cattle at very extravagant prices and then butchering them and selling the meat for much less than it was worth to any and every person who would buy from him, and to persons wholly unable to pay for it.[9]

Their concern was that these irrational forms of farm work were endangering John's property and, by extension, the wellbeing of his wife and three children. In the case of John McIntire, witnesses clearly linked the inability to conduct productive work with mental derangement. According to his father, McIntire was 'frequently offering to sell or give away all his property', but he was also erroneously convinced that 'his family are taking away all his property'.[10] Moreover, 'John frequently starts off from home under an idea that he must attend to business, but does not appear to know where he is going and some person must always attend him to bring him back again'.[11] The constant supervision required to prevent John McIntire's irrational work practices from damaging his property or from causing self-harm, along with his tendency to 'abuse' his wife and eight children, led to a lunacy trial that found him *non compos mentis*.[12]

In similar fashion John Bertholf petitioned that his father, John, 'wanders about doing no business … that he talks a great deal about buying farms and horses … [and] that he offers to buy and give his notes for the same old horses, sleds, wagons, or other property without regard to price, worth or value.'[13] Of greater concern was that when John occasionally 'meets with a man who is unacquainted with his deranged state of mind – or with persons disposed to take advantage of it – he makes bargains with them greatly prejudicial to his estate'.[14] This situation was likely exasperated by the fact that a year before the petition for a *writ de lunatico inquirendo*, John Bertholf had sold his farm to his oldest son for $2,500. It is possible that the sale of the farm was partly motivated by the failing of John Bertholf's mental health. Another contributing factor may have been the death of his wife, about six months before witnesses in court dated his first symptoms. If he had control of the money that he was given from the sale of his farm, the irrational way in which he was spending it on farming activities likely would have been distressing to his twelve children.

In the trial of Daniel Higgins, witnesses framed a raft of symptoms of madness in terms of his loss of capacity in farming work. Starting in 1821, Higgins' first symptoms of 'derangement of mind' were described by his brother Lewis Higgins as 'hallowing aloud, and complaining of pain, while he would at the same time be at work – and nothing appeared to ail him, as to real pain or sickness'.[15] This went on for some time until Higgins stopped working, and began to run about the neighbourhood 'talking to himself constantly, and making rhymes and saying that he was going to the Devil, that destruction was come upon him, and that everybody wanted to destroy him'.[16] At this stage he also became 'ill natured', hitting and threatening further violence to family members and friends. As winter approached, concern that his violence would do serious harm and that in his wanderings he might 'perish by exposure to the weather' led family and friends to construct a 'pen or partition' in his own house where he was confined. One neighbour described 'taking hold of him' through the grating of the pen and endeavouring to 'get Daniel to talk with him', but to no avail. The pen was situated 'where the family sit, and near the fire so as to make him as comfortable as possible'.[17]

All witnesses placed these symptoms of madness in the context of Higgins' ability to work. For example Moses Rogers, a neighbour who claimed to have known Higgins for sixteen years, noted that he 'used formerly to be a very industrious and prudent man about his business' but that early in the last summer he discovered that there was a great alteration in the said Daniel – that he quit all kind of work, and appeared to be wild and crazy'.[18]

The connections between ineffective labour and mental trouble was also evident in the trials of women. The content of the work and the context of the problem reflected contemporary understandings of women's roles in rural New Jersey settings. For example, in 1829 William Probasco in Kingswood Township, Hunterdon County, a next-door neighbour and friend of Rebecca Large, noted that her 'intellectual faculties' had been 'impaired' for the last eight years.[19] Probasco and other witnesses explained that, as the only child of Samuel Large who died in 1825, she inherited a 100-acre property with a house. However, since her father's death, 'she takes no care of her person or property about her house'.[20] Moreover, Large apparently 'will not cook her own victuals or make her own bed' necessitating the assistance of neighbours who 'have to wash and cook for her'.[21] In this case it is clear that the lunacy trial was initiated in order to make some formal arrangement whereby Large's property could be taken care of, with the income from it being used to arrange for her welfare. Although brief, the trial evidence also suggests a similar description of mental incapacity as related to the typical tasks of women in early nineteenth-century New Jersey as that attributed to men in the majority of trials. Large was found to be a lunatic for two years, her property being placed into the guardianship of her uncle.

In testimony at the trial of Phebe McPherson, accounts of both her habits and her delusions seem to demonstrate the close connections between work and madness. In his 1853 petition for a trial in lunacy, Samuel McPherson considered his mother to be deprived of her reason for eighteen months. Trial witnesses described her irrational insistence that:

> [S]he and her family had nothing to eat and were all starving and had nothing to wear and were going naked and exposed and had nothing to live or subsist upon or to clothe themselves with when in fact she and the family had plenty to eat and to wear and were comfortable.[22]

Along with these delusions of domestic deprivation, according to witnesses, 'Phebe does not pretend to take any charge of her affairs or to employ herself at any occupation whatever'. Nor could McPherson muster the energy to take care of herself, 'but is dressed and washed and minded to entirely by her daughter', Hester, and a neighbour.[23] In effect, not only was McPherson's insanity manifested by her inability to tend to her domestic work, and by her delusions that her family was starving and unclothed, it is clear that her expressions of mental distress required that the domestic labour of other women be employed to compensate. On one level this was no different to the extra labour required of women as principal care givers in New Jersey when men became dysfunctional as the result of mental illness. In both cases, in a society in which such a premium was placed on productive labour, and labour for subsistence, lunacy investigation law fitted rather well with verdicts of *non compos mentis* that were tied to the inability to govern self and property broadly defined.

Idiocy and effective work

The inability to work effectively was at the core of trials that focused on those who were considered to be 'idiots' or mentally incompetent from an early age, or from birth. With such individuals the event precipitating the use of lunacy investigation law was usually the death of a principal caregiver. Jacob Wood, a twenty-year-old who lived on his father's farm in the township of Greenwich, Cumberland County, was thrown into the care of his aunt and uncle when his father died in 1825. Wood stood to inherit his father's farm, but with his aunt as his legal representative. In order to provide guardianship for their nephew (in the form of a monthly allowance) and to legally ensure that the farm was looked after properly, Wood's aunt and uncle issued a petition in the form of a *writ de idiota inquirendo*. The evidence in the ensuing trial was very much wrapped up in Wood's inability to do the work of a person his age and gender. Joseph Allen, a farm hand on the farm, stated that he:

> [C]ould not trust [Wood] to perform those acts usually performed by boys of ten years of age – that he cannot count 12 – cannot distinguish between hoy and gee – that this affirmant last spring ... put him to ploughing – but he was not able to accomplish it not understanding how to plough – that this affirmant hath directed him to reap corn, to put four grains on a hill, but he could not do that correctly, sometimes putting in many more, sometimes less.[24]

Moreover, at harvest time, Wood was unable to 'carry the sheaves together in shocks of 12'. Neighbouring farmer George Mitchell agreed that Wood could not conduct the normal tasks of farm work, also pointing out, as in many cases of idiocy, that he could not count, measure, or recognise the value of money.[25]

The trial of Nathaniel Allen suggests that not all those in New Jersey who were considered in their local communities to be idiots were by definition deemed unfit for productive work. According to witnesses, 'under the charge of his father, Joshua Allen', Nathaniel was able to work effectively enough.[26] But around 1832 Nathaniel's father died, leaving his forty-year-old son an inheritance of a fifty-acre farm, but without the strong guidance of his father to keep him to task. Eight years later, Nathaniel's stepmother with whom he lived petitioned that with no 'guardian to take charge of him and his estate' he was being taken advantage of.[27] Neighbouring witnesses agreed, noting that Nathaniel was 'perfectly harmless and willing to labour', but that he 'is wholly without mind sufficient to contract bargains or to procure chattels and other necessities'.[28] In this situation, they argued, 'the avails [of his inheritance] cannot be collected for want of a competent authority' to manage his affairs.[29] The value of Nathaniel's inheritance, based at least in part on his own labours under the strict supervision of his father, was now under threat by altered familial circumstances. The use of lunacy investigation law was an attempt to re-establish a more stable relationship between mental incompetence and productive labour.

Work and mental decline

Another reason for initiating the law of lunacy investigation in New Jersey was the reorganisation of property in the face of the 'mental decline' of an ageing head of household. The lengthy legal case of Abraham Rogers demonstrates how legal and informal traditions overlapped and collided in the familial struggles over the mental and physical decline of an ageing farmer from

East Windsor Township in Mercer County. In January 1843, the husband of Abraham Rogers' niece, Daniel Carson, petitioned for a *writ de lunatico inquirendo* to investigate Roger's mental capacity. The testimony appeared convincing. One witness noted that he had known Rogers for fifty years and that in the past fifteen months Rogers 'hath altogether given up transacting business … and that his whole deportment manifests utter imbecility of mind'.[30] Another witness had much the same things to say, elaborating that the imbecility of mind was partly demonstrated by Rogers' incontinence and his tendency to stay in bed most of the time.[31] The lunacy investigation, held at the beginning of February, found that Rogers had been *non compos mentis* for about twenty-two months. In due course, responsibility over the Rogers' farm was delegated to Daniel Carson.

For a couple of weeks it appeared that Daniel Carson had moved on to the property to fulfil his guardianship obligations.[32] However, on 16 February Rogers' wife, Elizabeth Rogers, filed a 'caveat against further proceedings' in the clerk's office of the court.[33] Soon thereafter, on 6 March, Abraham Rogers petitioned to traverse the earlier decision, noting that he was 'greatly aggrieved and prejudiced by the finding' of his insanity. Within days of Rogers' appeal for traverse, Abraham and Elizabeth Rogers signed a legal agreement with Aaron Eldridge whereby Eldridge agreed to look after the needs of the elderly Rogers in exchange for a portion of their property. This led to Daniel Carson filing a counter charge that Eldridge was taking advantage of Abraham Rogers' lunacy in order to exploit the couple's property by 'cutting down, felling and carting off the wood and timber standing and frowing [sic] upon the premises … and in committing other and further waste and destruction upon the said premises' to Carson's 'manifest wrong and injury'.[34] The resulting conflict led to further testimony from witnesses that helps to put the relationship between the mental decline from ageing and the ability to labour in interesting perspective.

Witnesses testifying on behalf of Abraham Rogers who were called upon to testify to his mental soundness noted that his mental soundness was intact despite physical infirmities. Wilson Eldridge, uncle to Aaron Eldridge, noted that Rogers was 'weak in body but as strong in mind as he ever was'.[35] William Tindale, the legal authority that issued the will that the Rogers signed vesting authority of their farm to Aaron Eldridge summarised the situation in this way:

> I asked him [Rogers] what his notion was for making Aaron Eldridge a deed for his property – he said that they were alone and it was necessary to have somebody to take care of them – I read the deed over to them and told them that it was a deed conveying to Aaron Eldridge the farm and wood lot on condition that he would maintain them and find them everything. He and Mrs. Rogers appeared to be satisfied.[36]

Rogers' physician, Dr George Robbins, used his medical expertise to confirm his patient's sanity. He (like other witnesses) noted that Rogers suffered from 'general paralysis weakening the whole system'.[37] Not only did this make it hard for him to 'be on his feet much', but it also caused him to 'pass off' his urine 'without being able to prevent it'. This condition at one point in the spring of 1840 led Rogers to take 'a large quantity of laudanum' that rendered 'his mind ... unsettled'.[38] This Dr Robbins assured the jury, was quickly corrected with an 'emetic, which threw it off his stomach' after which 'he soon recovered and has been in his right mind since'.[39]

Rogers' wife Elizabeth was the last witness to speak on behalf of her husband's sane mental state. In her view Rogers appeared unsound in mind for a brief period when Daniel Carson was first appointed guardian of their farm.[40] She argued that the reason for it was Carson's insistence that he be treated by drinking 'cup full after cup full' of cold water, which aggravated his condition to the point of mental incompetence. However, after Dr Robbins' interventions along with the services of a nurse, 'he has always been sensible ... talking sensibly and answering sensibly in every instance'.[41] Elizabeth Rogers' explanation for the switch of arrangements from Carson to Eldridge was that Carson had not been taking care of them properly. Thus, the decisions to enter into legal arrangement with Eldridge and to place a legal 'caveat' against the proceedings of the lunacy investigation were strategically made to improve their situation. She concluded by noting that, 'for the last three years I have had the control of the property here pretty much – my husband did not feel very strong and as I was pretty smart he gave it up to me'.[42]

Unsurprisingly, witnesses testifying on behalf of Daniel Carson argued that the same physical symptoms went hand in hand with a failing mental capacity to conduct the everyday work of Rogers' farm. For example, in his very long testimony, neighbouring farmer John Hutchinson noted that although he was 'formerly a capable business man', within the past two years Rogers had not possessed 'mind enough to make a bargain' without the assistance of his wife.[43] Later in his testimony, on cross-examination, he stated that 'there was some doubt as to whether [Rogers] understood' the business of his farm, and that 'for four or five years past he has given up his business more or less to his wife'.[44] During the past few years, Hutchinson and others saw Rogers' disregard for his state of nudity when needing to 'pass urine' along with his tendency to 'cry without hiding his features, like a baby' at unusual times, as further signs of mental incapacity. Witnesses could get very specific about the details when cross-examined. When the court judge questioned Abraham Hutchinson about Rogers' insane behaviour he put it this way:

> I made up my opinion of his insanity from his general appearance and behaviour – He was greatly altered from what he had formerly been – This silence which I

have mentioned did not appear to proceed from bodily pain – I have seen other things which have impressed me with the idea that he was not in his right mind – I have seen him walk about the house before all his family with his private parts exposed – it made no difference who was there – the night I was there he would when he was on the chair take a cob and wipe himself with it – he would then play with the cob awhile with it in his hands, and then wipe himself with it again and put it in the basket under the bed – another thing indicating insanity is that he would take the basin provided for him to make water in and walk about the room with his privates in the water.[45]

These more anatomically oriented signs of mental frailty were accompanied by witnesses' assertions that Rogers had not in fact been mentally aware of the business of his property, nor had he been capable of working his farm, for a considerable time. One witness noted that, 'he has not gone out with his team as formerly for the last four or five years'. Another, William Robbins, stated that 'the olde [sic] man has had no say in regard to his business – when his business has been talked over in his presence he never said any thing and never appeared to me as if he was paying any attention to it'.[46]

For the jury, the burden of evidence pointed to a situation in which Abraham Rogers was not able to manage his property. On 9 March 1843, the jury thus upheld the earlier judgement of *non compos mentis* of the original inquisition in lunacy and concluded that Eldridge had been 'taking advantage of the imbecility of the said Abraham Rogers' in order to exploit his property 'contrary to equity and good conscience'.[47] The court thus forbade any further 'waste and destruction in or upon the premises' of the Rogers' farm, though the extent to which Daniel Carson afforded Abraham and Elizabeth Rogers the good guardianship that the law of lunacy investigation in theory provided is not clear from the surviving records.[48]

In the equally long trial process of Daniel Van Auken, the same ingredients of ageing, labour and mental capacity were at play, but with an entirely different outcome. In mid-April 1854 Mark Ayers petitioned the court that his father-in-law, Daniel Van Auken, had been insane for two years. The subsequent trial found that Van Auken had been *non compos mentis* for two years, mainly attributed to failing mental powers as evidenced by several instances of a loss of memory relating to his property and to the identity of some of his close neighbours.[49] However, on 31 May 1854, Van Auken petitioned to traverse this decision citing several reasons for the fact that the lunacy trial had been wrongfully conducted. These reasons included the fact that the trial had not been held in the same township as Van Auken's place of residence and that there had been only two days of notice for preparing a defence.[50] Van Auken also objected that the witnesses in the first trial 'were not medical men or experts in questions of lunacy, as to the lunacy of your petitioner and his competency to transact business without confirming the testimony of said witnesses to [the] facts'; that the definitions of 'dementia' that were considered sufficient proofs of lunacy to reach a verdict of *non-compos mentis* were not defined clearly enough; and that evidence showed 'nothing more than a partial failure of memory, mere forgetfulness, and did not prove a failure of judgement or of the reasoning faculties of your petitioner, nor any improper management of your petitioner's person or property'.[51] Van Auken's argument that rigorous medical evidence was necessary to reach a verdict of *non compos mentis* was unusual at mid-century in New Jersey, although the use of medical experts was increasing. Ironically, the subsequent trial of traverse was no more medically laden than the original trial had been.

Van Auken's petition led to a very long trial of traverse that included over sixty pages of testimonials from neighbours and family. This trial was held in Van Auken's town of residence, Wantage, in Sussex County, NJ, and was filled with detailed accounts that gauged his abilities in conducting the work of a proprietor farmer. Jasper Younger, whose farm was next to Van Auken's, described him as well capable of conducting:

> [H]is haying last season – that he would go at it pretty strong handed and would therefore be able to get through with it … and within the past two or three years has noticed his stacking his hay in haying season and that he moved and stacked hay … with as much judgement and understanding as any man.[52]

William Roy, a practising physician acquainted with Van Auken for about twenty years, noted that 'he has not had much occasion for the service of a physician on account of his bodily health'. Nevertheless, Dr Roy noted that Van Auken's memory was no longer as sharp as it was previously, citing specific examples relating to the purchasing of property and the inability to properly identify neighbours. He, like many other witnesses, also noted that, 'the business of the farm is carried on by the sons'.[53]

Most witnesses took pains to explain that Van Auken's instances of memory loss and repetition in conversation were no impediments to his successful conduct of his farming business. A local cooper, Nelson Crane, noted that he had done a considerable amount of work for Van Auken during which time they both spoke about farming and that there was 'nothing that appeared loony in the old man'.[54]

In a telling testimonial Crane noted that:

> [I]n a conversation with him about a year ago, he remarked to me that his memory was not as good as it had been – that he was getting forgetful and that he did not like to go away from home much any more for he would often in the same conversation ask the same question two or three times – which made him appear bad.[55]

Crane added that he 'noticed that Van Auken for the past two or three years seems to be somewhat forgetful, and has noticed it by his sometimes in the course of a single conversation asking the same question two or three times'. However, Van Auken's 'horses, cows, hogs and his farming [practices] all appeared to be conducted with judgement and skill' and 'his conversation is always rational and to the point except the repetition of the same question in some of his conversations'.[56]

Witness Jasper Younger recounted a conversation with Van Auken that perhaps put the dynamics of the original trial of lunacy and the struggle for a traverse into perspective. Younger noted that in conversation, Van Auken:

> [C]omplained very much about the course his son in law Mark Ayers had pursued toward him – and remarked that if they would only let him alone they would soon have his property for he was an old man. And in the last conversation this deponent had with him in relation to this proceeding against him Daniel Van Auken's wife was present and she complained and seemed to be very much affected about the matter, she cried over it – and Daniel Van Auken said to her not to take it to heart so much as they could not help it and he supposed would have to put up with it although it was hard for them in their old days.[57]

As with the trial of Abraham Rogers and several others, the decision to put Van Auken's mental capacity on trial was tied up with familial struggles over inheritance and the passing of wealth and property from one generation to the next. In this case, every witness in both legal proceedings acknowledged that Van Auken was becoming repetitive in his conversations, and also forgetful. Most witnesses claimed that he still had the knowledge, skill and physical capacity to conduct the myriad tasks of his busy farm properties. And some – those who were keen to expedite the transfer of his property to their advantage – argued that his mental decline rendered him incapable of operating his farming business without the guardianship afforded by the process of lunacy investigation law. In this case, the fact that Van Auken's two sons were actively engaged in compensating for his loosening grip on the business end of his farming work, along with the burden of evidence in the traverse proceedings and the deceptive nature of the original trial in lunacy, likely accounted for the final verdict of the courts. On 25 October 1854, the lunacy trial was traversed and Van Auken once more gained legal control of his property and person.

Working towards recovery

In trials involving younger individuals, evidence of the return to effective and productive work was considered a sign of recovery. At the lunacy trial of Lukas Hogland in April 1831, held in the house of James Taylor, the innkeeper of the township of Hillsborough, witnesses determined that 'trouble of the mind' on account of 'religious concerns' had rendered Hogland insane for about three months.[58] However, by January 1833, Hogland found himself sufficiently recovered in mind to petition for a *supercedas* of the earlier decision. In fact, in his petition Hogland explained to the New Jersey Chancellor that he had for some time already taken back 'the management and oversight of his farm and all his affairs that he transacts all his own business and also public business as executor, administrator, etc.'[59] However, as 'some portion of his property such as bonds, notes of mortgages' were still under the control of John Vroom, his guardian, he thought it best to formally apply to the courts for a *supercedas*.[60]

In his testimony of support at Hogland's trial, neighbouring farmer John Lawns noted that Hogland now 'manages his farming business himself and has done so from within two months of the time when he was declared a lunatic'.[61] Moreover, according to Lawns, Hogland:

> [M]anages his affairs as well as any of the farmers in the neighbourhood – his fences and everything about him appear to be kept in good order and he seems to be prosperous in his circumstances ... he takes his family to church ... and attends regularly. He has always taken his own grain to market during the last eighteen months and disposes of it himself.[62]

In this case, agricultural prosperity, the rational organisation of farm business and productive work were bundled together as sure signs of mental recovery. As in other cases, witnesses delved into the detail of work tasks successfully and coherently achieved in order to prove mental competence.[63]

The case of Peter Drummond suggests that this relationship between effective work and soundness of mind was recognised to have an informal rehabilitative quality in some local communities in New Jersey. In 1834, Edmund West, Drummond's brother-in-law, along with neighbours Rolph Conover, Joseph Barclay and Joseph Daly, provided evidence in a lunacy trial indicating that Drummond had been insane for several months. Drummond, a twenty-five-year-old bachelor with considerable farm holdings, was exhibiting signs of violence. When Edmond West was sent to Drummond's house, he discovered that Drummond had 'knocked the plastering off the room in which he was and had broken up a table and the shutters off the house'.[64] His friends thus resorted to hiring a full-time male caregiver 'to take charge of him and prevent his doing mischief to himself and others'.[65] Joseph Barclay testified that his wife (who was also Drummond's cousin) who would sometimes 'set him some dinner', observed that, 'after eating he took a cake knife and took a gun in the room and took it to pieces and when asked what he was doing he said he was cleaning it, and rubbed and scraped it with the knife'.[66] When Joseph Barclay asked him 'what he done with the knife he answered he kept it for opening people that he had opened several and intended to open others that it was a disagreeable business but he said he must do it and the next one he would open was Edmund West'. These and other bizarre forms of behaviour made it clear to the courts that Drummond was insane.[67]

Remarkably, seventeen years later in 1851, Drummond petitioned to traverse the 1834 decision. In the evidence of the subsequent legal proceeding, witnesses noted that he had once more regained his ability to perform the tasks of a successful farmer. The most fascinating testimony was from Rulif Smith, a tenant hired by the guardians of Drummond's estate to work Drummond's farm. Smith testified that Drummond had been working for him as a hired hand over the course of an eleven-year period and that in this capacity Drummond had gradually recovered his ability to successfully work a farm. In particular, Drummond had:

> [D]one considerable work for me for the last five or six years on the farm and more or less ever since I have lived on the place. He has helped me plant corn and potatoes[,] husk corn, dig potatoes – kill hogs – and all other kinds of work that I have had to do pretty much … I have seen him work alone without any body's being with him. He has worked for me alone frequently – In performing this work for the past few years I have discovered nothing like insanity or derangement in him. In my judgement I should think that he was now capable of taking charge of his farm and managing it himself.[68]

When cross-examined, Smith noted that Drummond had not worked the kinds of full-time hours that he expected of his other hired hands. Nevertheless, Smith explained that, 'in hay and harvest I paid him what I paid other folks and for other work I paid him 41 or 51 a day, whatever wages were at the time'.[69] In Smith's opinion, if Drummond was 'restored to his property now I believe from the present tone of his mind that he would take care of it'.[70] In this and other trials, accounts of the journey of insane individuals back to a sane state of mind were closely tied to the close monitoring of improvements in the ability to conduct farm labour. Though perhaps not a form of conscious rehabilitation, a kind of custom developed in which some space was created for individuals who might recover to reacquaint themselves with the multiple aspects of their former work, and property management.

Asylum work

If effectiveness at work was one pivot around which the determinations of madness and mental recovery revolved in the rural and town settings of New Jersey, how did this compare to the consideration of patient work in a nineteenth-century lunatic asylum? As earlier works and many of the contributions to this volume demonstrate, there is no shortage of material with which to consider the role of work as a form of therapy, rehabilitation, discipline and coercion in the asylum. But before we add these considerations to our discussion here, it is worth pointing out that psychiatrists of public (and some private and semi-private) mental institutions in the United States, including the New Jersey State Lunatic Asylum, were rather critical of the pre-admission domestic context of management and care that I have described thus far. This critique formed part of the promotion of the asylum as the best bet for the successful treatment of the mad.

As part of his characterisation of the asylum as the best option for the insane, John Buttolph, the first superintendent of the New Jersey State Lunatic Asylum noted that public asylums were better places of treatment than:

> [P]rivate families, or even private institutions, where the objects of interest and diversion are less numerous, and where the architectural arrangements and the general system of moral discipline and management are less perfectly adapted for the guidance of the erring and the control of the wayward and violent.[71]

Along with superior medical treatment, Buttolph argued that the advantage of his asylum's moral treatment was 'the removal [of the patient] from home and the sources of irritation there existing, to the care of strangers who should be intelligent kind and conscientious, and who have tact and experience to aid them in the performance of their particular duties'.[72] Finally, in an asylum setting it was possible to arrange for:

> [S]uch occupation and amusements as are adapted for their benefit in view of their previous habits and pursuits, and the form and stage of disease under which they are labouring ... as a means of enlisting their feelings, and of directing their attention from themselves and the morbid trains of thought in which they are inclined to indulge.[73]

In 1863, Buttolph reiterated his point, noting that:

> [I]n many cases of mental disorder ... caused or perpetuated by unfavourable circumstances and influences connected with home life ... no time should be lost in removing the patient from the sphere of noxious influences that have caused or continued his disorder, and in such cases a well regulated institution for the insane is generally the most favourable for his comfort and restoration.[74]

Colleagues at other American institutions echoed Superintendent Buttolph's remarks on the superiority of the asylum over home care.[75]

In his first annual report, under the heading 'Occupation and Amusements', Superintendent Buttolph made the familiar argument that physical exercise was 'important in many, especially chronic cases, by assisting to restore a healthy state of the physical functions, by promoting appetite and digestion, and above all, by securing cheerfulness and contentment during the day, and quiet and refreshing sleep at night'.[76] Although mentioning 'riding, walking, and various games' along with other amusements in the list of exercises, physical labours such as farming did not appear on the list. Yet in almost every year in his annual reports, from 1850 to 1860, Buttolph noted the productivity of patient work in farming and gardening, to the twin advantages of his patient's mental health and the institution's financial health.

A brief examination of Buttolph's statements about patient work in the New Jersey asylum brings to the fore many of the elements of work, occupational therapy, and mental health under consideration here, and establishes some basis for comparison with these same elements explored through the records of New Jersey's lunacy investigation law. As in other institutions, Buttolph took pains to explain that patient work on the farm and in the garden was profitable to the asylum. In 1851 he asserted that the 'results of the farming and gardening operation for the year have realised our just anticipations', but the main aspiration in this case was 'a clear gain to the institution of eight hundred and nine dollars and thirty-seven cents'.[77] Just as often the superintendent clearly articulated the links of farm and garden work, institutional prosperity, and mental health. He noted in 1855:

> The products of the farm and garden, as in former years have aided materially, by supplying the house with wholesome vegetables in their seasons, while the labor expended thereon, by patients, have served the double purpose of lessening the cost of production, and of aiding the effect of other means, in securing their comfort or recovery, or both.[78]

Within the first twelve years of the New Jersey Asylum's existence, Buttolph was claiming that for:

> [A] large number of the patients[,] useful employment is regarded as a valuable, if not the most valuable means of strengthening and restoring the physical system, and of diverting the mind from such morbid trains of thought and feeling, as are habitually indulged by the insane.[79]

Occasionally, the superintendent was more specific about why physical labour was claiming first place in the pantheon of 'activities and amusements' that the asylum provided for its patients. In 1852 he noted that:

> The grounds about the building ... have been improved as much during the past year by grading, the laying of walks and planting of trees and shrubbery, as the means at our disposal would permit. In this work many of the patients have cheerfully joined, and thus rendered to the institution valuable assistance, while they secured to themselves the great benefits, physical and moral, attendant upon useful labor, and not to be expected from exercise for mere amusement.[80]

'Useful labour' – work that would provide for the material needs of the asylum, and reduce institutional costs – was best designed for mental improvement. Although other forms of exercise and amusement would be of constitutional benefit to asylum patients, they could not match the powers of productive labour.

Conclusion

In both asylum and community in nineteenth-century New Jersey there were clearly strong connections between the understandings of and responses to work and madness. Yet, a wide gulf separated the work/madness relationship as understood and practised in each setting. The relationship between work and mental status that formed part of lunacy investigation law was centuries old. Nineteenth-century New Jersey legal officials would have found the central aspects of lunacy investigation, as it was practised in England in the seventeenth century, remarkably familiar to them. Lunacy trials were, by definition, inquiries as to whether an individual was fit to govern self and property. As part of that definition, the ability to pursue work rationally, whether that work entailed running the family fortunes of a large landed estate, a retail business, a factory, or a farm, was central to the definition of mental health. Lunacy investigation law thus thrived and adapted remarkably intact in a variety of economic settings over a long historical period, including the predominantly agricultural setting of nineteenth-century New Jersey. Like elsewhere, and in previous eras, the preoccupations of lunacy investigation law were the same – whether or not those who had property at stake could still maintain it rationally in the face of apparent signs of mental decline.

In townships in nineteenth-century New Jersey, lunacy investigation law was used to protect the property interests of those showing signs of mental alienation, the property concerns of those standing to inherit from them, and the immediate needs of family. Trial witnesses frequently described in detail the capacity of the defendants to work productively at the everyday tasks of farm and other forms of work in small town and rural settings. As we have seen, this legal process sometimes entailed conflict in instances when differences of opinion arose about the extent to which productive work was compromised by the mental state of individuals in question. Witnesses placed a very high value on unproductive work as a sign of madness and productive work as a measure of mental recovery. This consideration of madness in relation to productive labour was context specific, depending, for example, on the age of the individuals, the point at which inheritance intersected with their incapacity to work effectively, or the manner in which their work habits were perceived as a threat to their property. Furthermore, testimonials from New Jersey lunacy trials strongly suggest that some individuals who were considered no longer mentally capable of working their property rationally were given some space for recovery. In these cases incremental improvements in their capacity to work effectively was considered as a measure of mental restoration.

This outlook on productive work as a salutary sign of mental soundness, contrasts sharply with the ways in which work was understood therapeutically and organised institutionally for patients in an asylum setting. The work/

madness relationship in an asylum setting was new to New Jersey compared to the much older understanding of this relationship that had developed through civil law. The extent to which alienists understood either lunacy investigation law, or the familial and local understandings of madness in relation to productive labour, is difficult to assess. Nevertheless, superintendents like New Jersey Asylum's John Buttolph were openly hostile to the idea of familial care of the mad as compared to asylum care. In the asylum setting patient work was in theory more 'medicalised' than it was in the community. It was meant to promote more rational behaviour among patients through the repetition of familiar tasks, through the stimulation of the body in the service of the brain, and by keeping morbid thoughts at bay. Yet, from the beginning patient work in asylum settings was also about shoring up asylum budgets and helping to guarantee the smooth running of the institution. For Superintendent Buttolph the value of productive labour was as much about the financial wellbeing of his institution as it was about the mental recovery of his patients. In the asylum patients were not working their own farm property or the property of neighbours, nor were they demonstrating through productive work that they had regained the right to take back legal ownership of their farms. The relationship between productive labour and the easing of mental symptoms was certainly pointed out by Buttolph, but it is unclear if patients who worked productively in the asylum were considered likelier to be discharged as improved or recovered. Those who were admitted to the asylum were introduced to a very different world – one in which farm, garden and some domestic work may have been the most familiar element. But their co-workers would not have been familiar and the other aspects of asylum life would scarcely have looked to its patients like life back home. In both settings the work/madness relationship was of major concern, but the travails of madness played out very differently in each.

Notes

1 Discussions of patient work in asylum settings can be found in: Patricia D'Antonio, *Founding Friends: Families, Staff, and Patients at the Friends Asylum in Early Nineteenth-Century Philadelphia* (Bethlehem: Lehigh University Press, 2006), pp. 108–29; Steven Cherry, *Mental Health Care in Modern England: The Norfolk Lunatic Asylum/St. Andrew's Hospital c. 1810–1998* (Suffolk: Boydell Press, 2003), pp. 53–82; Ellen Dwyer, *Homes for the Mad: Life Inside Two Nineteenth-Century Asylums* (New Brunswick, NJ: Rutgers University Press, 1987); Nancy Tomes, *A Generous Confidence: Thomas Story Kirkbride and the Art of Asylum-Keeping, 1840–1883* (Cambridge: Cambridge University Press, 1984), pp. 188–263, passim; James Moran, *Committed to the State Lunatic Asylum: Insanity and Society in Nineteenth-Century Quebec and Ontario* (Kingston, ONT: McGill Queen's University Press, 2000), pp. 92–5.

2 Geoffrey Reaume, 'Patients at work: Insane asylum inmates' labour in Ontario, 1841–1900', in James Moran and David Wright (eds), *Mental Health in Canadian Society: Historical Perspectives* (Montreal: McGill Queen's University Press, 2006). Reaume's advocacy work related to patient labour is exemplified in Geoffrey Reaume, 'Why words on the wall?', *Voices: Newsletter of the Psychiatric Survivor Archives of Toronto*, 1:1 (2010), 2.
3 Reaume, 'Patients at work', p. 90.
4 Andrew Scull, *The Most Solitary of Afflictions: Madness and Society in Britain, 1700–1900* (New Haven, CT: Yale University Press, 1993), p. 35.
5 *Ibid.*
6 As a host of recent writings in the field have demonstrated, despite the obvious influence of the asylum, and its increasing patient population up to the mid-twentieth century, a great many people considered as mentally troubled were not cared for in an asylum institutional setting. See, for example, David Wright, 'Getting out of the asylum: Understanding the confinement of the insane in the nineteenth-century', *Social History of Medicine*, 10:1 (1997), 137–55; Peter Bartlett and David Wright, *Outside the Walls of the Asylum: The History of Care in the Community, 1750–2000* (London: Athlone Press, 1999).
7 See James Moran, *Non-Compos-Mentis: Madness and Civil Law in Trans-Atlantic Historical Perspective* (Rochester: Rochester University Press, forthcoming); James Moran, 'Asylum in the community: Managing the insane in antebellum America', *History of Psychiatry*, 9:34 (1998), 217–40. For a history of the use of trials in lunacy in early modern England see Richard Neugebauer, 'Mental illness and government policy in sixteenth and seventeenth century England' (PhD dissertation, Columbia University, 1976). For an excellent study of trials in lunacy in early nineteenth-century England see Akihito Suzuki, *Madness at Home: The Psychiatrist, the Patient, and the Family in England, 1820–1860* (Berkeley, CA: University of California Press, 2006).
8 The New Jersey trials in lunacy documents are held in the New Jersey State Archives (hereafter NJSA), Chancery Court Lunacy Case Files, 1796–1912, SCH00020.
9 Trial of John Barron, NJSA, Chancery Court Lunacy Case Files, 1826.
10 Trial of John McIntire, NJSA, Chancery Court Lunacy Case Files, 1807.
11 *Ibid.*
12 *Ibid.*
13 Trial of John Bertholf, NJSA, Chancery Court Lunacy Case Files, 1838.
14 *Ibid.*
15 Trial of Daniel Higgins, NJSA, Chancery Court Lunacy Case Files, 1822.
16 *Ibid.*
17 *Ibid.*
18 *Ibid.*
19 Trial of Rebecca Large, NJSA, Chancery Court Lunacy Case Files, 1829.
20 *Ibid.*
21 *Ibid.*
22 Trial of Phebe McPherson, NJSA, Chancery Court Lunacy Case Files, 1853.
23 *Ibid.*

24 Trial of Jacob Wood, NJSA, Chancery Court Lunacy Case Files, 1825.
25 *Ibid.*
26 Trial of Nathaniel Allen, NJSA, Chancery Court Lunacy Case Files, 1841.
27 *Ibid.*
28 *Ibid.*
29 *Ibid.*
30 Trial of Abraham Rogers, NJSA, Chancery Court Lunacy Case Files, 1843.
31 *Ibid.*
32 *Ibid.*
33 *Ibid.*
34 *Ibid.*
35 *Ibid.*
36 *Ibid.*
37 *Ibid.*
38 *Ibid.*
39 *Ibid.*
40 *Ibid.*
41 *Ibid.*
42 *Ibid.*
43 *Ibid.*
44 *Ibid.*
45 *Ibid.*
46 *Ibid.*
47 *Ibid.*
48 *Ibid.*
49 Trial of Daniel Van Auken, NJSA, Chancery Court Lunacy Case Files, 1854.
50 At this first trial, Van Auken's two sons did make it to court to testify on their father's behalf in opposition to Mark Ayers (Van Auken's son-in-law) and Van Auken's brother, who were attempting to find him insane.
51 *Ibid.*
52 *Ibid.*
53 *Ibid.*
54 *Ibid.*
55 *Ibid.*
56 *Ibid.*
57 *Ibid.*
58 Trial of Lukas Hogland, NJSA, Chancery Court Lunacy Case Files, 1831.
59 *Ibid.*
60 *Ibid.*
61 *Ibid.*
62 *Ibid.*
63 See, for example, the trial of Moses Allen, NJSA, Chancery Court Lunacy Case Files, 1833.
64 Trial of Peter Drummond, NJSA, Chancery Court Lunacy Case Files, 1834.
65 *Ibid.*

66 *Ibid.*
67 *Ibid.*
68 *Ibid.*
69 *Ibid.*
70 *Ibid.*
71 John Buttolph, 'Annual Report of the New Jersey State Lunatic Asylum', 1848, p. 30.
72 *Ibid.*, p. 29.
73 *Ibid.*, p. 29.
74 John Buttolph, 'Annual Report of the New Jersey State Lunatic Asylum', 1863, p. 14.
75 Moran, 'Asylum in the Community', pp. 230–40.
76 John Buttolph, 'Annual Report of the New Jersey State Lunatic Asylum', 1848, p. 30.
77 John Buttolph, 'Annual Report of the New Jersey State Lunatic Asylum', 1851, p. 13.
78 John Buttolph, 'Annual Report of the New Jersey State Lunatic Asylum', 1855, p. 18.
79 John Buttolph, 'Annual Report of the New Jersey State Lunatic Asylum', 1860, p. 15.
80 John Buttolph, 'Annual Report of the New Jersey State Lunatic Asylum', 1852, p. 22.

4

From blasting powder to tomato pickles: Patient work at the provincial mental hospitals in British Columbia, Canada, 1885–1920

Kathryn McKay

This is the first year that the patients have been allowed to work ... On days when the weather would not permit them working outside, they [the patients] framed pictures and did light carpentry work in the house. If we are allowed to take in another ten acres of ground to the back of us we will be able to grow enough vegetables for our table ... Of course the female patients all worked at sewing &c.[1]

The necessity and wisdom of liberally providing means of diversion for the insane is so generally admitted that the question is scarcely, if at all, in the field of controversy ... Encouragement has been given them to work in the shops, in the gardens, on the lawns and in various departments of the farm. We have found that work, and especially work in the open air and in open and healthy surroundings, is of the utmost value to mental patients. Being a factor in the production of health and happiness, it also becomes a means of cure.[2]

This chapter examines how medical superintendents presented patient work within the larger narrative structure of the annual reports submitted to the Provincial Secretary. While critics such as patient advocates and labour organisations considered patient work to be evidence of exploitation, proponents maintained that it allowed mental hospital inmates the opportunity to develop and maintain a sense of accomplishment in a safe and secure setting.[3] Through an analysis of a variety of public and private sources, I argue that superintendents and medical authorities were well aware of the contentiousness of patient work and devised a number of strategies to address the tension between exploitation and therapy. Their strategies involved not only the placement of the statistics outlining patient labour in relation to the social and economic conditions in British Columbia but, importantly, also included discussions of gender and race. To this end medical authorities focused on the constructive nature of male labour over the consumptive character of female work. Further, racial stereotypes, such as the Chinese laundryman, frequently informed the organisation of patient labour.

British Columbia

Situated on the coast and isolated from the rest of the country by the Rocky Mountains to the east, British Columbia was known as the 'west beyond the west'.[4] This physical isolation from the population centres in the east deeply influenced the historical trajectory of the province. While the colonial settlement of eastern Canada began in the seventeenth century, most of the developments in British Columbia, excluding those of the First Nations,[5] only began in the early nineteenth century.

Geographer Cole Harris contends that: 'time seems telescoped in British Columbia ... the long story of emerging modernity, extending back through European millennia, is compressed into 100 years or so'.[6] The history of state formation in British Columbia, as it transitioned from a territory defined by the fur trade to a province in the Dominion of Canada in the space of twenty-five years, was also accelerated. Thus, the development of the asylum in British Columbia differed from those established in the east. Most of the asylums in eastern Canada came into existence during the reform movements of the mid-eighteenth century and were situated in, or close to, established urban centres with well-developed physical and social infrastructures.[7] In contrast, with the exception of three cities in the south-western portion of the province, British Columbia in 1872 contained neither large urban centres nor a developed system of roads.[8]

The first asylum, opened in 1872, although situated in the capital city of Victoria was located on land that had only recently been removed from an Indian reserve.[9] In 1878, when the asylum was relocated to the city of New Westminster, the site was still being hewn from the landscape.[10] While much of eastern Canada was characterised by agricultural settlements, British Columbia relied on resource extraction, employing mobile groups of able-bodied men rather than sedentary family units for its economic base.[11] Thus, in 1885, the first year of this study the male to female ratio in the hospital was 5 : 1,[12] while males represented just under 75 per cent of the non-Aboriginal population.[13] By 1920, the final year of this study, the ratio had shifted to approximately 2.5 : 1.[14] The 1921 census indicated that males represented 58.5 per cent of the non-aboriginal population.[15]

The institutions

Although physically proximate, mental institutions in Canada and the United States of America followed very different models of development. Asylums and hospitals in the United States tended to be private and granted more autonomy to their superintendents. In contrast, provincial governments in Canada administered most of the mental institutions as part of a system of publicly funded health and welfare. Medical superintendents functioned as public servants who were responsible to the provincial government.[16] In British Columbia, then, the annual report delivered to the Provincial Secretary provided information not only to the government, but also functioned as a means to highlight the positive measures undertaken at the institution and broadcast them to the entire province.

In his annual report for 1901, the newly appointed medical superintendent, Dr George H. Manchester (1872–1956), reflected on the history of asylums in British Columbia. He maintained that prior to the gold rush of 1858–59 insanity was rare in British Columbia. Manchester attributed the increase in the incidence of 'break down' to the 'strain and hardship' experienced by many of the newcomers.[17] Most of the afflicted were either sent to asylums in the state of California, the location of the closest institution, or placed in local jails.[18] While it is clear that some were merely being repatriated to the United States, Manchester also noted that although the Californian authorities offered to take British Columbia's insane for a price, the colonial government rejected this offer and continued to house the insane in jails.[19]

Citing moral principles, the newspapers in the capital city of Victoria frequently argued for governmental action to segregate the insane from the criminal element. In 1869 an editorial in the *British Colonist* maintained that lunatics, unlike criminals who were deemed to be responsible for their actions, required specialised medical care which was beyond the capabilities of a jailer.[20] In 1870 the *Colonist* again appealed to social mores when raising concerns regarding the confinement of three sisters, considered lunatics, who were held in the city jail: 'There are now three females compelled to herd with black guards, felons and murderers and for no other cause than that they have been so unfortunate to lose their reason!'[21] Despite these emotional arguments, it was not until 1872 that the province finally opened its first mental institution known as the Victoria Lunatic Asylum. Located in a former pesthouse across the harbour from the centre of Victoria on Vancouver Island, the building was ill-suited for use as an asylum. Small and in bad condition, locals considered it a 'poor excuse for an asylum'.[22] However, faced with numerous tasks of state development, the provincial government did not consider the management of the insane to be a pressing problem in the early 1870s.[23]

The Victoria Lunatic Asylum predated by one year the passage of the Insane Asylums Act 1873, which provided for the establishment of public asylums that would be controlled by the provincial lieutenant-governor in Council.[24] This initial act did not include provisions for detailed record keeping and required little more than the collation of admission documents. Twenty-four years later, the act was replaced by the Hospitals for the Insane Act of 1897. This revised legislation reflected growing concerns with the treatment of the insane as well as with the proliferation of bureaucratic practice in medicine.[25]

In 1878 the province closed the asylum in Victoria and opened a purpose-built institution in New Westminster, close to the mainland city of Vancouver. This was followed, in 1913, by the establishment of Essondale Hospital, initially known as the Hospital of the Mind, a state of the art establishment, located less than fifteen kilometres away in Port Coquitlam.[26] In 1919 the province acquired Colquitz, located on Vancouver Island approximately ten kilometres north of Victoria, as a forensic hospital for the criminally insane. By 1920, these three mental hospitals were operating in British Columbia, making provision for 1,417 male and 608 female patients from a variety of national and cultural backgrounds.[27] The initial focus will be on the asylum in New Westminster and, after 1913, will shift to the newly opened hospital at Essondale.[28] During the period under study both Essondale and Colquitz Hospitals were male-only facilities. It is important to note that once Essondale opened, the medical superintendent shifted his narrative to discuss the opportunities for patient labour at this hospital at the expense of the hospital in New Westminster. Thus, his discussions privileged male labour over that of female patients.

Work: Benefiting the patient and the province

From 1885 until the 1920s, the annual reports of the provincial asylums, later hospitals, of British Columbia contained narrative and statistical information regarding all aspects of institutional management, including patient work. These reports not only reflected the gendered and racialised facets of settler colonialism in British Columbia, but their emphases also shifted in accordance with the economic and social circumstances of the province, wider attitudes towards patient work, and the changing precepts of state policies.

During the early years of the asylum, from 1872 to 1900, the complexity of the annual reports increased steadily. The earliest reports featured a one- or two-page narrative that outlined the general state of the asylum. In this section the medical officer or superintendent discussed the overall change in the number of patients and the conditions, both positive and negative, of the institutions.[29] A statistical section followed, providing data on patients' occupation, place of residence and type of illness. It also provided a tabulation of the yearly expenses and always closed with the list of garden products grown at the asylums. The reports generally followed this template until 1901.

Although early reports mentioned the importance of exercise for patients, the 1882 report for the Asylum for the Insane in New Westminster was the first to argue that patient work could offer a benefit to the province. In his report, the medical officer, Thomas R. McInnes (1840–1904), speculated on the probable benefits of fencing and cultivating four acres in front of the asylum. He posited:

> This would not only add materially to the appearance of the institution, but would have a most beneficial effect on a large portion of the patients ... and I am confident, by utilizing patient work, more vegetables could be grown than would supply the institution, thereby saving at least six hundred dollars per annum.[30]

With an outlay of $5,400 for consumable goods, $600 would represent a significant saving. McInnes made it clear that the asylum, given the proper resources, could not only provide a benefit to the patients, but also ameliorate the cost to the province.

However, there was no indication in the annual reports that patients participated in any type of work until 1885, when the medical superintendent, Dr Richard I. Bentley (1854–1909), remarked:

> This is the first year that the patients have been allowed to work, and to see them at it proves that they enjoy it thoroughly. They have done a great deal, although they only go out to work on fine days, and then only for five or six hours. It is entirely voluntary.[31]

A critical examination of Bentley's comment reveals a number of important points. By using the words 'allowed' and 'enjoy' he suggested that the patients considered labour a privilege. Further, as this labour occurred only on 'fine days' and for a short while, Bentley pre-empted any potential allegations of exploitation and harsh conditions. Finally, stressing the voluntary nature of the labour, he promoted the idea that the patients were active participants, concerned with both their own improvement and that of the institution.

Gendered work

During this early period, superintendents tended not to assign monetary values to either male or female work, but merely specified the types of tasks carried out. By doing so, they revealed contemporary gender norms in regard to work considered suitable for men and women. For example, in the scant report for 1885 Superintendent R. I. Bentley dedicated two paragraphs to the various activities carried out by patients, such as planting an orchard, building a cow shed, and light carpentry work. Bentley further stressed that male workers were occupied with building, clearing and ploughing land, and producing crops and livestock. In contrast, women worked by the piece, making tape yards and dusters, and repairing trousers and undershorts. In the Report for 1888, he remarked that patient work had contributed not only to the production of eighteen and a half tons of potatoes, but also cleaning one half mile of water pipe, building a sidewalk, and clearing five acres of stumps and underbrush. 'These works kept all the patients who could be trusted to work out of doors occupied ... The female patients get through a lot of sewing, mending and &c., as may be seen in Table No. 14.'[32]

This regime reflected the work practices of the era; it also reproduced the economic model of society. Although most of the male work was actually consumed by the catch-all category of 'ward work', the overall narrative in the reports focused on the larger building and clearing projects, and thus reverberated with the wider settlers' trope of making the land inhabitable. Men went out to work and their work contributed to the construction of a new society. Women stayed at home and performed domestic tasks, such as sewing and putting up tomato pickles. Unlike the long-term, permanent projects of settlement, female work was intended for short-term consumption and repairs.

Work and its benefit to all

The tension between treatment and work was evident in the report for 1895, when statistics in the report listed for the first time the number of man-days worked. The superintendent at New Westminster, George F. Bodington (1828–1902), explained that although the men were actively employed for a combined total of 21,564 days, these were not full eight-to-ten-hour work days, as was then the norm in British Columbia. He explained further:

> It must be remembered that a day's work for these patients only amounts to four or four and one-half hours, and that the men employed are, for the most part, in a languid or feeble bodily condition, and the quantity of work per hour done by them is considerably less than the average done by an ordinary able-bodied worker.[33]

According to the report, 172 men had been resident in the asylum during the year. If all of them each worked equally, the result would be 123 days per man. Clearly, as not all of the men were capable, some must have worked quite steadily. Thus, the superintendent's assertion that their labour was valuable, but not as valuable as that of the 'average man' outside the institution, may have been designed to alleviate accusations of exploitation, yet still promote the notion of patients' contribution to public finances.

The following year, in 1896, Bodington expanded his discussion of patient work, arguing that the efforts of some benefited all. He noted that patients, under the direction of an attendant, had almost completed the fencing of the grounds. Once the fencing was complete, and means of escape thwarted, patients would be able to use the grounds for walks and other forms of exercise.[34] The gains were twofold. First, working patients benefited from being engaged in meaningful activities. Second, their fellow inmates could enjoy the results of their labours. In his report for 1897 Bodington remarked: 'My aim and object is to bring as much land as possible under culture [sic], whereby the Asylum may not only have its own wants supplied, but a profit may, I doubt not, in the course of time, be made by the sale of superfluous garden products.'[35] Again he reiterated the dual benefits of patient labour in the production of healthy food for both the asylum table and for sale.

From 1885 to 1900, the narratives focused mainly on structural improvements such as the construction of buildings and the clearing of land. While the medical superintendent stressed that the institutions were striving towards self-sufficiency, rather than being a drain on the public purse, he also began to discuss labour as an effective therapeutic regime. For example, in 1896 Bodington stated that: 'Nothing contributes more to the recovery of insane patients, and also to their happiness and contentment, than plenty of exercise in the open air. The dull monotony of the wards is depressing and detrimental.'[36] He continued in his 1897 report that: '[W]hile the cultivation of land is made remunerative, at the same time the occupation will be most beneficial to the patients, for whom such labour ... is a most valuable means of medical treatment'.[37] By discussing patient labour as both remunerative and therapeutic, Bodington addressed the historically important financial issues and also indicated the shift in medical thought regarding this practice.

During the later part of the nineteenth century, the production statistics that referred to patient work were listed in the annual reports immediately after the overall statement on spending and expenditure and were thus separated from the bulk of the patient data. Although the tables did not include detailed monetary information, their placement emphasised the financial nature of this information. While not all that significant in relation to the overall balance sheet of the ever-expanding institutions, the work undertaken by patients clearly contributed to their financial soundness. The asylum, initially only half-heartedly supported by the government, had to present itself as a valuable component in the development of the province. By indicating fiscal responsibility through the use patient work, medical officials could argue that the institution would not prove an unnecessary drain on the provincial budget and would also offer a positive model for the treatment of the insane. Although patients remained inmates of an asylum, under the tutelage of the medical and other staff, at least some of them were deemed productive members of society.

Work: 'An absolute necessity'

During the second period, from 1901 to 1920, both the narrative and statistical sections in the reports became increasingly lengthier. While the structure of general description followed by hard data remained the same, the medical superintendents bolstered their discussions with reflections on new areas of interest, such as laboratory reports, dentistry, and coroners' statements. As before, the statistical section provided information on patient numbers, morbidity and mortality, length of stay, types of illness and the like. Details on the ever expanding roster of agricultural activities were added to the statistics, as well as photographs of the institutions and the grounds, blueprints for proposed additions, numerous depictions of the prizewinning livestock, and artistic reproductions of therapeutic devices, such as the hydrotherapy cabinet.[38] While dependent upon developments in the technology of publishing and the willingness of the province to utilise these expensive techniques, the reports evolved from simple accounts of finances and patient statistics to a persuasive tool illustrating the modernity of the institution and, by extension, the province.

In the annual report for 1901, the new medical superintendent of the provincial mental hospital,[39] Dr G. H. Manchester, changed the position of the statistical tables.[40] He included discussion of income and expenditure, and of the monetary value of goods produced on the grounds in the narrative section, together with the quantitative data. The section entitled 'Statistical Tables' consequently provided information on the patients only. A particularly intriguing change in regard to work was the inclusion of the heading 'Treatment' in the narrative section of the report. In 1902, Manchester noted:

> Employment for the insane was an absolute necessity, and of its beneficial results there can be no question. Without it the life of many patients would be simply intolerable ... I have always considered the provision of occupation for the patients under my care as one of my foremost duties, and I know that in this I am only following the footsteps of the leading alienists of the day. That there are many difficulties and dangers attendant upon the employing of the insane I will admit, but these must be surmounted in the interests of the patients themselves.[41]

This statement highlights a shift from patient work as a means of cost reduction to one of treatment. Manchester clearly suggested that patient work benefited the patient more than it did the institution. Nevertheless, Manchester still remained fully aware of the monetary value of patient labour. He noted in a passage titled 'Work':

> [A] fine maple desk for the chief attendant's office, a typewriter cabinet for the Medical Superintendent's office ... all of which are beautifully constructed and

worth a good sum of money ... This work was previously done in the City, and so a saving has been effected with benefit to the inmates.[42]

Using the categories of treatment and work, Manchester argued that patient work reduced institutional expenses as well as constituting an important part of modern treatment. The placement of the production tables in the section concerning the patients highlighted the role of work as a therapeutic regime as it directly connected it to the statistical data on patients such as mortality and cure rates rather than the institutional finances. Pairing production tables with patient outcomes not only implied a direct connection between the two, but also suggested that patients were not a burden on society, but contributed to the greater good in the province. The production tables provided a kind of positive closure to this section and presented the hospital as a site of patient activity rather than a place where patients were locked away, deprived of distraction and useful occupation.

Manchester focused expansively on the operation of the hospital and innovations designed to improve the lives of the patients. He proudly stated:

> I saw that there were enough trustworthy patients, who, if gathered together, would fill one ward, which they might be able to take care of themselves with some oversight, and at the same time have the privilege of open doors; accordingly the 'open-door ward' was established and has proved successful, so that two less attendants were required on the staff. These patients were also allowed to remain up at night until 10 p.m. for reading and social games.[43]

At first glance this statement indicates that Manchester introduced a modern, liberal approach to patient care by granting a certain amount of autonomy to 'trustworthy patients', thus encouraging their progress. However, it was also designed to address the primary concerns raised by Dr Charles K. Clarke (1857–1924)[44] in the 1901 Commission of Inquiry.[45] Clarke's report had contended that: 'One of the most serious questions to be dealt with at New Westminster is that of the enormous per capita cost.'[46] Clarke suggested that: 'there is not the slightest reason why a very great reduction cannot be made by means of a complete reorganization of the staff'.[47] He also maintained that patients should be enlisted to engage in tasks currently performed by staff members and that having a full-time teamster or driver of a team of animals on the staff was a luxury when 'there is no doubt an intelligent patient who has had experience with horses, can under the direction of attendants, be found to do this work efficiently and satisfactorily'.[48] Thus, what appears on a first reading of the report to have been a measure aimed at improving patients' freedom of action and work satisfaction, was fuelled by concerns to enhance the balance sheet of the institution. The rhetoric of work as treatment was strongly intertwined with the language of financial prudence.

Manchester's 'open door ward' at the New Westminster hospital was most probably mainly dedicated to English speakers. The superintendent listed 'reading and social games' as one of their privileges. Each year the annual report closed with 'acknowledgements' dedicated to the various newspapers and people who had provided reading material to the hospital. All of the newspapers listed were English-language publications.[49] The working ward was clearly male as women worked indoors and Manchester noted that the inmates 'went out to work every fine day'. Gender was also a factor in relation to amusements: 'Two more billiard tables were secured and placed on the male wards, where they have been greatly appreciated and enjoyed ... For the women a piano was purchased and this has made a great change for those patients.'[50]

Gendered views were reflected also in Tables 22 and 23. The former recorded the type of employment that the male patients followed during the year and also listed the number of days they worked. Generally, men's activities were arranged by trade, such as work with the gardener, tailor, and blacksmith, and tabulated on a 'per day' basis. Although there were a number of trades mentioned, the bulk of the work done by men was the undetermined 'working on the wards' at 29,684 days. The next most frequent occupation was working with the farmer at 6,805 days. Table 23 recorded the articles made and repaired in the wards and in the workshops during the year. It primarily listed the piecework done on the female wards. In 1901 the list included all manner of clothing and furnishings, such as rugs and curtains, as well as two billiard table covers. The table concluded with articles produced in the tailor's and shoemaker's workshops. In contrast to women's activities, men's were recorded twice: in relation to the generic types of work pursued and the products resulting from them.

Work as treatment

The *Rules and Regulations of the Public Hospital for the Insane* published by the province in 1901, highlighted the role of work in the treatment process as well as reiterating its financial importance. The manual stated that it was the duty of the chief attendants to assign and select patients for work. There were three principles: 'All should do something!! None should do too much!! Avoid danger!!' Emphasis was on how work could benefit patients.[51]

By the early 1910s, patient work had been part of the institutional regime at New Westminster for twenty-five years and the superintendents were increasingly more inclined to discuss its economic importance, especially during a period of economic downturn in the province.[52] In the 1912 report the medical superintendent reflected on the construction of a second hospital that had been begun in 1908:

> In the spring of the following year [1909] ... we started to clear land in earnest; over forty patients, many of whom were excellent axe-men, with the assistance of two donkey-engines, also manned ... by patients, managed to clear ... some 80 acres. In 1909 ... the temporary quarters were enlarged until we could accommodate some sixty-five of our best working patients. The manner in which our patients took hold of this work surprised me, one patient alone during one month handling 17 tons of blasting powder.[53]

From today's point of view it may strike us as remarkable that mental patients were trusted with axes and blasting powder. Lacking information on their mental condition, it is difficult to gauge if such trust was well judged and due attention was given to the principle 'Avoid danger!' There is some information though on the temporary arrangements made for the patients during construction work and the value of their labours. In a private letter written in 1947 to the office of the Provincial Secretary by Gowan S. McGowan, the long-serving bursar of the institution. He recorded that in 1906 'the patients were put out in canvas camps and enjoyed the outing a great deal, but the pleasure of the occasion was often spoiled during the rainy weather by the intense leaking'.[54] By 1908, the patient force had cleared over eighty acres and 'well informed men estimated that clearing an acre of this land was worth $250.00 so that the work already done to this time by patient work represented some $20,000.00 to the Province'.[55]

The new state of the art hospital was due to open on the day following publication of the *Annual Report* of 1912, which was liberally festooned with photographs of its construction. The superintendent was able to illustrate that patient work was a crucial component in the realisation of the province's public building projects. The report also included a nearly page-long quotation from Dr Eugenio Tanzi's (1856–1934) *Textbook of Mental Diseases* of 1909, in which the author advocated the establishment of colonies of workers within the hospital.[56] Tanzi maintained that work in the open air and in healthy surroundings was of the utmost value for mental patients. He stated: '[T]he spirits of the patients are brightened, the work of those who attend them is ameliorated, and the mission of the State, provinces and communes, which thus provide not only for the custody but also for the recovery of their patients is ennobled.'[57]

By reproducing a section from Tanzi's text that discussed the beneficial effect of work on patients and their contribution to 'the mission of the State', the superintendent presented patient work as a 'win-win' situation, and effectively dismissed any potential challenges against this unwaged form of work.[58] Further, transforming the men from patients in a mental hospital to 'colonies of workers' confirmed the hospital as a place of recovery and activity rather than, as was suggested by Scull, a 'warehouse' for the unfit.[59]

The following year, when building work was nearly finished, the superintendent refocused on agricultural pursuits. He included a section of an article from the newspaper *Chicago Inter Ocean* in his annual report for 1913, which reported the success of livestock raised at the new hospital during an international agricultural show:

> When the judges pinned the blue ribbon on Nerissa [a mare] at the International Livestock Show … they recorded a victory for the new method of treating insanity which is being worked out in the Province of British Columbia … Nerissa and her companions … are the product of the care and labor of insane patients at the Mental Hospital at Coquitlam, where agriculture and stock-breeding have proved a self-sustaining means for curing insanity, and which last year netted the Province $40,000 instead of being a heavy expense to the taxpayers, as such hospitals usually are. The result of this hospital's revolutionary methods may mean world-wide changes in the administration of State institutions for the care of those who are in the twilight state of mental derangement.[60]

Reproducing two full pages of a reporter's unedited hyperbole, the superintendent suggested that British Columbia was the innovating force in the use of agriculture and stock breeding as a new, cost-saving method of treating insanity. The rhetoric had shifted from work as merely beneficial to patients' condition to the assumption that work was a curative agent.

Alas, presenting work as an important part of treatment may well have been economically rather than medically motivated. By 1915 the focus on farming was so intense that other means of treatment were unapologetically dismissed. The acting superintendent at Essondale hospital stated:

> We are at present in a position, by having at our disposal considerable acreage consisting of our farm, nursery, and lawns, to offer employment to our patients which is not only congenial but curative, in that the great majority after a short time show an interest which no indoor occupation would stimulate to the same degree. Having these opportunities relieves us of the necessity of indoor instructions, such as schooling and mechanical training, that is now in vogue in many institutions.[61]

This was a highly problematic statement. The resettlement of British Columbia did not rely on agriculture. The province has always been known as a site for the extraction of resources. Mining, logging, and fishing were the economic drivers of the province. Thus, a machine workshop or mechanic's training would have benefited any curable male patients far more on discharge than farming, nursery or lawn work.[62]

Chinese patients and work

According to the case files, there were many patients who objected to work.[63] However, the only explicitly negative comments in the *Annual Reports* were directed against Chinese inmates. This reflected wider social perceptions in British Columbia that specifically vilified Chinese people.[64] Although encouraged to immigrate in the 1870s as expendable labourers on the railway, public opinion soon turned against this population.[65] In 1884 the provincial government in British Columbia passed the *Chinese Population Regulation Bill* taxing all Chinese persons over the age 10.[66] In 1885 the province reintroduced the *Chinese Immigration Act*. Although both of these attempts to restrict the Chinese population were disallowed as they interfered with federal jurisdiction, once the railway was complete, the federal government imposed a head tax of $50 on all incoming immigrants.[67] By 1903 this legislation had been amended a number of times and the tax had grown from $50 to $500.[68] Within this wider context, mental hospital superintendents frequently presented Chinese patients as an unnecessary drain on society.[69] Further, the medical superintendents continued their diatribes against the Chinese well into the twentieth century.

In 1901 the superintendent at New Westminster reported that the laundry, despite the lack of appliances, was quite productive. He noted that: '[M]uch credit is due to the laundryman, who has so skilfully handled his gang of Chinamen, whom it is not always easy to keep in good washing humour.'[70] This statement may have been made tongue in cheek, but as such drew upon the cultural stereotype of the 'Chinese laundryman' and seemed to question Chinese patients' inclination to engage in hard work. Chinese men were not particularly drawn to laundry work, but neither was anyone else. With few options besides railway work, in the mid-1800s Chinese men saw the opportunity and took it.[71] While it cannot be established whether medical staff actually believed that Chinese men were natural laundry workers, it is clear that it was an unpleasant task relegated to this particular group of patients.[72] This was not the kind of work in the open air that was considered so beneficial for patients. It seems that racial prejudice, prevalent in wider society, managed to penetrate the walls surrounding mental institutions.

Chinese patients were disadvantaged in various ways. For example, while numerous workplace incidents from cuts and burns to serious bodily injuries were mentioned in the patient files, the only workplace injury described in the annual report of the hospital at New Westminster during the first decades of the twentieth century involved Chinese patients. This episode also highlights a wider problem of communication between staff and patients from non-English-speaking backgrounds. The superintendent reported that, while working on the grounds, one Chinese patient attacked another without warning. He noted: 'The Chinese are peculiar, and we suffer from the disadvantage of not knowing their language, so are ignorant of what friction may occur between them.'[73] If lack of language expertise on the part of staff members had an adverse impact on workers' safety, how could Chinese patients have benefited from any treatment during their confinement in the institution?

Despite the decline in the population of Chinese patients, medical superintendents continually singled out the Chinese population during the early twentieth century.[74] In his report for 1899 Bodington stated:

> None of these patients pay for their maintenance, and though some of them work in the gardens and grounds and laundry, yet they are not all able to work at all, being too much broken down in body and mind, and in the main the cost of their maintenance falls upon the revenues of the Province ... It certainly seems to be a hardship upon the taxpayers of the Province that they should be compelled to maintain these decrepit and unprofitable Chinese lunatics for such prolonged periods.[75]

Manchester, in his 1901 report noted that he never missed an opportunity to 'deport an Asiatic and have succeeded in getting rid of a great number'.[76] These comments both reflected and bolstered the anti-Chinese sentiments so prevalent in the province.

Just as the annual reports reflected the gender norms of society in British Columbia, they also conveyed the racial order of settler colonial society. In a settler colonial society the settler polity replaces the purportedly weak indigenous population with that of an exogenous other who is recruited as a labour force.[77] However, once the task is accomplished, or is essentially altered, perception shifts casting the exogenous population as racially dangerous.[78] In British Columbia, authorities bypassed First Nations' labour and recruited Chinese persons to work on the westward expansion of the railway during the 1880s. With the railway completed, the province began to fashion legislation to remove or marginalise the Chinese population. While the patient case files suggest that the medical authorities frequently organised working groups on the basis of race, it is important to note that Chinese labour was the only type discussed in the annual reports and that this mention was always negative. These comments made by the medical superintendents served to highlight the perceived inadequacies of the Chinese as a labour force.

Conclusion

It is clear that medical superintendents tailored their discussions of patient labour in the annual reports to address shifting governmental positions regarding mental asylums and hospitals. During the early years, from 1885 to 1900, authorities primarily focused on aspects of fiscal responsibility, in an era when the asylum had to primarily justify its existence, and secondarily responded to accusations of exploitation. From 1900 to 1920 the annual reports focused on patient work as a therapeutic regime that incidentally contributed to the fiscal wellbeing of the institution. In both instances the medical superintendents presented work as a crucial element in the efficient management of the patient population. Importantly, these discussions reflected the social complexity of the province and represented the institution not as excluded from but rather as an integral component of a rapidly expanding British Columbia.

Notes

1 British Columbia Sessional Papers (hereafter BCSP), *Annual Reports for the Asylum (Hospital) for the Insane*. (Victoria: Richard Wolfenden, 1885–1920). The *Annual Reports* were generally dated for the year they reported on but were published in the following year. There was one year, 1920, when the reporting period shifted from December to March. The citations hereafter give BCSP report year, author, publication year and page number. At times these page references appear as just a number, as in this case, at other times they are preceded by a letter indicating the place in the overall sessional publication. BCSP 1885, Richard I. Bentley, 1886, 391.
2 BCSP 1918, Charles Doherty, 1919, V9.
3 Judith Friedland, *Restoring the Spirit: The Beginnings of Occupational Therapy in Canada, 1890–1930*. (Montreal: McGill Queen's University Press, 2011), p. 20.
4 Jean Barman, *The West Beyond the West A History of British Columbia* (Toronto: University of Toronto Press, 2nd edn, 1996), p. 2.
5 'First Nations' is the name used when discussing the indigenous inhabitants of Canada. In the United States the term 'Native American' is used. These terms replace the word 'Indian'.
6 Cole Harris, *The Resettlement of British Columbia: Essays on Colonialism and Geographical Change* (Vancouver: University of British Columbia Press, 1997), p. 104.
7 Thomas Brown, 'The origins of the asylum in Upper Canada, 1830–1839', *Canadian Bulletin of Medical History*, 1 (1984), 27–58; Daniel Francis, 'The development of the lunatic asylum in the Maritime Provinces', *Acadiensis: Journal of the History of the Atlantic Region*, 6:2 (1977), 23–38; James Moran, *Committed to the State Lunatic Asylum: Insanity and Society in Nineteenth-Century Quebec and Ontario* (Kingston: McGill Queen's University Press, 2000), pp. 49–51.
8 John Belshaw, *Becoming British Columbia: A Population History* (Vancouver: University of British Columbia Press, 2009), pp. 41–3; Harris, *Resettlement*, pp. 178–9.
9 Val Adolph, *In the Context of Its Time: A History of Woodlands* (Victoria: Government of British Columbia – Ministry of Social Services, c. 1996), p. 16.
10 *Ibid.*, p. 23.
11 Harris, *Resettlement*, pp. 178–80.
12 There were fifty-one males and ten females in care at the end of the year. BCSP 1885, Bentley, 1886, 392.
13 The 1881 census lists males at 74.4 per cent while the 1891 census records that men comprised 74.6 per cent of the population. Barman, *The West Beyond*, p. 385.

14 At the close of the fiscal year in March of 1921 there were 1,122 males and 444 females in residence at the three hospitals. BCSP 1921, H. S. Steeves, 1921, W15.
15 Barman, *The West Beyond*, p. 385.
16 Ian Dowbiggen, *Keeping America Sane: Psychiatry and Eugenics in the US and Canada 1880–1940* (Ithaca, NY: Cornell University Press, 1997), p. 20.
17 BCSP 1901, George H. Manchester, 1902, 464.
18 BCSP 1901, Manchester, 1902, 464.
19 BCSP 1901, Manchester, 1902, 464.
20 Gerry Ferguson, 'Control of the insane in British Columbia, 1849–78: Care, cure, or confinement?', in John McLaren, Robert Menzies and Dorothy E. Chunn (eds), *Regulating Lives: Historical Essays on the State, Society, the Individual, and the Law* (Vancouver: University of British Columbia Press, 2002), Ch. 2, pp. 63–96.
21 *Ibid.*, p. 81.
22 *Ibid.*, p. 83.
23 *Ibid.*, p. 83.
24 Adolph, *Context*, p. 18.
25 Robert Menzies, 'Historical profiles of criminal insanity', *International Journal of Law and Psychiatry*, 25 (2002), 379–404, 380, 383; Richard Noll, *American Madness: The Rise and Fall of Dementia Praecox* (Cambridge, MA: Harvard University Press, 2011), p. 30.
26 Adolph, *Context*, p. 69.
27 These are the figures for the patients under treatment during the fiscal year of 1919–20. On 31 March 1920 there were 1,033 male and 425 female patients in residence. BCSP 1920, Doherty, 1920, Y28.
28 In 1932 all patients were relocated to Essondale and the hospital in New Westminster became a residential centre for the 'subnormal'. The facility closed in 1982 and most buildings have since been demolished. Essondale Hospital, renamed Riverview Hospital in the 1960s, closed in 2013. There was a third facility, Colquitz Hospital on Vancouver Island, which housed the criminally insane from 1919 until 1964. This facility does not figure in this paper. http://historyofmadness.ca/index.php?option=com_content&view=article&id=52&Itemid=42&lang=en.
29 Prior to 1885, when the roles were combined, there was a medical officer as well as a medical superintendent.
30 BCSP 1882, Thomas Robert McInnes, 1883, 326.
31 BCSP 1885, Bentley, 1886, 391.
32 BCSP 1888, Bentley, 1889, 404. Following lists of information describing the patients, and all the expenditures for the year, 'Table 14' presented a list of the articles either made or repaired by the female patients. There were sixteen tables in this report.
33 BCSP 1895, George Fowler Bodington, 1896, 1062.
34 BCSP 1896, Bodington, 1897, 846.
35 BCSP 1897, Bodington, 1898, 1305.
36 BCSP 1896, Bodington, 1897, 849.
37 BCSP 1897, Bodington, 1898, 1305.
38 BCSP 1908, Doherty, 1909, D6–14.

39 This was also the year that the institution changed its name from the 'Asylum for the Insane' to the 'Public Hospital for the Insane'. BCSP 1901, Manchester, 1902, 463.
40 Manchester noted that a number of the tables he included in his initial report were new and others had been altered. According to his argument, these changes allowed for enhanced comparison of statistical information with similar institutions. As he maintained that this was an important use for the report, he concluded 'I trust that this will be sufficient explanation for the course I have adopted in altering the tables submitted'. BCSP 1901, Manchester, 1902, 471.
41 BCSP 1901, Manchester, 1902, 476.
42 BCSP 1901, Manchester, 1902, 478.
43 BCSP 1901, Manchester, 1902, 480.
44 Dr Charles K. Clarke had a long and respected career in Canadian psychiatry. At the time of the inquiry, he was superintendent of the Rockwood Asylum in Kingston, Ontario. Dowbiggen, *Keeping America Sane*, pp. 18–19.
45 This inquiry was a follow up to the 1884 Royal Commission for the Asylum for the Insane, which had found numerous problems with the institution. Clarke found that the Asylum for the Insane in New Westminster was still inefficient. Superintendent Bodington retired soon after the inquiry. Adolph, *Context*, pp. 56-7. In his report for 1901 Dr Manchester noted that Clarke 'came under instructions from your Department to inspect the Institution … After a most searching investigation … Dr. Clarke recommended that certain changes should be made in the system, with a view to introducing greater economy of supplies'. BCSP 1901, Manchester, 1902, 479.
46 BCSP 1900, Charles Kirk Clarke, 1901, 229.
47 BCSP 1900, Clarke, 1901, 229.
48 BCSP 1900, Clarke, 1901, 231.
49 BCSP 1901, Manchester, 1902, 492.
50 BCSP 1901, Manchester, 1902, 477.
51 Government of British Columbia, *Rules and Regulations to the Employees of the Provincial Hospital for the Insane* (Victoria: Richard Wolfenden, 1901), p. 18.
52 Barman, *The West Beyond*, pp. 194–5.
53 BCSP 1912, Doherty, 1913, G37-8.
54 British Columbia Archives, Victoria (hereafter BCA), GR 647 Box 1:16, letter to Provincial Secretary from Gowan S. McGowan, 1947, p. 2.
55 BCA, McGowan, 1947, p. 3.
56 Eugenio Tanzi was an Italian alienist who advocated patient labour. According to Kelm, then Medical Superintendent, Dr C. Doherty greatly admired his work. Mary-Ellen Kelm, 'A Life Apart: The Experience of Women and the Asylum Practice of Charles Doherty at British Columbia's Provincial Hospital for the Insane, 1905–15', *Canadian Bulletin of Medical History*, 11 (1994), 335–55, 350.
57 BCSP 1912, Doherty, 1913, G8.
58 Neither the Annual Reports nor the case files indicate any monies paid for patient labour. However, the individual case files suggest that those patients who worked may have received intangible benefits such as access to the outdoors and recreational facilities.

59 Andrew Scull, *The Insanity of Place, the Place of Insanity: Essays on the History of Psychiatry* (London: Routledge, 2006).
60 BCSP 1913, Doherty, 1914, H10.
61 BCSP 1915, James G. McKay, 1916, L9.
62 Belshaw, *Becoming British Columbia*, p. 14; Harris, *Resettlement*, pp. 179–80.
63 Reaume presents a detailed discussion of the patients' complaints concerning labour in the asylum in Toronto, Ontario. Geoffrey Reaume, *Remembrance of Patients Past: Patient Life at the Toronto Hospital for the Insane, 1870–1940* (Don Mills: Oxford University Press, 2000), pp. 133–80. In my own review of patient files, I found similar complaints.
64 Ban Send Hoe, *Enduring Hardship: The Chinese Laundry in Canada* (Gatineau: Canadian Museum of Civilisation, 2003), p. 5; Patricia Roy, *A White Man's Province: British Columbia Politicians and Chinese and Japanese Immigrants, 1858–1914* (Vancouver: University of British Columbia Press, 1989), p. 13.
65 Roy, *A White Man's Province*, p. 14.
66 *Ibid.*, p. 45.
67 *Ibid.*, p. 66.
68 *Ibid.*, pp. 69, 156.
69 For example, the report for 1900 contained a chart listing the Chinese patients and reporting how long each had been resident in the hospital. No other group experienced this level of scrutiny. BCSP 1900, Bodington, 1900, 1048. In his discussion of deaths during this same year, Bodington singled out a long-term resident as 'a Chinaman ... is also recorded on the death roll, who has been in residence over 25 years'. BCSP 1900, Bodington, 1900, 1034.
70 BCSP 1901, Manchester, 1902, 488.
71 Hoe outlines how legislation and racism denied many opportunities for other types of employment to the Chinese in British Columbia. Hoe, *Enduring Hardships*, pp. 5–6.
72 Manchester continued his discussion of Chinese laundry workers noting that 'the Chinese patients do the washing by hand, but very few of them are willing to do it, because they receive no remuneration, and when they refuse they cannot be compelled like convicts. In the face of these facts ... it is simply wonderful what is accomplished ... under the skilful handling of the laundryman'. BCSP 1901, Manchester, 1902, 488.
73 BCSP 1901, Manchester, 1902, 473.
74 In 1885 both China and England provided four each of twenty-one admissions. BCSP 1885, Bentley, 1886, 392. In 1895 Chinese represented five of sixty-two admissions and fifteen came from England. BCSP 1895, Bodington, 1896, 1072. In 1905 there were ten Chinese admissions and twenty from England from a total of 123. BCSP 1905, Doherty, 1906, G21.
75 BCSP 1899, Bodington, 1900, 897.
76 BCSP 1901, Manchester, 1902, 473.
77 Lorenzo Veracini, *Settler Colonialism: A Theoretical Overview* (New York: Palgrave Macmillan, 2010), pp. 25–7.
78 *Ibid.*, pp. 30–1.

5

'Useful both to the patients as well as to the State': Patient work in colonial mental hospitals in South Asia, c. 1818–1948

Waltraud Ernst

This chapter focuses on the organisation of patient work in the mental institutions established by the British for both Europeans and Indians in South Asia. It explores the changing and plural meanings of work in relation to prevalent medical ideas and practices in different institutional settings in British-held territories from the early nineteenth to the middle of the twentieth centuries. Different aspects of work will be discussed, such as work as therapy; means to combat idleness; patients' empowerment; institutional profit; and forced labour. The incentives used by staff to induce patients to engage in physical labour and the punishments employed in cases of non-compliance will be scrutinised. It will be shown that gender, social and caste prejudices and sentiments affected the types of activity patients were expected to engage in, and how, with the emergence of professionalised occupational therapy from the early twentieth-century patient, work became increasingly acceptable also with regard to European patients. The link between intensive work regimes and the concomitant decreased use of other treatment methods such as sedation, prolonged rest and hydrotherapy from the 1920s onwards will be explored.

The chapter shows that ideas on and practices of patient work in therapeutic and institutional contexts were closely informed by varied European and North American psychiatric paradigms. At the same time, work regimes in the different provinces were seen to require certain local modifications on account of broader cultural beliefs, social and racial prejudice, and attitudes towards work within colonial settings. Individual superintendents' medical preferences, social preconceptions and passion for asylum reform as well as institutional conditions, such as overcrowding, under-staffing and spatial restrictions determined the ways in which patient work was organised in diverse ways in institutions in British India.

The main primary sources for this chapter consist of government correspondence and annual reports of lunatic asylums or mental hospitals, from c. 1818 to 1940, with particular emphasis on the mental hospitals in Bengal, Bihar, Orissa and Madras.

The context

Lunatic asylums in South Asia were established by the British in the late eighteenth century in the main provinces under colonial control, in Madras (Chennai), Calcutta (Kolkata), and Bombay (Mumbai).[1] These were privately run, small establishments with no more than twenty to thirty inmates, geared towards the confinement of mentally ill Europeans and Anglo-Indians (Eurasians) and a few Indians. Most of the patients had formerly been employed by the East India Company or were found wandering at large by the police. By 1820, the East India Company had established asylums for Europeans in Calcutta, Bombay and Madras, alongside eleven institutions reserved for Indians only. These provided for between 35 to 170 patients on average.[2] During the course of the nineteenth century, the previously privately managed facilities were replaced by larger, state-run institutions in the different provinces of the expanding British territory in South Asia. This mirrored developments in England and Wales. By the first half of the twentieth century about twenty or so mental hospitals provided different levels of medical care and institutional facilities. Several hundred people were confined in each of these institutions. The largest during the 1930s and 1940s was the Ranchi Indian Mental Hospital, with capacity for about 1,200 to 1,400 patients.[3] Along with the extension of the asylum system, patient work came to figure increasingly in most of the institutions from about the middle of the nineteenth century.

Therapy: 'Work is a pleasant pastime and is undoubtedly curative'

Evidence of the assumed link between work and therapy, in particular 'moral therapy' as advocated at the York Retreat in England, can be dated to the second decade of the nineteenth century. In its report on asylums in Bengal, the medical board argued that work and occupation were part of moral therapy and would help to 'reclaim [patients] to the enjoyment and exercise of reason' as well as providing a way for the superintendent to 'gain their confidence'.[4] How these aims were to be achieved in practice, was not elaborated on. However, a number of activities in which patients were engaged were listed, such as spinning of hemp, and cultivation of rice, tea, tobacco, etc.[5]

Work increasingly became an important part of asylum management and an indicator of a good-quality institution, as can be discerned from official correspondence in 1847. Assistant surgeon F. P. Strong was accused of running a regime of treatment and care at the Rasapagla Asylum that was 'inadequate'.[6] In his defence he pointed out the various employments and amusements in which the inmates were involved: spinning, weaving, cleaning, gardening, cultivation, and music, dancing, cards ('after their own fashion'). He maintained that the inmates raised 'coffee, cotton, sugar-cane, mulberry, … tapioca, sapan-wood, alva plant (for rope making)'.[7] Surgeon G. Paton of the Delhi Asylum even considered mental and physical occupation to be the chief means of cure, noting in 1853: 'It leads to a diversion of the mind from its morbid channel of thought and thus favours the restoration of the faculty or faculties of the mind which have been at fault'.[8]

Throughout the nineteenth and into the early twentieth century work was seen as an intrinsic part of the therapeutic regime in mental hospitals. Dr Jal E. Dhunjibhoy of the Indian Mental Hospital at Ranchi proclaimed in 1926: 'Work is a pleasant pastime and is undoubtedly curative.'[9] He went on to explain that, 'The spotless cleanliness found in this large hospital, the pride of the staff and wonder of the visitors, is largely the result of the help of willing patients.'[10] Dhunjibhoy had also become attuned to the medical and managerial jargon that was common in Western countries during this period, as evidenced in his report of 1928:

> Patients are principally occupied in remunerative work which is mainly directed towards remoulding the more primitive manipulative capacities and which makes very little demand on the more complex mental processes at the same time. The patients are chiefly engaged in gardening, weaving, cane and bamboo work, smithy, carpentery [sic], tailoring and miscellaneous domestic works, while some are engaged also in mending clothes, cobbling, lace-making, knitting, office work, etc. So that the patients' labour is fully utilised towards supplying the needs of the hospital, which apart from its therapeutic effect on patients themselves, serves to keep down the rates of the institution.[11]

What exactly the 'therapeutic effect' consisted of was not explained. Colleagues at Madras were similarly opaque when they reiterated contentions such as:

> The latest methods of treatment are aimed at in so far as is possible with the limited resources which are available. General treatment such as fresh air, sunlight and liberal dieting are adopted for all cases; and rest, sedatives, hydrotherapy and tonics in selected cases. In recovering cases occupation is found to have a more beneficial effect than any other treatment. Occupation therapy is found to be useful to the chronic, degenerated and demented patients who had formerly been regarded as incurable and unemployable.[12]

The financial benefits of patient work were more tangible, as these could be set off against expenses and thereby supported the institutions to a considerable extent.

Finances: 'Besides benefiting the patients, [work] helps finance'

Patient work not only contributed to the internal economy of hospitals and helped to keep institutions spotlessly clean, as Dhunjibhoy so proudly noted in 1926, it also provided produce for the local and global market. As early as the 1830s, assistant surgeon F. P. Strong commended patients in the Rasapagla asylum, pointing out that 'their coffee in 1832 was highly approved by the London brokers'.[13] The products of patients' labour had become part of India's export economy.

At the 'native lunatic asylum' in Delhi, in 1853, surgeon G. Paton was 'happy to say' that of seventy-eight male patients 'every one of them excepting 16 is working with a good will in the Garden'.[14] He also expected his plan to employ the female patients in the spinning of cotton thread to become a similar success. To ensure profitability, the superintending matron had been authorised to retail the goods, whereby she was expected to become interested in the production.[15] This measure did of course open up the potential for abuse and corruption as she and her subordinates may have done more than simply gently encourage the help of 'willing patients'. Profiteering was rife in colonial institutions in India, as a number of examples show.[16] The staff's structural position of power enabled them to withhold food and treats or privileges in case of patients' non-compliance. Paton himself was known for his minimalist diet regime and the high mortality rates resulting from it; non-compliant patients starved to death.[17]

In the early twentieth century, Dhunjibhoy at the Ranchi mental hospital confirmed the continued monetary benefits of patients' work: 'So far we have been dealing with work of definite economic value for, besides benefiting the patients, it helps finance'.[18] Patient work in Indian institutions was also commended by international bodies. For example, in 1928, by which time the number of working patients at Ranchi had 'gradually increased', Dr Yves M. Biraud, a representative of the health section of the League of Nations, visited the institution and judged it in very positive terms:

> We were most interested to see the work which you are carry[ing] out at this hospital and especially that of your occupational treatment. We were also struck by the efforts which you are making to utilise the labour of your patients towards the supplying of the needs of the Institution. Public Health Officers regard such work as distinctly beneficial to the community as it enables public funds to be utilised for purposes of prevention as well as for curative measures.[19]

As such, Biraud emphasised another aspect of the potential benefit of patient work, namely the freeing up of funds for other public health-related purposes. This would have worked if the ensuing profit and savings were indeed invested in such measures. Desirable as this may have sounded in principle, it is doubtful that this was the case in practice. Dhunjibhoy himself lamented the lack of funding for preventative, institutional and legal mental healthcare measures in India, underscoring in particular, in 1933, 'the necessity for mental hygiene movement in India' and, in 1936, the 'absence of proper homes for mentally defective children as well as of the Mental Deficiency Act for India'.[20]

Did institutions make a profit from patient labour? Superintendents were clear that patients contributed towards the maintenance of the institution, in particular with regard to food, clothing and furniture, and daily domestic household tasks. These are difficult to quantify and evaluate. Although financial statistics were provided for every institution on a yearly basis, it is unlikely that the monetary effect of patients' work could be fully identified from these. An assessment of the accounts for the three mental hospitals in the province of Madras of 1948, the first year after Indian Independence, shows that the value of stores received from the manufacturing department (less cost of raw materials) was specified at Rs 17,239-7-11. The sale of manufactured articles and of garden produce had brought in Rs 79-7-6 and Rs 421-10-3 respectively. The monetary value of manufacturing and gardening appears minor if considered in relation to the charges for electricity, for example, which amounted to Rs 10,014-0-0.[21] Figures for 1938 at the Ranchi Indian Mental Hospital, where 80 per cent of patients were employed in work, were of a similar magnitude. Dhunjibhoy listed the value of produce from the garden and poultry farm at Rs 22,323-2-9, while the total expenditure that year amounted to Rs 463,509-2-1.[22] Institutions clearly profited from the products of patient work, in particular domestic chores that did not find monetary expression in the accounts. However, mental hospitals did not produce big enough monetary gains to induce the colonial administration to maintain these institutions on profit grounds alone.

Whatever the impact of patient work on institutions' internal finances and the public good may have been, there was clearly much external acknowledgment of the standard of work achieved by patients, for instance when the occupation therapy department at Ranchi was awarded four first prizes in 1934 in a local exhibition for their lace, baskets, mats and bed-sheets.[23] The following year, they secured nine first and one second prize. At a local flower show in 1936, the hospital won 'a beautiful Silver Cup for the best roses grown in Ranchi and 3 First Class certificates for the Annuals and other flowers'.[24] Dhunjibhoy was proud of his patients' achievements and the likelihood that at least some of the patients shared the superintendent's sentiments should not be dismissed.

Discipline and punish: 'Discourage idleness and malingering'

During the early nineteenth century, the rhetoric of patient work was intrinsically linked with 'moral therapy' and, to a certain extent, the expectation that mechanical restraint could be avoided if the mentally ill were productively occupied and their mental and physical energy channelled in positive ways. Combating idleness, too, was part of moral therapy, and became a prominent trope in Indian and Western psychiatrists' reports during the 1930s in particular.

The means by which idleness was to be sanctioned did not always have a salubrious effect, leading in some cases to high mortality rates. This was so in Delhi in 1853, for example, where Dr G. Paton considered the restriction of patients' food provision as 'an easy and unobjectionable means … to encourage exertion, and to discourage idleness and malingering in Hospital'.[25] However, conditions were not always detrimental to patients' wellbeing. At other institutions at the time and at the Ranchi Mental Hospital during the twentieth century, patients were well fed, not least because the agricultural produce grown by them made the institution self-sufficient in vegetables. In 1935, the cultivated area at Ranchi was increased by another twenty acres and dedicated to *paddy* (rice), of which eighty-nine *maunds* (a little over three tons) were produced. Fish that had been stocked in the large tanks or water reservoirs supplied the hospital with 146 kg of high-quality protein, while the poultry farm provided 2,942 eggs.[26] The Ranchi hospital had clearly diversified into an adjunct agricultural enterprise.

The prevention of idleness was a catch-phrase also used by Dhunjibhoy on his return from a study tour in Europe. The date of his Europe visit, 1936, is important. He had visited the 'famous occupational therapy centres in Europe and England', such as the Devon Mental Hospital at Exminster, which he reckoned had 'a great name', as did 'the famous Santpoort Hospital in Holland and in Germany the famous hospital at Guetersloh'.[27] During the 1930s, emphasis on work, in preference to rest and sedation, in the management of the mentally ill and 'defective' was widespread among psychiatrists in Europe and northern America. Dhunjibhoy put contemporary views in a nutshell: 'Occupation is recognised as an important therapeutic agent and has been defined as the organisation of suitable employment for the purpose of combating idleness.'[28]

This emphasis fitted in with the increased level of activity at Ranchi and had a strong affinity with contemporary schemes, for example, in Germany, where Hermann Simon promulgated his 'more active treatment' of the mentally ill, as highlighted by Dhunjibhoy.[29] Like other psychiatrists in India and in Western countries, Dhunjibhoy emphasised positive aspects such as the breaking up of the 'routine institutional life of the Hospital', its relief of 'monotony' and the 'busy activity with resulting cheerfulness and hope of recovery'.[30] However, to what extent involvement in work became itself part of the dreaded 'routine institutional life of the Hospital' is difficult to judge, not least in view of some ambiguous statements by Dhunjibhoy to the effect that occupation may for some patients mean 'tearing coir for mattresses as a contrast to tearing up their own clothing'.[31] At the time of this statement, in 1937, 80 per cent of patients were employed in what Dhunjibhoy called an 'intensive system'.[32] At the mental hospital in Madras, only about 42 per cent of inmates were reported to have been employed.[33] Dhunjibhoy may have faced some criticism about the extent to which he discouraged idleness, as he kept stressing that patients were allowed to choose their own occupations, asserting that he was 'confident that "picking threads" out of rags is much better for [the introspective type of patient] than sitting about and "day-dreaming"'.[34]

Dhunjibhoy considered work as the 'sheet-anchor of our treatment in this hospital'.[35] The scope of work was soon extended further by the provision of indoor 'occupational classes'. He noted:

> While employing out-of-doors is recognised as being of the greatest value, there are many patients who cannot or will not take part in work of the hospital garden or even in domestic occupations and for them provision has been made by the establishment of occupational classes where instructions in various arts and crafts are given by experienced instructors.[36]

In Madras, too, arts and crafts were practised, but here they were referred to as 'hobbies' and listed under the rubric of 'amusement and physical training', alongside entertainments such as performances by His Excellency the Governor of Madras's Jazz Band (see figure 5.1).[37]

The line between proper labour and mere busyness was not drawn in a uniform way by the different superintendents. Although staff at Madras gained inspiration regarding up-to-date treatments during their visits to the European and Indian Mental Hospitals at Ranchi, they also championed certain initiatives such as in regard to the treatment of mentally defective children from the late 1930s onwards in a small cottage separate from adult wards, where they benefited from educational input, physical and fun activities as well as training in handicrafts such as weaving, carpentry and spinning, mat and rope making.[38]

An important question in relation to these occupational ventures is how staff went about encouraging patients to engage in work and occupational classes rather than being idle. In 1853, Dr G. Paton aimed for the asylum at Delhi to become self-sufficient as well as pleasant to look at by employing patients not only in vegetable gardening and fruit cultivation but also having them tend the grounds and gardens. When he introduced a number

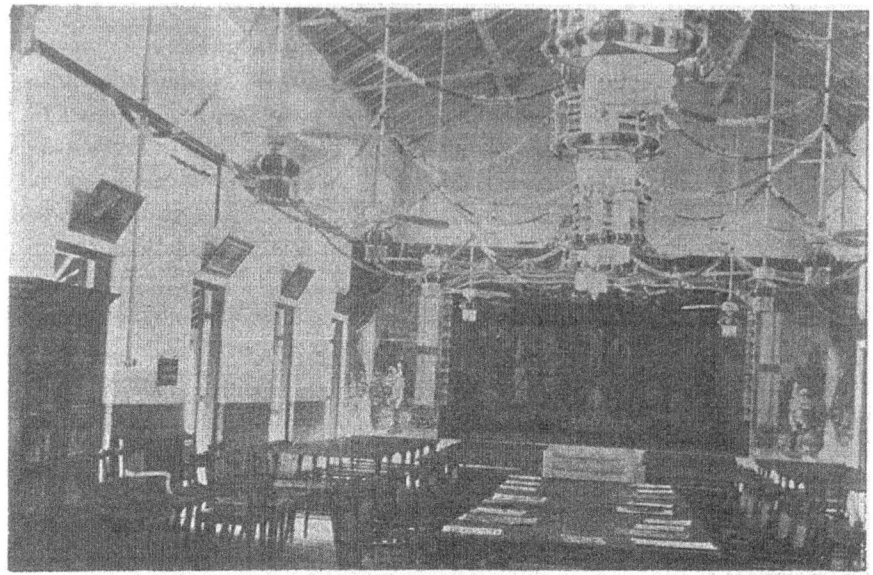

5.1 Interior of the recreation hall with stage in the background, Madras, c. 1940.

of changes in 1853, he also listed the 'diversification' of the diet regime as a recent innovation. This meant that considerably less food was allowed for those 'idle, unwilling or unable' to work.[39] Furthermore, tobacco was in future to be 'given as a reward for good behaviour only'.[40] Paton was clear about the role of diet in disciplining patients and inducing them to work. He said that it provided 'an easy and unobjectionable means by which to enforce Discipline among the patients … and to encourage exertion, and to discourage idleness and malingering in Hospital'.[41]

Paton at Delhi may not have been representative of everything that was happening in Indian lunatic asylums during the early nineteenth century. There is evidence of great diversity in regard to employment of patients. In the 1850s, at Rasapagla and Patna only a few patients were employed, while even at Delhi, as well as at Dacca and Murshidabad, it was observed that 'a great deal remains to be done'.[42] In Benares it was found impossible to 'attempt anything systematic in this respect'; Bareilly, in contrast, employed its lunatics 'extensively'.[43] Dilapidated buildings and confined space were major problems for many institutions at the time, affecting the practicability of patient work.

A particular kind of occupation that worked as an inducement for patients if used as a rationed privilege was cooking. On account of religious and caste prescriptions that involved avoidance of pollution of food and water by impure human agency, patients had clear preferences about who provided the catering and, in many cases, self-catering was preferred. Superintendents were aware of this, considering the 'process of cooking' also 'an excellent test and aid of convalescence'.[44] In 1854 the members of the medical board of Bengal noted: 'This is one of the few resources possessed by those who are in charge of Asylums in India which are not enjoyed by those who treat insanes in European ones.'[45] Like the withholding of tobacco, limiting the access to firewood and cooking facilities constituted a means of disciplining patients. Practices varied in the different institutions. In Patna and Delhi 'some of the best men cook for all'; in Dacca no patient was permitted to cook, while in Benares and Bareilly at least a few were allowed to cook their own food.[46]

During the early twentieth century, too, incentives were commonly used to encourage patients to engage in work. At Ranchi monetary rewards were given; there were 'small monthly rewards which are collected and with which [patients] are allowed to buy any useful articles they desire from the shops at Ranchi'.[47] From the early 1930s, efforts were also made to engage the 'refractory' and 'turbulent' who had previously been exempted from work. The professed aim was to 'make them happier and more tractable'.[48] Apparently this 'experiment' was successful and, in Dhunjibhoy's view, proved that 'practically every ambulant patient can be employed and is infinitely better and more easily controlled when he is employed'.[49] Those in charge of 'turbulent patients' had noticed that they developed 'a good appetite, eat well and look much fitter and better than before and [have] put on weight'.[50] It was also noted that patients enjoyed the 'extra gifts', such as 'cigarettes, tobacco and other comforts of life' and their share in the sum of Rs 600 which was annually divided among 'hardworking patients'.[51] Dhunjibhoy noted that 'patients look forward to this reward and spend [their money] as they like and some of them even send this money to their family at home'.[52] In those cases, engagement in work may indeed have empowered patients. However, if we compare Dhunjibhoy's and Paton's approaches, it is clear that patients' compliance may have guaranteed them a plate full of food at dinner time and even some treats, but those resisting work routines or unable to participate in them may have been starved in some institutions. Given that the Bengal Government demanded an explanation from Paton for the high-rate mortality among patients under his care during the 1850s, the way in which he struck what he referred to as a balance between 'kindness and firmness' clearly caused considerable suffering.

That not all inmates willingly joined into institutional work regimes is clear from one of Dhunjibhoy's statements: 'When persuasion has been applied to every fit patient to induce him to engage in useful service (compulsion is barred), there is a remnant who refuse to bestir themselves, some are lazy, others obstinate and others perverse.'[53] Conditions at Ranchi were generally very favourable and death rates low, but it remains difficult to assess even with regard to Dhunjibhoy's managerial approach where the line between 'persuasion' and 'compulsion' was drawn. The only cases explicitly exempted from work until 1933 were the 'sick, old and infirm and refractory patients'. This made it possible for about 50 per cent of the hospital's population to be employed in 1927.[54] For the Madras Mental Hospital, patient work was not formally specified in annual reports until 1932, when 'industries and employment' first appears as a separate rubric.[55] However, 'an industrial workshop' appears to have existed in 1927 at Calicut, one of the two other institutions in this southern province.[56] During the 1920s, the 'reorganisation of the existing mental hospitals in this Presidency so as to convert them into hospitals for the scientific treatment of mental disorders' was still 'under consideration' and provision for work therapy was apparently limited.[57] Yet, even in 1933, the surgeon-general of Madras observed:

> We cannot yet claim that our institutions for reception of the insane are mental hospitals in the best sense of the word: they still retain the features of lunatic asylums where the primary consideration was the protection of the outside public from a possible danger rather than the treatment of individual mental patients.[58]

Conditions and the extent to which patient work could be implemented in institutions in South Asia therefore varied greatly. In institutions such as Ranchi, where patients did work, views on the therapeutic benefits that could be derived from agricultural labour were divided. According to one of Dhunjibhoy's locums at Ranchi only 'mild states of excitement' could be allayed by outdoor work. This did not deter him from enforcing a culturally insensitive, if not racially flawed, work regime. He reported: 'Even though a large number of the patients are agriculturalists to whom this work is suited, those who are not, are also sent.'[59] Like any other medical treatment or institutional procedure, patient work was subject to varied styles of implementation and, potentially, abuse.

Race and mechanical labour: 'Injurious to Europeans' and 'most adapted' for Indians

The perceived cultural and political acceptability of work to particular social communities constituted a difficult problem in British India. For example, in 1821 the medical board of Bengal identified Indian culture as an impediment to patient work. 'Employment would be most desirable,' it noted, 'but besides their mental unfitness there are the prejudices of Cast [sic], of which many seem perfectly sensible.'[60] As the case of Paton at Delhi showed, such 'prejudices' were, however, at times overcome by more or less gentle persuasion. Paton had no qualms about assigning what he called 'most healthful' work tasks to Indian patients. Agricultural labour and cleaning of cells were considered by him more appropriate for Indian patients than educational or recreational pursuits. He argued: 'It would be desirable to introduce the school master into the Asylum, but the patients are not of that class to benefit by or take advantage of intellectual improvement. Mechanical work seems most adapted for them.'[61]

In contrast to Indian patients, Europeans in the institutions in Madras, Calcutta and Bombay and, later, at the European Mental Hospital at Ranchi, for example, fared much better, especially those considered to belong to the higher classes. They were not deprived of the facilities and comfort their social position was assumed to demand. Their accommodation was superior, as was their diet, and numerous entertainments were laid on for them.[62] For European second-class patients conditions were more variable, depending mainly on the various superintendents' approaches. For example, in Calcutta, a patients' library, equipped with a *punkah* or fan to provide a cool breeze during the hot season, was available during the early nineteenth century for first-class patients. Reading material included *The Illustrated News*, *The Times* and *Punch*, and chess, draughts, backgammon, dominos, kaleidoscopes and, occasionally, music, were provided. Second-class rooms were more spartanly furnished, with un-matted floors and simple wooden bedsteads similar to those used in European barracks and hospitals.

Regardless of social class, however, superintendents agreed during the nineteenth century that patient work was contra-indicated in the case of Europeans. The reasons assigned during this period were allegedly environmental, related to the climate. For example, in 1836, the medical board of Bengal pointed out that: 'Remedial employment [was to be considered] utterly inapplicable in tropical India, where the climate renders farming, gardening and occupation in the Kitchen [sic], laundry or bakehouse impracticable, if not injurious to Europeans.'[63] The rationale underlying this argument was ultimately one of race, as Europeans, unlike supposedly inferior races, were seen to thrive in temperate climes and to suffer if exposed to overexertion and the tropical sun. The allegedly detrimental effect of manual labour was one of the few, if not the only, peculiarly colonial factors that cut across the lines of social class, which were otherwise strictly enforced. The medical board emphasised this in 1856: 'To the Majority of the Patients at [the European Lunatic Asylum], Soldiers, Sailors and Gentlemen' alike, mechanical labour was 'uncongenial'.[64] For them employment was considered to produce exactly the opposite effect to that in Britain. Besides, the premises of colonial rule implied, at least at the level of political rhetoric, that the colonised were to serve and labour while the colonisers were to rule and, if Britons were to suffer hardship, it was to be due to the white man's burden of attempting to civilise their subjects at high personal costs.

While work was considered counter-indicated for Europeans from all walks of life, surgeon T. Cantor mused in 1856 about different Asian races' amenability to work. He had succeeded, after 'some five months perseverance', in 'introducing a system of moral treatment' into an Indian lunatic asylum near Calcutta, 'not by compulsion, but by persuasion and well timed rewards'.[65] His patients, 'some 300 of the poorer classes of Bengallees' [sic], were made to pluck hemp or coir, make ropes, swabs and rugs, spin wool for blankets or work in the kitchens and gardens.[66] However, in contrast to asylum inmates in South East Asia, where Cantor had previously been on duty, Indian patients were in his view less amenable to such 'moral treatment'. Cantor found the introduction of 'voluntary manual labour' to have been a 'task less easy to accomplish at [the Indian institution] than it proved in the Lunatic Asylum at Pinang in 1843', where the patients had been 'Malays, Chinese, Klings, Burmese, Siamese, Chochin-Chinese and Hindostanees' [sic].[67] According to Cantor, they 'took kindlier to a variety of light work than has been found the case with the Bengallees'.[68] As Mrinalini Sinha has shown in her work on *Colonial Masculinity*, Bengali men were increasingly represented by the British as 'effeminate' and contrasted with 'the manly Englishman' during the late nineteenth century.[69] Similarly, mixed-race or Eurasian patients were thought to loathe manual labour. According to common British stereotypes they were 'scribblers', or 'crannies', dedicated to secretarial work, and therefore they 'despised all trades, save that of the desk'.[70] Eurasian inmates in the Calcutta asylum, who were seen to 'evince their habitual propensity to scribbling', were therefore supplied with slates in order 'to save paper and walls'.[71]

The logistics of implementing patient work were complex in Indian mental hospitals as superintendents had to deal not only with patients' personal idiosyncrasies and mental conditions but also to consider real and alleged sentiments of caste and social standing. The observation that, however deranged patients may have been, they were still frequently sensitive to prescriptions of caste and social class was made throughout the nineteenth century by British doctors.

Occupational therapy:
'Organised on a scientific basis and conducted methodically'

Work regimes in mental hospitals became more easily justified and implemented across the racial divide from the turn of the nineteenth to the twentieth century. By the second decade of the twentieth century, 'occupational therapy' (OT) had become the standard term for patient work in many institutions in Europe and North America, and Western-trained psychiatrists in India did their best to show their familiarity with the regimens and fashions of modern hospital management. This made it more acceptable and indeed desirable for European patients, too, to be employed in a range of activities in mental hospitals in India. The sister institution of Dhunjibhoy's Indian Mental Hospital, the European Mental Hospital at Ranchi, which was dedicated exclusively to the treatment of Europeans and higher-class Eurasians, introduced OT in 1918 and from 1922 employed an expert 'occupational therapist', A. K. Mukherji. He established OT, as he pointed out, 'on a scientific basis', and conducted it 'methodically', drawing on ideas and initiatives developed by the American Occupational Therapy Association under the leadership of 'Mrs Slagle' (Eleanor Clarke Slagle, 1870–1942).[72] The aim was to rehabilitate patients or, as he put it, for them to become again 'whole men and women'. Occupation was designed to achieve this.[73] Staff, he noted, were:

> [T]o instill [sic] into the patients who have been bereft totally or partially of their mental functions, thinking capacities or creative faculties, the will to get back into their old places as active self-respecting citizens and not as objects of charity, and to enable them to function once again as whole men and women – physically, socially, educationally and economically.[74]

The range of activities pursued was exhaustive and in line with what was done in institutions in Western countries: 'weaving, carpentry, varnishing, blacksmithing, cane work, book-binding, cobbling, cement and brickwork, sericulture, Braille work, coir-rope and doormat making, mattress making, carpet, rug and Kalimpong mat making, crotchet work, needle work, tailoring, cooking, leather work, raffia work, bead work, drawing and painting, etc.'[75] A similarly exhaustive array of sports and leisure activities were offered and destructive and non-compliant behaviour was dealt with by 'stopping [patients'] daily supply of cigarettes or forbidding their participation in some of the amusements'.[76] Habit formation charts were 'carefully kept' and the weekly progress of each patient was recorded.[77]

Racial and cultural objections to Europeans being set to work were clearly no longer issues of concern as the wholesomeness of occupation had now become a dominant albeit not entirely uncontested discourse around the globe and a central part of treatment in institutions that considered themselves 'modern' and up to date with developments in Western countries. This does not mean that race was no longer a systemic problem. The Ranchi Mental Hospital for Europeans was privileged in contrast to the neighbouring institution dedicated to Indians, in terms of funding and scale. In the latter, only about 200 patients were accommodated, while at Dhunjibhoy's institution of 1,200 to 1,400 inmates overcrowding constituted a continual problem. Staffing was also more congenial to modern treatment at the European institution. For example, while Dhunjibhoy was clearly proud of his work regime at Ranchi and its success, he was well aware of the lack of specialist staff at the institution for Indians, especially as by the 1920s OT in Western countries had become increasingly professionalised. Dhunjibhoy noted: 'This institution is not fortunate enough to possess the services of occupational therapists for both the [male and female] sections of the hospital.'[78] However, he added, 'the patients quietly carry on very useful work.' A few years later, when work therapy had been extended further, he was more assertively defensive: 'It is a mistake to suppose that occupational therapy is impossible without the employment of a few costly and highly trained occupational therapists.'[79] Dhunjibhoy was at pains to turn a deficiency into a virtue. His defensiveness may have been due to the fact that Mukherji, of the neighbouring European hospital, had published his article on OT in the American journal *Occupational Therapy and Rehabilitation*, referring to two occupational therapists and twenty-five male and female instructors being employed at his institution.[80]

In contrast to Dhunjibhoy, his locum, Dr J. N. J. Pacheco, who helped out both at the European and the Indian Mental Hospital, was a believer in professional expertise. He argued that the 'need for a trained occupational instructress' was 'keenly felt' in the female section.[81] In his view, without 'a qualified and enthusiastic worker' it was very difficult to 'train patients or stimulate their interests from lethargy and indolence to useful and helpful occupation with a view to rehabilitation'.[82] Pacheco rubbed salt into the wounds of a superintendent whose consistent attempts to gain authorisation from government for more expert staff were regularly thwarted. Like Pacheco and Mukherji, Dhunjibhoy, too, was aware of the role the professionalisation of auxiliary medical services played during this period. His colleagues in Madras did not have the funds to support a trained occupational therapist either, but during the late 1930s they managed to advertise their facilities for OT (and other institutional measures provided) by means of a series of photographs appended to the annual reports.

The first set of these, in 1938, provided impressions of facilities such as the recreation hall and a bus for drives available at the institution at Madras and of male patients doing exercises or being 'at drill' on a sports field, and female patients engaging in 'musical drill'. An 'indigenous oil mill' was shown to be worked by a team of male patients. At the Calicut Mental Hospital women posed during badminton games and an egg and spoon race, and were shown engaged in rope making (see figure 5.2) and curry powder preparation. Men were shown participating in a *chattie* or earthen pot race. On a photo labelled 'mad musicians' melodious music', patients were shown walking in proces-

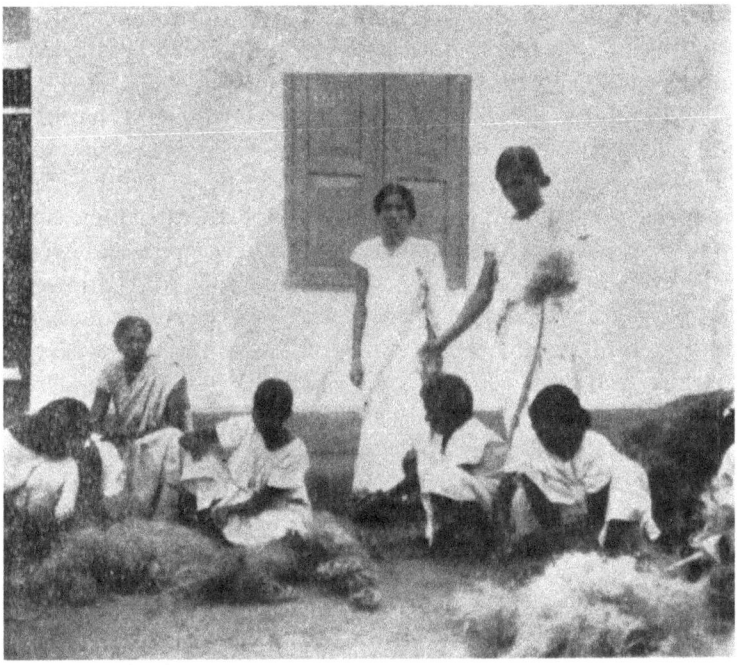

5.2 Rope making, Government Mental Hospital, Calicut, c. 1938.

sion behind a drummer. They posed with their instructor during needlework training at Calicut and while starching yarn at Waltair.

Gender:
'Looseness of morals consequent on the unlimited communication of mad persons of both sexes'

Shortly after the revelations of the 1815–16 Select Committee on the Better Regulation of Madhouses in England, and only about one decade after the introduction of native lunatic asylums in Bengal, a committee was set up to inquire into the 'state and internal management of lunatic asylums' in Bengal. The areas under scrutiny were similar to those investigated by the select committee in England. One of these concerned the lack of gendered segregation in private and public institutions. The medical board of Bengal proclaimed that during the investigations in England:

> [N]o feature amidst the numerous scenes of gross mismanagement there brought to light, appears to have been productive of more serious consequences or to have excited deeper regret, than that of the looseness of morals consequent on the unlimited communication of bad persons of both sexes.[83]

The reference to 'bad persons' was duly rectified in the original proceedings by an attentive proof reader to 'mad persons'. It was clear that there had been cause for concern, as patients in various asylums in Bengal were described as not segregated into different classes such as violent, dirty, harmless, convalescent, and men and women were allowed to mingle in improper and immoral ways. At the Dacca Asylum, for example, thirty to fifty patients were reported to 'have been promiscuously huddled together in a hired house' and at Murshidabad 'scenes of the utmost licentiousness' were said to have prevailed.[84] Following these revelations, attention had to be paid to the separation of the sexes and, 'if practical', male and female wards were recommended.

By the middle of the nineteenth century, sexual segregation appears to have been common and work activities, too, were allocated on a gendered basis. This was in line with practices in institutions in Western countries, where work activities were clearly gendered in accordance with the sociocultural premises prevalent at particular times and places. The example of Madras during the early twentieth century illustrates this for the 1920s to the mid-1940s, when between 40 and 45 per cent of patients were involved in some kind of work – about half of them in manufacturing (such as mat plaiting, broom-making, weaving, sewing, knitting etc., see figures 5.3 and 5.4) and the other half in 'unskilled labour' (such as gardening, sweeping and cleaning of foodstuffs).[85]

Available records do not reveal whether the proportion of patients involved in activities varied on the basis of gender. They do report, however, in the case of the Waltair mental hospital, for example, that:

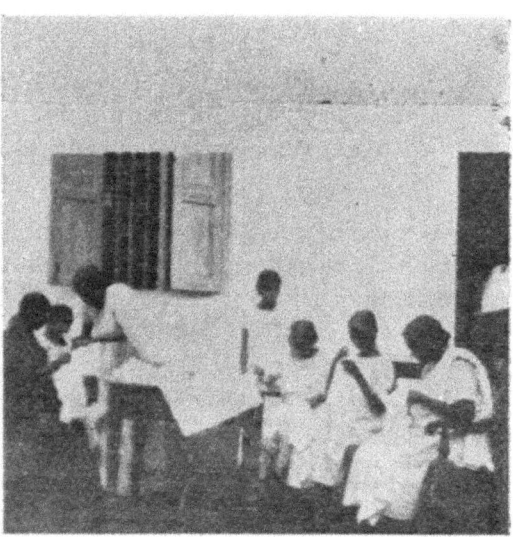

5.3 Embroidery class, Government Mental Hospital, Calicut, c. 1939.

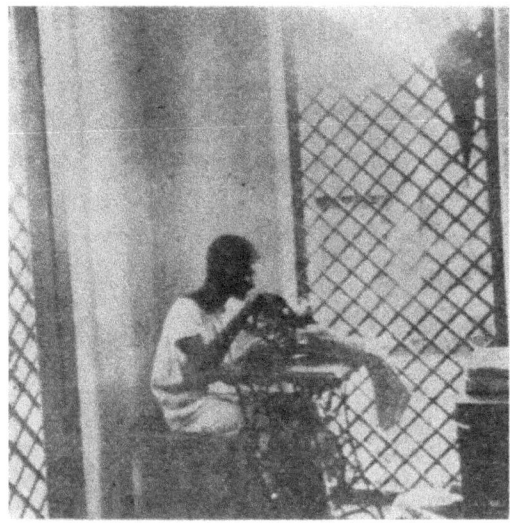

5.4 Tailoring, Government Mental Hospital, Calicut, c. 1939.

As the bulk of the population here is rural, agriculture, cattle tending, weaving and gardening are the principal occupations followed by the male patients while women are put on to work which they are accustomed to in their houses. Some of them do spinning at charkas [spinning wheels] as well.[86]

Both women's and men's labour was important for the internal economy of the mental hospitals, as in many cases 'most of the requirements' of the institutions were covered internally. These included bedding and clothing, for which the weaving department at Madras, for example (see figure 5.5), 'supplied all the clothing needed for the whole institution with more than 1,600 patients' in 1945, while women helped to mend worn-out sheets and dresses.[87]

Only at one institution in British India was gender segregation abolished. At the European Mental Hospital at Ranchi, the psychoanalytically inclined O. A. R. Berkeley Hill was in charge of the institution. Here 'free social intercourse' was allowed between male and female patients.[88] The hospital's first qualified occupational therapist, Mukherji, pointed out this 'distinguished feature', contending that the 'unrestricted association has a very healthy influence upon [patients'] minds in that it raises their moral standards and keeps alive in them their social duties and responsibilities'. He even contended that there were cases 'on record where this form of companionship has effected permanent cures'. Certain activities were still undertaken by men or women only, such as cobbling by men and needlework by women, but others, such as weaving and cane work, were found to be 'congenial occupations' by both

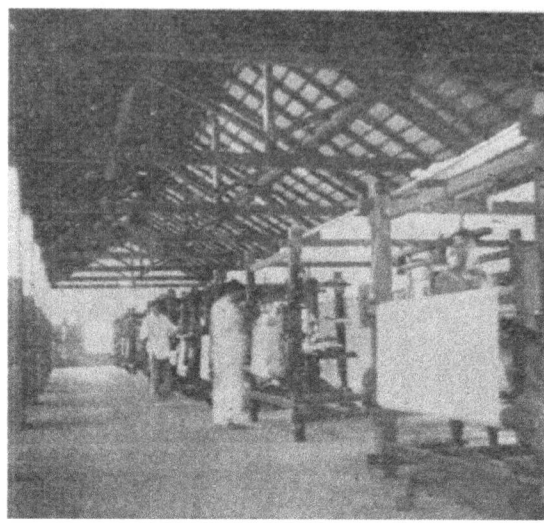

5.5 Weaving section, Government Mental Hospital, Calicut, c. 1939.

males and females. The European Hospital at Ranchi was, however, unusual in many ways within the British Indian context and remained controversial during Berkeley Hill's leadership. Mukherji, however, was a loyal member of staff, referring to his superior as 'a man of international reputation', who had 'not only the imagination and vision to conceive great ideals but also the courage and ability to translate those ideals into action'.[89] He even suggested that 'the European population of India does indeed owe a great debt of gratitude and thanks to the genius of this remarkable man'.[90] During the twentieth century, superintendents at institutions for Indians, such as Dhunjibhoy at the neighbouring mental hospital at Ranchi, would not, on account of sociocultural preferences among patients and their families, have been able to desegregate men and women on any large scale as was done by Berkeley Hill.

Medical treatment: 'The number of hypnotic draughts given at night is considerably reduced'

Work was one of a range of interventions and treatments made use of by doctors at different periods. During most of the nineteenth and, even, the early decades of the twentieth centuries, medication was restricted to sedatives and drugs for physical conditions. Work, alongside water therapy, therefore had an important role to play in mental institutions. From the late nineteenth century, European and North American doctors' enthusiasm for bed rest, sleep cures and sedation put constraints on the implementation of work regimes. Hermann Simon, medical director at the Gütersloh Mental Hospital in Germany, highlighted how rest cures inhibited patients' level of activity, social engagement and the likelihood of improvement. He advocated a 'more active therapy' and perfected work therapy to a degree that was, as Mukherji had noted, scientifically based, methodically conducted, and overseen by trained staff.[91]

The reported benefits of intensive work regimes extended also to cost savings in relation to drugs. This was welcomed by accountants and may also have had positive consequences for patients as they were less likely to be subdued by the pharmacological strait waistcoat and the range of shock treatments popular among psychiatrists during the 1930s and 1940s. In British India, work was mainly used in the case of chronic and quiet patients. However, Dhunjibhoy's 'experiment' in 1933 of extending it to refractory and turbulent patients appeared to result in the improvement of their bodily health and an increased level of alertness and fitness. They even slept better at night, 'which they never did before without hypnotics'.[92] Dhunjibhoy reconfirmed this in 1936, when he noted that the 'number of hypnotic draughts given at night is considerably reduced'.[93] Notwithstanding the many concerns and controversies around patient work in the British territories in this time period, the fact that patients so employed were spared continued sedation and shock treatments, may go some way to see it in a less negative light. As with hydrotherapy, it constituted a way for patients to experience daily life without the haze induced by medication.

Looking back on the experiment of making refractory patients, too, contribute to their own upkeep and remain active, Dhunjibhoy mused that his only regret was that he had not tried this earlier. He gave the example of ward no. 11, in which 'highly excited' patients were kept:

> The whole atmosphere … is now completely changed. This was a noisy, dirty and destructive ward before and since the introduction of active outdoor garden work every patient on an average has put on 2 to 3 lbs. in weight, they sleep better, there is no noise in the night or day and no sleeping draughts are now required.[94]

The functions of occupation and the effects of work were clearly multifaceted. It would be simplistic to suggest that early twentieth-century mental hospitals in British India and their nineteenth-century predecessors were 'no more than forced labor houses producing goods for the British Empire'.[95]

Conclusion

The available records for British India show that patient work played an important role in asylums from the early nineteenth century onwards. As in the colonial motherland, there was a persistent emphasis on its financial benefits to the state and the positive impact on patients' minds and bodies. Shifts in the meaning of labour can be identified. Work during the early nineteenth century was invariably embedded in the rhetoric of 'moral therapy', with emphasis on kind and humane treatment of the insane. From the late nineteenth century the continued role of work within the framework of moral treatment tended to accentuate in particular the prevention of 'idleness'. During the early twentieth century, patient work became more firmly set within a medical paradigm and coexisted alongside an array of other practices (such as hydrotherapy, sedation, tonics, and shock treatments). It was reconceptualised in the scientific terms of the period and, with the emergence of newly professionalised auxiliary medical disciplines, refashioned as 'occupational therapy'. During most of the period discussed above, work figured alongside, yet was considered separate from, leisure and pastime activities. Recreational pursuits and 'special treats' were offered in the better-equipped institutions as part of hospital life, but also had a role in the disciplinary regime that provided incentives and rewards for patients willing to work, and were withheld from those reluctant to do so. The separation of leisure and work appears to have continued well into the twentieth century in institutions reserved for Indian patients, and even in the European mental hospital at Ranchi from the 1920s, when occupational therapy was meant to re-form patients as 'whole men and women – physically, socially, educationally and economically'.[96]

Although the rhetoric and organisation of work as therapy was based on European and North-American blueprints, there were certain limits to the transnational transfer of concepts and practices. The politics of colonialism and the social hierarchies and cultural sentiments of Indian society impacted on the ways patient work could be implemented within different institutional settings. Issues of race and caste were prominent factors in the choice of suitable work activities, with Europeans of all social classes being exempt from exerting themselves in the colony during most of the nineteenth century. With the increased conceptualisation of active occupation in science-based, medical terms in the early twentieth century, work became an acceptable therapy also for Europeans. The shift in British India from work as moral therapy during the nineteenth to OT in the early twentieth century engendered, in principle, the universal applicability of a more active treatment of the mentally ill of all social and cultural backgrounds. Differences of race, social class and caste no longer necessitated selective exemption from work, but, depending on superintendents' style of management, diversification of work activities in line with social parameters and patients' sensitivities were still common. Patient work inside institutions in British India was determined in varying ways over the period by the wider organisation of colonial labour and the politics of colonial relationships as well as shifting medical ideas on the place of work and occupation within institutions for the mentally ill.

Acknowledgement

Many thanks to Jennifer Laws, who provided many useful comments on an earlier draft of this chapter.

Notes

1 Waltraud Ernst, *Mad Tales from the Raj. Colonial Psychiatry in South Asia, c. 1800–1858* (London: Anthem, 2nd edn, 2010; first published by Routledge, 1991).
2 Waltraud Ernst, 'The establishment of "Native Lunatic Asylums" in early nineteenth-century British India', in Gerrit Jan Meulenbeld and Dominik Wujastyk (eds), *Studies on Indian Medical History* (Delhi: Motilal Banarsidass, 2nd edn, 2001; first published by Egbert Forsten, 1987).
3 Waltraud Ernst, *Colonialism and Transnational Psychiatry. The Development of an Indian Mental Hospital in British India, c. 1925–1940* (London: Anthem, 2013).
4 British Library, London (hereafter BLL), Rules, Bengal Judicial Proceedings, 28.8.1818, p. 55; BLL, Summary of Correspondence relating to the Calcutta Asylum for Insane Patients (hereafter Summary of Correspondence), 30.10.1847; BLL, Board's Collections, 1852, 2494, 141.296, p. 52.
5 BLL, Rules, Bengal Judicial Proceedings, 28.8.1818, p. 55; BLL, Summary of Correspondence.
6 BLL, Summary of Correspondence.
7 *Ibid.*
8 BLL, Civil Surgeon to Medical Board (hereafter Civil Surgeon), 11.2.1853; BLL, North West Provinces General Proceedings (hereafter General Proceedings), 15.6.1853, 150, p. 16.
9 Jal Edulji Dhunjibhoy, *Report on the Working of the Mental Hospitals for Indians in Bihar and Orissa for the Years 1924–27* (Patna: Government Printing, 1928), p. 5.
10 *Ibid.*
11 *Ibid.*, p. 8.
12 [John Wallace Dick Megaw], *Annual Report of the working of the Mental Hospitals in the Madras Presidency for the Year 1928* (Madras: Government Press, 1929), p. 5.
13 BLL, Summary of Correspondence.
14 BLL, Civil Surgeon, 11.2.1853; BLL, General Proceedings, 15.6.1853, 150, p. 16.

15 BLL, General Proceedings, p. 17.
16 With regard to army hospitals, the East India Company's Court of Directors observed in 1818 that 'an arrangement by which the interest of the Surgeon was put in opposition to his duty, and by which there was too much reason to believe that, on some occasions at least, the health and life [of the patients] was sacrificed to the avarice of the Surgeon'. Court of Directors Despatch to Bengal, Military Department, 26.8.1818, 147. During the second half of the nineteenth century, corruption was still reported – and censored by the authorities – as, for example, in the case of James Wise's institution at Dacca. Wise, a knowledgeable medical doctor whose work provided the ethnographic data for Herbert Hope Risley's *Ethnographic Survey of Bengal, 1885–1891* and *Tribes and Cases of Bengal*, had been unaware of the fraudulent practices committed by his subaltern staff.
17 See the discussion on diet and mortality rates in Ernst, 'Native Lunatic Asylums', in Meulenbeld and Wujastyk (eds), *Studies*, pp. 169–204.
18 Dhunjibhoy, *Report on the Working of the Mental Hospitals for the Years 1924–27*, p. 5.
19 Jal Edulji Dhunjibhoy, *Annual Report on the Working of the Ranchi Indian Mental Hospital, Kanke, in Bihar and Orissa* [hereafter *Annual Report Ranchi*] *for the Year 1928* (Patna: Government Printing, 1929), p. 6.
20 Jal Edulji Dhunjibhoy, *Triennial Report on the Working of the Ranchi Indian Mental Hospital, Kanke, in Bihar and Orissa, for the Years 1930–1932* (Patna: Government Printing, 1933), p. 12; Jal Edulji Dhunjibhoy, *Annual Report Ranchi for the Year 1936* (Patna: Government Printing, 1938), p. 7.
21 [A. S. Mannadi Nayar], *Annual Report on the Working of the Mental Hospitals in the Madras Presidency* [hereafter *Annual Report*] *for the Year 1948* (Madras: Government Press, 1949), Statistical Appendix, pp. 10–11.
22 Jal Edulji Dhunjibhoy, *Annual Report Ranchi for the Year 1938* (Patna: Government Printing, 1940), pp. 18, 36–39. Total expenditure exclusive of amounts received from paying patients and miscellaneous receipts.
23 Jal Edulji Dhunjibhoy, *Annual Report Ranchi for the Year 1934* (Patna: Government Printing, 1935), p. 15.
24 Jal Edulji Dhunjibhoy, *Annual Report Ranchi for the Year 1936* (Patna: Government Printing, 1938), p. 17.
25 BLL, Civil Surgeon, 11.2.1853; BLL, General Proceedings, 15.6.1853, 150, pp. 10–11.
26 BLL, General Proceedings, p. 15.
27 Dhunjibhoy, *Annual Report Ranchi for the Year 1936*, p. 10.
28 *Ibid*.
29 Hermann Simon, 'Aktivere Krankenbehandlung in der Irrenanstalt', *Allgemeine Zeitschrift für Psychiatrie*, 87 (1927), 97–145. Hermann Simon, 'Active therapy in the lunatic facility (1929)', in Greg Eghigian (ed.), *From Madness to Mental Health. Psychiatric Disorder and its Treatment in Western Civilisation* (New Brunswick, NJ: Rutgers University Press, 2010), pp. 271–5.
30 Dhunjibhoy, *Annual Report Ranchi for the Year 1936*, p. 9.
31 *Ibid*.

32 Jal Edulji Dhunjibhoy, *Annual Report Ranchi for the Year 1937* (Patna: Government Printing, 1939), p. 12.
33 [Norman Methven Wilson], *Annual Report for the Year 1937* (Madras: Government Press, 1938).
34 Dhunjibhoy, *Annual Report Ranchi for the Year 1937*, p. 12.
35 Jal Edulji Dhunjibhoy, *Annual Report Ranchi for the Year 1930* (Patna: Government Printing, 1932), p. 9.
36 Jal Edulji Dhunjibhoy, *Annual Report Ranchi for the Year 1933* (Patna: Government Printing, 1934), p. 17.
37 [Norman Methven Wilson], *Annual Report for the Year 1939* (Madras: Government Press, 1940), p. 3.
38 [Hugh Stott], *Annual Report for the Year 1940* (Madras: Government Press, 1941), p. 3; [Wilson], *Annual Report for the Year 1937*, p. 8; [F. P. Connor], *Annual Report for the Year 1936* (Madras: Government Press, 1937), p. 4: 'It is satisfactory to note that a beginning has been made by the Superintendent' with regard to the training of mentally defective children.
39 BLL, Civil Surgeon, 11.2.1853; BLL, General Proceedings, 15.6.1853, 150, pp. 6 and 8.
40 BLL, General Proceedings, p. 9.
41 *Ibid.*, pp. 10–11.
42 Medical Board to Lieutenant Governor, 10.10.1845; North West Provinces Public Proceedings, 12.12.1854, 87, p. 6.
43 *Ibid.*, p. 7. Even less activity was reported with regard to amusements in the various institutions.
44 *Ibid.*, p. 9.
45 *Ibid.*
46 *Ibid.*
47 Dhunjibhoy, *Annual Report Ranchi for the Year 1926*, p. 5.
48 Dhunjibhoy, *Annual Report Ranchi for the Year 1933*, p. 17.
49 *Ibid.*
50 *Ibid.*
51 *Ibid.*, p. 18.
52 *Ibid.*
53 Dhunjibhoy, *Annual Report Ranchi for the Year 1926*, p. 5.
54 Jal Edulji Dhunjibhoy, *Triennial Report Ranchi for the Years 1927–29* (Patna: Government Printing, 1931), p. 6.
55 [C. A. Sprawson], *Annual Report for the Year 1932* (Madras: Government Press, 1933), p. 2.
56 [F. H. G. Hutchinson], *Annual Report for the Year 1927* (Madras: Government Press, 1928), p. 2.
57 *Ibid.*
58 [Sprawson], *Annual Report for the Year 1932*, p. 3.
59 Julian Norman Joseph Pacheco, *Triennial Report on the Working of the Ranchi Indian Mental Hospital, Kanke, in Bihar, for the Years 1933, 1934 and 1935* (Patna: Government Printing, 1936), p. 14.

60 Medical Board to Government of Bengal, 6.6.1821; Bengal Judicial Proceedings, 21.8.1821, 4, no par.
61 BLL, Civil Surgeon, 11.2.1853; BLL, General Proceedings, 15.6.1853, 150, p. 16.
62 For further details, see Ernst, *Mad Tales*, pp. 58–67.
63 Bengal Asylum Report, 14.6.1856.
64 *Ibid.*
65 *Ibid.*
66 *Ibid.*
67 *Ibid.*
68 *Ibid.*
69 Mrinalini Sinha, *Colonial Masculinity. The 'manly Englishman' and the 'effeminate Bengali' during the late nineteenth century* (Manchester: Manchester University Press, 1995).
70 *Ibid.*
71 *Ibid.*
72 A. K. Mukherji, 'Occupational therapy in the European Mental Hospital, Ranchi, India', *Occupational Therapy and Rehabilitation*, 9:6 (1930), 323–30, pp. 323, 326.
73 *Ibid.*, p. 323.
74 *Ibid.*
75 *Ibid.*, p. 324.
76 *Ibid.*, p. 328.
77 *Ibid.*, pp. 328–9.
78 Dhunjibhoy, *Annual Report Ranchi for the Year 1928*, p. 6.
79 Dhunjibhoy, *Annual Report Ranchi for the Year 1933*, p. 17.
80 Mukherji, 'Occupational therapy', p. 328.
81 Pacheco, *Triennial Report Ranchi for the Years 1933, 1934 and 1935*, p. 14.
82 *Ibid.*
83 Medical Board to Government of Bengal, 22.7.1818; Bengal Judicial Proceedings, 28.8.1818, 53, p. 35.
84 *Ibid.*, pp. 50 and 35.
85 [Norman Methven Wilson], *Annual Report for the Year 1938* (Madras: Government Press, 1939), p. 3.
86 [Connor], *Annual Report for the Year 1936*, p. 3.
87 [J. P. Huban], *Annual Report for the Year 1946* (Madras: Government Press, 1947), p. 2.
88 Mukherji, 'Occupational therapy', p. 329.
89 Mukherji, 'Occupational therapy', p. 329.
90 Mukherji, 'Occupational therapy', p. 329.
91 For more details on Hermann Simon's approach see Chapter 11, by Monika Ankele, in this volume.
92 Dhunjibhoy, *Annual Report Ranchi for the Year 1933*, p. 17.
93 Dhunjibhoy, *Annual Report Ranchi for the Year 1936*, p. 9.
94 Dhunjibhoy, *Annual Report Ranchi for the Year 1934*, pp. 14–15.
95 Kymberly Cancilla Brumlik, 'Lunacy for profit: The economic gains of "native-

only" lunatic asylums in the Bengal presidency, 1850s–1870s', *Journal of South Asian Studies*, 2:1 (2014), 1–10.
96 Mukherji, 'Occupational therapy', p. 323.

6

'A powerful agent in their recovery': Work as treatment in British West Indian lunatic asylums, 1860–1910

Leonard Smith

Following William Ellis's (1780–1839) pioneering endeavours at the West Riding Lunatic Asylum between 1818 and 1830, the organised labour of patients became acknowledged as a key element in the effective operation of British public institutions for the insane.[1] Ellis's achievements gained him a prestigious appointment in 1830 as medical superintendent of the large new Middlesex County Asylum at Hanwell, where he consolidated his programme and further enhanced his reputation. His methods were gradually adopted at several of the other early English county asylums.[2] By the time that the substantive legislation of 1845 laid down the framework for a national network of public asylums, employment was regarded, alongside 'non-restraint' and 'classification' of patients, as an essential aspect of a modern, progressive treatment regime.[3] The overall system that became known as 'moral management' adapted the ideas and doctrines associated with 'moral treatment' to a large, purpose-designed, structured institution. Moral management provided the practical operating basis of these asylums for at least half a century. Within it, the employment of patients came to be regarded as the most effective therapeutic tool that a public lunatic asylum could offer.

As part of the activities intended to further its credentials as an enlightened colonial power, Britain disseminated its models of managing the insane throughout the empire.[4] In carrying this out, the principles and practices of moral management appeared particularly applicable in taking the ideals of the 'civilising mission' to the colonies. The order and structure inherent within the system appeared appropriate for the direction of institutions where large numbers of disorderly and unpredictable people were gathered together. Arrangements whereby much of patients' time was occupied in organised labour were a considerable aid to discipline. Furthermore, engagement in work served as an important tranquillising aspect in the asylum regime.

The most significant means for transmission of the relevant ideas and practices to the empire was via the emigration of British doctors, many of whom had acquired specialist knowledge and expertise within the public lunatic asylum system.[5] These men had usually spent several years in subordinate capacities, but saw their opportunities for advancement within the sector as limited. Migration to the colonies offered new challenges and possibilities, as well as the significantly higher salary associated with appointment as medical superintendent of a colonial lunatic asylum. As elsewhere, the role of such men was pivotal in the West Indies, especially in the important colonies of Jamaica, British Guiana and Trinidad, which form the main focus of this chapter.

The moral management system's emphasis on work accorded well with imperial perceptions of the main roles of colonised peoples, particularly those who were not white. This clearly applied in the islands and other territories that comprised the British colonies in the West Indies, which had been forged through the capture, forced transportation, and enslavement of African people.[6] Indeed, the whole rationale for the existence of the Caribbean colonies was the labour-intensive, large-scale production of cheap sugar and other crops for consumption in Europe and America, whereby substantial profits were amassed for planters, landowners, and British mercantile interests. Although more than two centuries of enslavement of black and 'coloured' people formally ended in 1838,[7] the exploitative plantation-based economic model persisted.[8] Work on the plantation, with its established methods, structures and racially based hierarchies, continued to be the main source of livelihood for the majority of the West Indian population. The resemblances to a well-ordered plantation were quite striking in lunatic asylums where moral management systems based around patient work prevailed.

In the aftermath of emancipation in 1838, one of the planters' main preoccupations was to ensure an adequate supply of cheap labour. In Jamaica, and particularly in the under-populated colonies of Guiana and Trinidad, where there were large areas of uncultivated land, many formerly enslaved people chose to leave the estates and become peasant farmers, rather than work for low wages.[9] The planters, supported by the colonial and imperial governments, responded by encouraging immigration from other Caribbean islands, Africa, Madeira, China, and particularly the Indian subcontinent. By 1920 about 430,000 East Indians, mostly indentured labourers, had come to the British West Indies, the great majority to Trinidad and British Guiana.[10] Here was another large group of people for whom work was the primary rationale for their presence in the colony. Not only did the immigrants dramatically alter the demographics, but their social and psychological casualties entered the lunatic asylums in considerable numbers.[11]

In societies where work had such central significance, its effectiveness as a method of treatment in the asylum was conceivably enhanced. Patients' advances towards 'cure' would be judged partly by their degree of willingness to engage in outdoor or indoor work, and the aptitudes, capabilities, and behaviours demonstrated while undertaking the tasks. Steady and consistent working, accompanied by socially appropriate behaviour, were important indicators of recovery and prospective readiness for discharge. More directly, labour and occupation in the asylum served as essential preparation for a person's resumption of family and community roles, together with the means to secure the basic necessaries of life.

Asylum populations

The administrative and legal arrangements for committal to West Indian lunatic asylums varied between colonies. English lunacy legislation was influential, though usually only implemented several years later. The requirement for certification by at least one medical officer and a magistrate's order emanated from accepted practice in England.[12] In Jamaica, legislation of 1861 provided for committal of any person 'so furiously mad, or so far disordered in his or her senses' that it might be dangerous for them to 'go abroad'. An amending act in 1873 extended this to allow for the detention of people 'wandering at large', even if not dangerous.[13] In British Guiana, following legislation in 1867, initial admission was to a general hospital for a probationary period, based on a single medical recommendation. A second certificate would then be provided by the hospital's medical officer, if the patient was subsequently transferred to the lunatic asylum.[14] In Trinidad, a law of 1844 provided only for admission of people indicted for a criminal offence or regarded as liable to commit a crime. Arrangements whereby 'dangerous lunatics at large' could be 'apprehended and kept in safe custody' were not enacted until 1877.[15]

The circumstances that led to an individual's committal to an asylum in the British Caribbean were generally not dissimilar to those in England or elsewhere in the empire.[16] The main criteria for admission were exhibitions of dangerous or otherwise challenging behaviours, either within the family or in a public place. The processes of committal usually involved police intervention, either through arrest or following representations made by distressed relatives. Manifestations of insanity would be distinguished from purely criminal behaviour by accompanying signs of derangement, in the form of shouting, gesticulating, confusion, excitement, destructiveness, sexual disinhibition, floridly delusional ideation or, at the other extreme, severe self-neglect and social withdrawal. Behind the immediate precipitants of admission were the economic, social, societal, and medical dynamics that underlay the onset of insanity. Many of those admitted to West Indian asylums exhibited overt signs of material deprivation, hunger, neglect, physical deterioration and associated bodily sickness.[17]

The profound social and psychological upheavals linked to transnational migration were influential factors in leading to asylum admission.[18] This was clearly reflected in the growing numbers and ratios of people of East Indian origin admitted to the British Guiana and Trinidad lunatic asylums.[19] Even in Jamaica, where the overall number of Indian immigrants was much lower, their proportionate presence in the asylum far exceeded that in the island's population.[20] Otherwise, the asylum's racial composition fully reflected the Jamaican populace, with black patients constituting the great majority. Those designated 'coloured' or 'brown' formed a significant minority, while there were always a small number of white patients.[21] For example, in 1886, out of 389 patients in the Jamaica Lunatic Asylum, 266 (79 per cent) were black, 68 (17 per cent) 'brown', and 13 (3 per cent) white, with 42 (11 per cent) described as 'Coolies'.[22] In Guiana and Trinidad, the asylum populations were consistently more mixed, reflecting the varied backgrounds of people in both countries. From 1870 onwards, the largest groups tended to be patients of East Indian origin, closely followed by black patients originating from the colony, elsewhere in the Caribbean, or from Africa. There were, in addition, smaller numbers of 'coloured' patients, as well as Chinese, Portuguese, and other Europeans.[23]

The Jamaican experiment

Jamaica was one of Britain's oldest colonies, and the largest and most populous in the Caribbean. Its first lunatic asylum was established around 1815, attached to the existing Public Hospital in Kingston.[24] Initially it catered almost entirely for white people, though by 1840 the racial composition of its patients had greatly altered. The Kingston Asylum was a deeply problematic institution, and in the late 1850s it became the focus of a major scandal, following revelations of appalling conditions that included insanitary and overcrowded buildings, incompetent medical staff, administrative corruption, and the widespread physical abuse of patients by staff. Pressure from British public opinion, articulated by Lord Ashley and the Commissioners in Lunacy, brought about a public enquiry, which was followed by dismissals of key staff and officers, and demands for far-reaching reform.[25] It prompted an empire-wide survey by the Colonial Office in 1863, into the state of hospitals and asylums throughout the empire, which showed many of the problems to be widely prevalent throughout the West Indies and elsewhere. The ensuing proposals for reform included an emphasis on the importance of employing and occupying insane patients.[26]

One direct consequence of the scandal was the long-delayed, though still only partial, opening between 1860 and 1862 of the new Jamaica Lunatic Asylum, in a sea-side location at Rae's Town near Kingston.[27] Among its regulations, drafted in 1862, was a requirement that the warden and matron should encourage the employment of patients in the grounds, the laundry and the kitchen.[28] However, the new institution experienced considerable difficulties from the outset, due to inadequate, deteriorating facilities and insufficient staff to manage the patients effectively. In late 1863, the acting medical superintendent Charles Lake acknowledged that there had been no employment in outdoor work during the year, claiming that a complete absence of classification of patients prevented any system of 'industrial occupation' within the asylum.[29]

Amid concerns that the new asylum was showing indications of the problems associated with its disgraced predecessor, the decision was taken locally to fund the appointment of a medical man with experience of working in an English public asylum.[30] The Colonial Office approached the Commissioners in Lunacy, who recommended Thomas Allen, assistant medical officer at the Lincolnshire County Asylum since 1854, where he received a modest £70 per year. Allen was duly appointed medical superintendent of the Jamaica Lunatic Asylum at the relatively huge salary of £600.[31] He arrived in October 1863, bringing with him the head attendant and head female nurse from Lincolnshire, to be warden and matron.[32]

Allen was deeply shocked to find the asylum in an extremely bad state, with dirty, dilapidated buildings, no classification of patients according to behaviours, inadequate sanitation, and vermin-ridden bedding. He was dismayed to witness a high level of disorder and violence, with small numbers of staff failing to control the many noisy and disorderly people.[33] He soon concluded that a 'large proportion of the patients', particularly among the women, were 'ungovernable, troublesome, dirty, and half savage in their habits, and others are but little removed from a state of barbarism'. They lacked the 'restraining influence' of education and 'civilising associations'.[34]

In confronting the perceived challenges, Allen utilised the knowledge and experience he had gained in Lincolnshire. He rapidly implemented a series of far-reaching reforms. A comprehensive work programme was at the heart of these, for, as he explained, there was 'nothing more important in the moral treatment of the insane' than mental and bodily employment, which tended to 'withdraw their attention from thoughts, & feelings, connected with their disordered state'. He regarded outdoor occupations providing 'opportunities of extended exercise' as especially beneficial, and by April 1864 there were twenty-eight men employed in the grounds, as well as a further seventeen on various types of indoor work, out of a total of seventy-six male patients. Up to forty women were occupied in needlework and cleaning duties.[35]

By late 1864, twenty-five acres of land had been weeded, cleared, and planted with vegetables, including sweet potatoes, cotton, pumpkins, and peas. Supervised by three or four attendants, male and female patients were reported to be 'cheerful and willing agents'. Men also cleared rubbish, dug trenches, built embankments, and made a 'carriage drive', while others worked at trades like carpentry, bricklaying, and painting. All the asylum's clothing and bedding was being made or repaired by patients. Many cleaned the wards and did other domestic work, while numerous women engaged in needlework. Allen had great plans for other enterprises. Significantly, he pointed out that, as well as directly benefitting patients, their work brought considerable financial savings to the asylum.[36] After only a year in post Allen was able to claim to Jamaica's Governor Edward Eyre that out-door work was having 'good effects in diminishing a Tendency to violence, improving the bodily health, and increasing tranquillity and cheerfulness among the Patients'.[37]

Two social investigators from England in 1866 were highly impressed with Allen's achievements, concluding that the asylum 'would compare with the best in the mother country'. They described him as 'full of resource' in devising occupation for the patients, showing a 'pardonable pride' in describing the amount of work done on the land.[38] Allen's considerable entrepreneurial skills were demonstrated in 1869 with the establishment of a commercial sea fishery, employing a large net made in the asylum. The undertaking proved very successful and profitable for several years. At its peak, in 1875, the annual catch exceeded 75,000 lb (33,750 kg). Curing rooms were set up within the asylum. As well as providing food for the patients and farm animals, sufficient remained to be sold off cheaply to Kingston's poor.[39]

Work remained central to the whole endeavour at the Jamaica asylum, as Allen made clear in 1880:

> The occupation of the Patients continues to be regarded as of the highest importance in their treatment, and it may be said that as a rule, every Patient in the Asylum from after breakfast up to one o'clock p.m. is required to do something, the only exceptions being the 'incapables' from old age, mental defect, or bodily infirmity.

He proudly summarised the range of trades and pursuits followed, which included 'needlework, coirmaking, tailoring, cocoanut oil manufacture, netting, hat-making, mat-making, farm and garden occupation', with patients also acting as 'clerks, porters, messengers, cooks, house cleaners, besides being painters, bricklayers, shoemakers, plumbers, carpenters and fishermen'. Some of the profits earned were used to pay for educational classes, and recreational activities such as an asylum band, weekly dances, picnics by the sea, and magic lantern shows.[40]

By 1880 Allen's regime in Jamaica had reached its zenith. His energy and enthusiasm were beginning to wane and distinct signs of decline were appearing in key aspects of the asylum's operation, including the work schemes.

The lucrative fishery enterprise was diminishing steadily, with only 33,000 lb (14,850 kg) of fish caught in the preceding year. Four years later it had to be abandoned as no longer sufficiently productive to justify the expenditure on nets and specialist attendants. Its demise was partially offset by a concurrent growth of dairy-cattle farming and beef production.[41] Nevertheless, changing fortunes were increasingly reflected in routine reports that dwelt more on financial savings than any therapeutic or social benefits for the patients.[42]

Thomas Allen retired in late 1886 and died a few months later. He was replaced by another British asylum-trained doctor, Joseph Plaxton, who had spent several years as medical superintendent of the Ceylon Lunatic Asylum.[43] Plaxton was also an advocate of organised patient employment, considering it to be 'the main holdfast in the treatment of the insane'. However, his efforts to encourage all the patients to occupy themselves were soon checked by the 'laughable, but intensely wearisome' attempts by the women to avoid work.[44] Plaxton nevertheless persevered and attempted to revive the asylum's fishing enterprise, among other activities.[45] The difficulties he faced were magnified by the dramatic rise in the average numbers of patients from 465 in 1890 to 844 in 1900.[46] The asylum became increasingly overcrowded, and there was insufficient land and workshop accommodation to provide work for all those eligible.[47] The erection of new buildings in 1898 only compounded the problems, especially as they remained unoccupied until 1906.[48] By 1914 the Jamaica Lunatic Asylum contained well over 1,300 people, and was demonstrating all the shortcomings of a large, overcrowded, under-resourced and stagnant institution.[49] Although some patients continued to be involved in various indoor and outdoor occupations, the impetus and energy behind the earlier development of the work programmes had long since evaporated.

Creative enterprise in British Guiana

Located on the South American mainland, British Guiana had been a British colony only since 1815. The first lunatic asylum was established nearly three decades after Jamaica's, in 1842. It adjoined the general hospital in Georgetown, Demerara. Conditions in the asylum were extremely poor. A shocked John Candler, until recently superintendent of the York Retreat, likened it in 1850 to a 'wretched' prison and described the patients' situation as 'miserable'.[50] A replacement building for fifty-five patients, opened in 1859, was evidently little better. The Colonial Office report of 1864 condemned every aspect, including its confined, unventilated cells and small exercise yards. There were no means of work or occupation for the inmates.[51] Two years later a new lunatic asylum was opened in a converted fortress on a river estuary near New Amsterdam, in the remote province of Berbice.

The asylum at Fort Canje had the great advantage of extensive available land. However, facilities remained crude for some time. In 1869 there was still little occupation or activity for its 100 patients, which the colony's Governor Scott attributed partly to the difficulty of amusing people from widely diverse racial backgrounds.[52] An inspection in 1872 highlighted the asylum's considerable defects and severe overcrowding. A new resident surgeon, Dr Cramer, was appointed in 1873. He was subsequently sent on an observation visit to other colonies' asylums, and particularly to study the 'many salutary improvements' carried out by Thomas Allen in Jamaica. Unfortunately, Cramer died immediately after his return.[53]

Cramer was replaced by a Scotsman, Dr Robert Grieve (1839–1906), appointed by the Secretary of State for the Colonies in 1875.[54] Grieve had previously worked under London's Metropolitan Asylums Board as medical superintendent of the Hampstead Fever Hospital, where he became a controversial figure. A move to the distant colonies probably offered both an escape route from a problematic situation and an opportunity to develop a new career. Before going out to British Guiana he spent several months visiting and studying the practices of various lunatic asylums around Britain, imbibing the doctrines of non-restraint and moral management.[55] Despite his apparent failures in London, Grieve proved a highly effective asylum medical superintendent. When he arrived there were 160 patients in an asylum that was defective in many ways. The building was permeated with custodial, prison-like features, mechanical restraint was used extensively, the accommodation was inadequate and sanitation poor. Grieve initiated a range of reforming measures, at the heart of which was the comprehensive programme of employment begun in 1876.[56] During his ten years in post Grieve pushed the system of patient work at least as far as Thomas Allen had done in Jamaica.

Robert Grieve was unequivocal about the centrality of work to the asylum regime; it was an essential part of the 'daily routine'. However, he went much further, arguing that it had a directly curative role:

> For of all the medicaments which 'minister to a mind diseased', there is none whose efficacy exceeds that of labour, when carefully proportioned to the needs and capabilities of the patient. Conducted, as medicine in hospitals always is, or ought to be administered, labour holds in the Lunatic Asylum a foremost place in its pharmacopeia.

In this analysis, work constituted an integral element in the institution's medical treatment of insanity. He claimed explicitly that, as in England, 'from the workshop and the farm proceed the larger number of our recoveries'.[57] Furthermore, in addition to these therapeutic benefits, work was an important means of maintaining order, especially in a colony like British Guiana where, according to Grieve, 'the lower classes are totally unfitted to employ any leisure they may have in intellectual pursuits or amusements, even of the simplest kind'. Without the opportunity to work, they would only 'sleep, eat and quarrel'.[58]

A wide range of work activities was established under Grieve's leadership. The extensive fertile lands around the asylum enabled large quantities of fruit and vegetables to be grown, including plantains, bananas, sweet potatoes, cassava, and coconuts. Livestock farming produced a good deal of pork and beef, as well as milk and eggs. Additional agricultural land was created by draining areas within the river estuary. Various indoor workshop-based trades were established, including carpentry, painting, tailoring and shoemaking, as well as a bakery and a printing office. Women were engaged in tasks such as sewing, laundry work, and chocolate making.[59] Much of this activity was meticulously recorded in the remarkable *Asylum Journal*, a monthly publication edited and largely written by Grieve himself, put together with the assistance of patients.[60]

The British Guiana asylum was moving steadily toward becoming a self-supporting community. By June 1882 slightly over 80 per cent of the 372 patients were reported to be working.[61] Grieve demonstrated marked entrepreneurial abilities, and new areas of work continued to be developed. His conviction regarding its importance remained unaltered. As he explained in his review of activities during 1882: 'The importance and value of suitable employment as a remedy in a large proportion of the cases of insanity which come under treatment here, becomes from year to year more apparent.'[62] During 1883 a new piggery was established for 150 pigs.[63] Male patients were increasingly being employed in constructing new buildings and facilities, as well as in alterations, adaptations, repairs and maintenance.[64] The profits and savings from the various enterprises were used to help finance the running of the asylum, thus reducing the costs of maintaining the patients. Some of the money was also used to pay for the array of regular organised entertainments, sports and leisure pursuits that characterised Grieve's regime. Grieve calculated that about one third of the gross cost of running the institution was earned by the patients' work.[65]

As in Jamaica it was becoming increasingly problematic to maintain the momentum, although the causes differed somewhat. Patient numbers continued to increase rapidly, reaching 456 by the end of 1885, and the asylum expanded in size accordingly. Grieve lamented in July 1883 that the 'task of devising or obtaining suitable employment for the people' was 'one of the greatest difficulties' in managing the institution.[66] In his annual survey he observed that the 'provision farm' was not large enough to accommodate all who could benefit from agricultural employment, and demand for clothing for the asylum and the adjoining Colonial Hospital was insufficient to 'fully occupy all able to sew'.⁶⁷ In July 1885 he complained that a shortage of materials meant insufficient work for the female patients. This particularly affected those from India, seemingly for cultural reasons:

> The coolie women cannot be allowed to labour in the fields, where indeed there is barely sufficient room for the men. They are unable to sew, the laundry is full, so that it is only in making cocoanut oil or similar work that they can be employed. But cocoanuts cannot be obtained in sufficient quantities, although full prices are offered for them.

Nevertheless, despite these problems and Grieve's evident disappointment, three quarters of the 439 patients were still being regularly employed.⁶⁸

In early 1886, Robert Grieve relinquished his post at the lunatic asylum. His appointment as surgeon-general for the colony was a recognition of the singular success he had achieved there.⁶⁹ His legacy was sufficiently strong for the system he had established to continue for some time to come. The new medical superintendent, George Snell, formerly Grieve's assistant, endeavoured to maintain operations as best he could. In 1900 he proclaimed his strong belief 'in the employment of the insane in producing contentment, and drawing their attention from the chief delusions under which they labour'. He had 'no doubt' about the advantages for health of suitable occupation, particularly if outdoors. However, there were clearly now some difficulties in achieving these goals, for Snell acknowledged that 'many of the patients are not able or disposed to look on occupation in the same light'.⁷⁰ By this time, patient numbers had risen to almost 700, and the British Guiana asylum was experiencing all the familiar pressures and challenges associated with a large institution.

Confronting adversity in Trinidad

Trinidad had been a British colony since 1802. The establishment of a lunatic asylum came relatively late. Prior to 1858, insane patients were kept in a designated section of the Royal Gaol in Port of Spain.⁷¹ In that year a purpose-built asylum was opened for forty people, located at Belmont in the hills outside the city. It soon proved inadequate, with buildings and facilities that were increasingly deficient. Little occupation or activity was provided for the inmates.⁷² Following the enforced retirement of its long-serving medical superintendent Dr Thomas Murray in 1877, the decision was made to follow Jamaica's example and recruit an experienced British man. Dr Alfred Martin (1849–81), who had worked at the Three Counties Lunatic Asylum at Carnarvon, was appointed.⁷³ He initiated some essential reforms, but before these could be consolidated he caught a fever and died, in the autumn of 1881.⁷⁴

The Trinidad government opted to bring in another British asylum doctor to succeed Martin. George Seccombe was duly appointed in July 1882, following recommendation from the Commissioners in Lunacy via the Colonial Office.[75] He had worked since 1875 as an assistant medical officer in the Metropolitan Imbecile Asylum at Caterham in Surrey, a very large, highly regimented institution that housed 2,000 chronic patients.[76] He arrived in Trinidad to find things half a world away from Caterham, in more ways than one. The asylum was seriously overcrowded, with crude sanitary arrangements, inadequate water supplies, and ramshackle buildings spread over the hillsides. The calibre of staff was poor, and there was a good deal of disorder among the inmates.[77] The extent of the challenge was only too apparent.

Like Allen and Grieve, Seccombe quickly implemented some fundamental reforms. Organised patient work was situated at the centre of these. On arrival he had found very few of the 300 patients occupied, apart from some women working in the laundry and others cleaning wards or carrying water from nearby creeks. He laid out his intentions clearly:

> This year I hope, partially, to remedy this state of affairs, by employing patients at several trades, such as Tailors, Bootmakers, Carpenters, &c. – in fact to make the Institution, as far as possible, self-supporting. It is by employment, and by employment alone, that we may hope to render these patients useful members of society. We have a large number of Coolies, both male and female, the majority of whom might, with advantage, be employed in the cultivation of land, rearing stock, &c., all of which means of employment have long been recognised in the Home Asylums as potent agents in the cure of Insanity.[78]

Seccombe's statement encapsulated several notable points. Patient employment would help the asylum's finances. It would enable people to resume their roles in outside society. Agricultural work would be particularly applicable to the many patients of East Indian origin. Perhaps most significantly, occupation was a direct means to bring about recoveries. As early as 1884 Seccombe was largely attributing the preceding year's unusually high number of discharges to 'the introduction of the various industrial departments'.[79]

The magnitude of the task faced by Seccombe was, in some ways, greater than that of Allen and Grieve. The asylum was relatively small, and its overcrowded buildings were becoming increasingly dilapidated, with little space to provide workshops. Due to its location among steep hills, with little adjoining land, there was limited scope either for expansion or for outdoor agricultural and horticultural work. Seccombe had to devote time and energy to laying his grievances before the colonial government regarding the asylum's many deficiencies, and demanding action toward the building of a new asylum. Nevertheless, despite the hindrances, he demonstrated considerable ingenuity in devising and organising various means to employ the patients. By the end of 1883, 172 people (approximately 60 per cent of the asylum population) were employed at tasks including gardening, water carrying, tailoring, needlework, furniture manufacture and repair, coconut fibre manufacture, laundry, and ward work.[80] Over the next few years 'industrial employment' was further developed. Clothing manufacture was expanded, and male patients were increasingly employed in various aspects of building and maintenance work, both indoor and outdoor, including some quite ambitious projects. Skilled tradesmen were recruited as attendants to supervise and work alongside them.[81]

In early 1888, with an average of 200 people employed daily, Seccombe reflected on the asylum's achievements since he took up office. He suggested that the establishment of 'industrial employment' was 'the greatest improvement of all', and claimed that 'we compare favourably with the more advanced Institutions at home'. He emphasised the importance of work 'as a means to their recovery and return to the outer world'.[82] He thought that more could be done, stressing not only the therapeutic benefits for individual patients but also the wider ramifications for peace and good order within the asylum:

> The industrial employment of our Inmates is still capable of expansion, and is admittedly a powerful agent in their recovery, and even where there is little hope of this result, a troublesome and excited patient is rendered more amenable to treatment when his surplus energies are usefully directed in assisting the Carpenter or Mason, than if left in his division where he will take every opportunity of either destroying his clothing, or assaulting his fellow patients. The tranquillity pervading the Institution of late years has been most marked.[83]

Other employments were still being developed, like making roads and levelling ground on the hillsides surrounding the asylum.[84] From 1896 onwards some male patients were clearing land and building roads around the new lunatic asylum being constructed at St Ann's, about two miles away.[85]

The impressive new Trinidad Lunatic Asylum finally opened in 1900, and just over 500 patients were relocated.[86] It was set on rising ground in a valley. In comparison to its predecessor there was ample land for outdoor employment. However, the numbers of patients employed hardly rose. In 1908, only 225 were employed, being only 35 per cent of the 638 in the asylum.[87] Something had clearly changed in the nature of the asylum's operation. In 1903, George Seccombe sought to account for what had become an established trend of admissions increasing faster than numbers employed. He associated it with the deteriorated physical condition of many of those being admitted, the consequence being that it was 'difficult to find patients capable of employment'.[88] Nevertheless, it was also evident that Seccombe had lost much of his drive and was becoming disillusioned. His complaints about the increasing numbers of chronic and incapacitated patients grew more strident.[89] The severe overcrowding endemic in the old asylum soon re-emerged, and in 1908 he lamented that it was 'almost impossible to maintain an environment suitable for the treatment of our inmates with a view to their recovery'.[90] In early 1909 Seccombe retired on grounds of ill health.[91] His successor George Vincent made valiant attempts to reinvigorate the employment system, and by 1914 the numbers of working patients had risen to 267, with a notable increase in those occupied in agriculture and gardening. However, this was still no more than a significant minority of the almost 700 patients in the Trinidad asylum.[92]

Conclusions

Work was at the centre of the therapeutic system in the better managed nineteenth-century colonial asylums, as it was in British public asylums. It was regarded as a crucial means of bringing about the recovery of mentally disordered people, and of preparing them to return to their families and communities as well as to productive employment. The routines and disciplines associated with structured work were considered to have a tranquillising role, helping the individual toward a more settled, amenable mental state. When applied to groups of patients, this contributed to the creation and maintenance of a settled and orderly institutional environment. In acknowledgement of these ostensibly therapeutic attributes, work became elevated to the status of medical treatment and consequently appropriate for control by doctors.

The transfer of ideas and methodologies from Britain was of great importance.[93] The role played by medical men who had worked within the British public asylum arena, albeit in subordinate capacities, was central. They went out to the West Indian colonies with a clear and adaptable model of how to manage a large institution that contained an assortment of deprived and disordered people. If they were also energetic, even charismatic, their abilities to implement a successful work-based moral management regime were enhanced. However, it became evident that the system worked successfully only while they retained their dynamism and enthusiasm. Once those qualities were affected, due usually to a combination of disillusion and exhaustion, the project was likely to enter a decline. These effects were compounded by the pressures and dynamics associated with increasingly large, impersonal and routine-bound asylums.

In the context of the colonial civilising mission, a work-orientated lunatic asylum had particular significance. Its pacifying processes helped to re-create orderly citizens who could reconnect with their assigned societal roles as subservient labourers. In the British West Indies, there was an additional parallel with the type of ordered, stratified plantation that many of the patients would have experienced prior to their admission to the asylum. However, whereas post-emancipation plantation labour was remunerated, albeit poorly, asylum patients rarely received direct payment for their work either in cash or kind. Any earnings derived either went to offset the institution's running costs or were, at best, set aside to pay for various educational, recreational or leisure activities for the patients.[94] Participation in work-based activity was conveniently deemed by asylum doctors as therapeutic in itself. Indeed, Dr Robert Grieve went so far as to claim that the asylum was one place where 'to toil' was experienced as a 'privilege' rather than a punishment.[95]

Race, ethnicity, and colour remained as fundamentally defining features of life patterns and opportunities in the post-emancipation societies of the British colonial Caribbean. Within the lunatic asylums white medical superintendents, assisted maybe by a white assistant medical officer as well as white matron and head male nurse, presided over institutions where the great majority of patients were black or 'brown'.[96] Here was another congruence with the plantation and other key colonial spaces and structures, albeit that men like Allen, Grieve and Seccombe adopted a largely paternalistic approach to their responsibilities. Perhaps without deliberate intention, the work regimes they implemented in the asylums both conformed to and reinforced the class, status, and racial hierarchies prevailing inside the institutions themselves as well as in wider West Indian societies.[97]

Notes

1 See Chapter 1 by Jane Freebody in this volume. She rightfully acknowledges the earlier achievements by Hallaran at the Cork asylum, but these were on a smaller scale than those at Wakefield.
2 Sir Andrew Halliday, *A General View of the State of Lunatics and Lunatic Asylums* (London: Thomas and George Underwood, 1828), pp. 19–24, 93; John Thurnam, *Observations and Essays on the Statistics of Insanity* (London: Simpkin, Marshall, & Co., 1845; reprinted New York: Arno Press, 1976), pp. 76–8; Samuel Tuke, 'Introductory Observations' to C. W. Maximilian Jacobi, *On the Construction and Management of Hospitals for the Insane* (London: J. Churchill, 1841), p. xxvii; Leonard Smith, *'Cure, Comfort and Safe Custody': Public Lunatic Asylums in Early Nineteenth-Century England* (London: Leicester University Press, 1999), pp. 208–9, 228–39.
3 Smith, *'Cure, Comfort and Safe Custody'*, pp. 192–4, 259–77.
4 Leland Bell, *Social and Mental Disorder in Sub-Saharan Africa: The Case of Sierra Leone, 1787–1990* (New York and London: Greenwood Press, 1991); Catharine Coleborne, *Madness in the Family: Insanity and Institutions in the Australasian Colonial World, 1860–1914* (Basingstoke: Macmillan, 2010); Waltraud Ernst, *Mad*

Tales from the Raj: The European Insane in British India, 1800–1858 (London and New York: Routledge, 1991); Lynette A. Jackson, *Surfacing Up: Psychiatry and Social Order in Colonial Zimbabwe, 1908–1968* (Ithaca, NY: Cornell University Press, 2005); Jock McCulloch, *Colonial Psychiatry and the 'African Mind'* (Cambridge: Cambridge University Press, 1995); Sloan Mahone and Megan Vaughan (eds), *Psychiatry and Empire* (London: Palgrave Macmillan, 2007); James Mills, *Madness, Cannabis and Colonialism: The 'Native-Only' Lunatic Asylums of British India, 1857–1900* (Basingstoke: Palgrave Macmillan, 2000); James E. Moran, *Committed to the State Asylum: Insanity and Society in Nineteenth-Century Quebec and Ontario* (Kingston, ONT: McGill Queen's University Press, 2000); Julie Parle, *States of Mind: Searching for Mental Health in Natal and Zululand, 1868–1918* (Scottsville, South Africa: University of KwaZulu Natal Press, 2007); Jonathan Sadowsky, *Imperial Bedlam: Institutions of Madness in Colonial Southwest Nigeria* (Berkeley: University of California Press, 1999); Ng Beng Yeong, *Till the Break of Day: A History of Mental Health Services in Singapore, 1841–1993* (Singapore: Singapore University Press, 2001).

5   Coleborne, *Madness in the Family*, pp. 32–6; Parle, *States of Mind*, pp. 43–5, 85, 95–7, 105–6; Yeong, *Till the Break of Day*, pp. 17–19, 40, 89, 103–6; Margaret Jones, *The Hospital System and Health Care: Sri Lanka, 1815–1960* (New Delhi: Orient Blackswan, 2009), pp. 181–3, 188–92; Elspeth Knewstubb, 'Medical migration and the treatment of insanity in New Zealand: The doctors of Ashburn Hall, Dunedin, 1882–1910', in Angela McCarthy and Catharine Coleborne (eds), *Migration, Ethnicity and Mental Health: International Perspectives, 1840–2010* (London and New York: Routledge, 2012), pp. 107–22; Jacqueline Leckie, 'Unsettled minds: Gender and madness in Fiji', in Mahone and Vaughan, *Psychiatry and Empire*, pp. 99–123; Shula Marks, 'The microphysics of power: Mental nursing in South Africa in the first half of the nineteenth century', in Mahone and Vaughan, *Psychiatry and Empire*, pp. 67–98; Sally Swartz, 'The black insane in the Cape, 1891–1920', *Journal of Southern African Studies*, 21:3 (September 1995), 399–415. A significant number of these men were Scottish.

6   Contemporaries included in the West Indies British Guiana (now Guyana) on the South American mainland, and British Honduras (now Belize) in Central America, both lying within the Caribbean region.

7   In this chapter, according to contemporary usage, the terms 'coloured' and 'brown' normally refer to people of mixed racial heritage, although 'brown' could also comprise people originating from the Indian sub-continent.

8   There is a vast literature on the history of the enslavement and emancipation of African people and their descendants in the British West Indies. For useful summaries, see James Walvin, *Britain's Slave Empire* (Stroud: Tempus, 2007); William A. Green, *British Slave Emancipation: The Sugar Colonies and the Great Experiment* (Oxford: Clarendon Press, 1976; reprinted 1981); Gad Heuman, 'The British West Indies', in Andrew Porter (ed.), *The Oxford History of the British Empire: Volume III, The Nineteenth Century* (Oxford: Oxford University Press, 1999), pp. 470–93; Hilary McD. Beckles, *Britain's Black Debt: Reparations for Caribbean Slavery and Native Genocide* (Mona, Jamaica: University of West Indies Press, 2013).

9 Green, *British Slave Emancipation*, pp. 170–6, 296–301; Bridget Brereton, *A History of Modern Trinidad, 1783–1962* (Port of Spain and London: Heinemann, 1981), pp. 69–70, 76–81; Douglas Hall, 'The flight from the estates reconsidered: The British West Indies, 1838–1842', *Journal of Caribbean History*, 10 (1978), 7–24.
10 Green, *British Slave Emancipation*, pp. 261–88; Brereton, *A History of Modern Trinidad*, pp. 96–113; Brian L. Moore, *Race, Power and Social Segmentation in Colonial Society: Guyana After Slavery 1838–1891* (London and Montreux: Gordon & Breach, 1987), pp. 161–88; Lomarsh Roopnarine, *Indo-Caribbean Indenture: Resistance and Accommodation, 1838–1920* (Kingston, Jamaica: University of West Indies Press, 2007).
11 Letizia Gramaglia, 'Migration and mental illness in the British West Indies 1838–1900: The cases of Trinidad and British Guiana', in Catherine Cox and Hilary Marland (eds), *Migration, Health and Ethnicity in the Modern World* (London: Palgrave Macmillan, 2013), pp. 61–82.
12 David Wright, 'The certification of insanity in nineteenth-century England and Wales', *History of Psychiatry*, 9 (1998), 267–90. Two medical certificates were normally required in Jamaica and British Guiana, but only one in Trinidad, where there was a marked shortage of medical officers.
13 Michael Beaubrun et al., 'The West Indies', in John G. Howells (ed.), *World History of Psychiatry* (New York: Brunner/Mazel, 1975), pp. 507–27; Frederick W. Hickling and Hari D. Maharajh, 'Mental health legislation', in Hickling and Eliot Sorel (eds), *Images of Psychiatry: The Caribbean* (Kingston, Jamaica: Stephenson's Litho Press, 2005), pp. 43–74; British Parliamentary Papers (hereafter BPP) 1875, vol. LI, Papers Relating to Her Majesty's Colonial Possessions, 1875, part 1, p. 11.
14 BPP 1871, vol. XLVII, Reports to Secretary of State on the Past and Present State of Her Majesty's Colonial Possessions, 1869, p. 49; *The Asylum Journal … . Conducted by the Medical Superintendent of the Public Lunatic Asylum for British Guiana* (Berbice (British Guiana): The Asylum Press, 2 May 1881), p. 18; *Ibid.* (15 November 1882), p. 74.
15 Beaubrun, 'The West Indies', pp. 510, 515; British National Archives, Kew Richmond, Surrey (hereafter BNA), CO 295/275, fos 242–9, 18 December 1875, Irving to Carnarvon; CO 295/276, fos 477–86, 7 April 1876, Irving to Carnarvon; CO 295/277, fos 624–30, 19 February 1876, Commissioners in Lunacy to Colonial Office; CO 295/278, fos 144–7, 9 March 1877, Des Voeux to Carnarvon; *Trinidad: Surgeon-General's Report on the Medical Department for the Year 1890* (Trinidad: Government Printing Office, Port-of-Spain, 1891), p. 23 (copy in Library of London School of Hygiene and Tropical Medicine).
16 Joseph Melling and Bill Forsythe, *The Politics of Madness: The State, Insanity and Society in England, 1845–1914* (London and New York: Routledge, 2006), pp. 73–175; Ernst, *Mad Tales from the Raj*, pp. 45–51; Jackson, *Surfacing Up*, pp. 62–109; Mills, *Madness, Cannabis and Colonialism*, pp. 67–102; Leonard Smith, 'Caribbean Bedlam: The development of the lunatic asylum system in Britain's West Indian colonies, 1838–1914', *The Journal of Caribbean History*, 44:1 (2010), 1–47. The factors associated with asylum admissions are considered fully in Leonard Smith, *Insanity, Race and Colonialism: Managing Mental Disorder in the Post-*

Emancipation British Caribbean, 1838–1914 (Basingstoke: Palgrave Macmillan, 2014).
17 Smith, 'Caribbean Bedlam', pp. 15–19.
18 McCarthy and Coleborne, *Migration, Ethnicity and Mental Health*.
19 *The Asylum Journal* (16 January 1882), p. 89; *Ibid*. (15 January 1886), p. 148; *British Guiana: Report of the Surgeon General for the Year 1899–1900* (Georgetown, Demerara: C. K. Jardine, 1900), p. 40 (copy in Library of the London School of Hygiene and Tropical Medicine); BNA, CO 298/40, Colonial and Criminal Lunatic Asylum, Trinidad, 1 May 1884, p. 12; CO 298/42, Colonial and Criminal Lunatic Asylum, Trinidad, 1 May 1886, p. 27; *Trinidad: Report of the Surgeon-General on the Medical Service and Medical Institutions of the Colony for the Year 1887* (Trinidad, Government Printing Office, Port-of-Spain, 1888), p. 23 (copy in Library of London School of Hygiene and Tropical Medicine).
20 *Daily Gleaner*, 22 November 1899. About 37,000 Indian migrants were brought to Jamaica, see: Roopnarine, *Indo-Caribbean Indenture*, p. 36.
21 BNA, CO 137/382, 12 December 1863, Lake to Trench, fo. 99; CO 140/186, Annual Report of the Jamaica Lunatic Asylum, Year Ended 30 September 1883, p. 174; CO 140/194, Annual Report, Year Ended 30 September 1887, p. 206.
22 BNA, CO 140/194, Report of Medical Superintendent, 1885/6, p. 45. 'Coolies' referred to people of East Indian or (occasionally) Chinese origin.
23 See note 19; *The Asylum Journal* (15 May 1883), p. 27.
24 BNA, CO 140/104, Votes of the Assembly of Jamaica, 9 December 1818, pp. 114–15, 11 December 1818, p. 137; Lewis Q. Bowerbank, *A Circular Letter to the Individual Members of the Legislative Council and of the House of Assembly of Jamaica, Relative to the Public Hospital and Lunatic Asylum of Kingston* (Kingston: publisher unknown, 1858), p. 43.
25 Margaret Jones, 'The most cruel and revolting crimes: The treatment of the mentally ill in mid-nineteenth century Jamaica', *The Journal of Caribbean History*, 42:2 (2008), 290–309; *The Lancet*, 23 October 1858, 3 September 1859; *The Times*, 8 September 1859; anon., 'The Jamaica Lunatic Asylum', *Journal of Mental Science*, 6 (1859), pp. 157–67; BNA, CO 137/366, fos 245–51, 'Report on the Management of the Public Hospital', 20 November 1861.
26 BNA, CO 885/3/4, 'Colonial Hospitals and Lunatic Asylums'.
27 BNA, CO 137/348, 10 January 1860, Darling to Newcastle, fos 12–13; CO 137/353, fos 47–9, 23 January 1861, Darling to Newcastle; CO 137/367, fos 272–3, 6 August 1862, Eyre to Newcastle. The Jamaica Lunatic Asylum had originally been projected around 1840.
28 BNA, CO 137/368, 'Rules and Regulations Lunatic Asylum Kingston Jamaica 1862', fos 527, 539.
29 BNA, CO 137/382, fos 83–93, 12 December 1863, Lake to Trench.
30 BNA, CO 137/364, fos 278–91, 22 February 1862, Darling to Newcastle; CO 137/372, fos 225–8, 22 May 1863, Eyre to Newcastle.
31 BNA, CO 137/372, fos 311–16, 8 June 1863, Eyre to Newcastle; Lincolnshire Archives, HOSP/ST JOHN'S 1/1/3, Minute Book of Visitors 1852/68, 12 October 1854, 29 July 1864.

32 BNA, CO 137/375, fos 187–9, 23 October 1863, Eyre to Newcastle; fo. 215, 2 November 1863, Eyre to Newcastle.
33 BNA, CO 137/382, 2 April 1864, Allen to Eyre, fos 306–29.
34 BNA, CO 137/382, fo. 378. Although Allen did not refer directly to race and colour, his implication was clear.
35 BNA, CO 137/382, fos 435–6.
36 BNA, CO 137/388, 21 October 1864, Allen to Austin, fos 95–102.
37 BNA, CO 137/388, fo. 97.
38 Thomas Harvey and William Brewin, *Jamaica in 1866. A Narrative of a Tour Through the Island, With Remarks on its Social and Educational Condition* (London: A. W. Bennett, 1867), pp. 5–6.
39 BNA, CO 137/484, Report of Medical Superintendent for 1875/76, fos 589–90; CO 140/186, fo. 167, Annual Report of the Jamaica Lunatic asylum, for the year ended 30 September 1883; BPP, 1873, vol. L, Report on Leprosy and Yaws in the West Indies, Addressed to Her Majesty's Secretary of State for the Colonies, by Gavin Milroy, MD, p. 50.
40 BNA, CO 140/183, Jamaica Assembly, Report of the Medical Superintendent and Director of the Jamaica Lunatic Asylum for the Year 1878/79, pp. 24–5.
41 BNA, CO 140/181, Report of the Medical Superintendent and Director, 1879/80, p. 197; CO 140/186, Annual Report, Year Ended 30 September 1883, p. 167.
42 BNA, CO 140/189, Annual Report, Year Ended 30 September 1885, pp. 65–6.
43 BNA, CO 137/527, 31 August 1886, fos 292–305; *Jamaica Gleaner*, 23 October 1886; CO 140/194, Annual Report, Year Ended 30 September 1887, p. 205; Margaret Jones, *The Hospital System and Health Care: Sri Lanka, 1815–1960* (New Delhi: Orient Blackswan, 2009), pp. 188–90.
44 BNA, CO 140/194, Annual Report, 30 September 1887, pp. 205–6.
45 BNA, CO 140/199, Annual Report, 30 September 1889, p. 162.
46 Annual Report on the Lunatic Asylum, p. 8, in *Annual Report of the Superintending Medical Officer*, Year Ended 31 March 1898 (Jamaica: General Printing Office, Kingston, 1898); Annual Report, p. 5, in *Annual Report of the Superintending Medical Officer*, Year Ended 31 March 1907 (Jamaica: General Printing Office, Kingston, 1907) (copies in Library of the London School of Hygiene and Tropical Medicine).
47 *Jamaica Gleaner*, 9 November 1892. Demands grew for provision of a second lunatic asylum.
48 *Daily Gleaner*, 16 December 1898, 22 November 1899, 14 September 1906.
49 *Daily Gleaner*, 27 August 1914.
50 Library of the Society of Friends, MS vol. S.22, John Candler: West Indies Journal 1849, 1850, fos 25–6, 12 Mon. 19; Joseph A. Borome, 'John Candler's visit to America, 1850', *The Bulletin of Friends Historical Association* (Philadelphia), 48:1 (Spring 1959), 21–62.
51 BPP 1861, vol. XL, Reports to Secretary of State on the Past and Present State of Her Majesty's Colonial Possessions, 1859, p. 43; BNA, CO 885/3/4, 'Colonial Hospitals and Lunatic Asylums', pp. 4, 5, 24.
52 BPP 1871, vol. XLVII, Reports to Secretary of State, 1869, pp. 47–9.

53 BNA, CO 111/394, 25 July 1872, 'Report on Lunatic Asylum. Gavin Milroy to Under Secretary of State for the Colonies'; BPP 1875, vol. LI, Papers Relating to Her Majesty's Colonial Possessions, part III, p. 67.
54 BPP 1875, vol. LI, Papers Relating to Her Majesty's Colonial Possessions, part III, p. 74.
55 Letizia Gramaglia, 'Colonial psychiatry in British Guiana: Dr Robert Grieve', in Kimberley White (ed.), *Configuring Madness: Representation, Context and Meaning* (Oxford: Inter-Disciplinary Press, 2009), pp. 191–206; Gramaglia, 'Dr Robert Grieve (1839–1906), an "Apostle of Science"', 'Introduction' to Robert Grieve, *The Asylum Journal* (Guyana: The Caribbean Press, 2010), vol. 1, pp. xiii–xxxii.
56 BPP 1875, vol. LI, Papers Relating to Her Majesty's Colonial Possessions, part III, pp. 74, 78; *The Asylum Journal* (1 March 1881), p. 2; *Ibid.* (1 April 1881), pp. 7–9.
57 *The Asylum Journal* (1 April 1881), p. 7.
58 *Ibid.*, p. 8.
59 *The Asylum Journal* (1 July 1881), pp. 34, 39–40; *Ibid.* (2 January 1882), pp. 87, 91; *Ibid.* (15 May 1882), pp. 31–2; *Ibid.* (15 September 1883), p. 63.
60 *The Asylum Journal* was first published in March 1881, and continued monthly for almost five years. As well as recording much information about the asylum's ongoing operations, it also contained material on aspects of insanity and its treatment as well as wider epidemiological and public-health issues in the colony. Grieve arranged for the journal to be distributed to asylum superintendents in Britain and elsewhere in the empire. (Copies are available in the British Library and in the Wellcome Library.)
61 *The Asylum Journal* (15 June 1882), pp. 38–9.
62 *The Asylum Journal* (15 January 1883), p. 92.
63 *The Asylum Journal* (15 February 1883), p. 6; *Ibid.* (15 June 1883), p. 38.
64 *The Asylum Journal* (15 September 1882), p. 62; *Ibid.* (15 November 1882), p. 78; *Ibid.* (15 January 1884), pp. 91–3; *Ibid.* (15 January 1885), p. 72; *Ibid.* (15 January 1886), p. 150.
65 Gramaglia, 'Colonial psychiatry in British Guiana', pp. 194–5, 199; *The Asylum Journal* (15 January 1885), pp. 71–3.
66 *The Asylum Journal* (15 July 1883), pp. 46–7.
67 *The Asylum Journal* (15 January 1884), pp. 91–2.
68 *The Asylum Journal* (15 July 1885), p. 112.
69 Gramaglia, 'Dr Robert Grieve (1839–1906), an "Apostle of Science"', pp. xix–xxi.
70 *British Guiana: Report of the Surgeon General for the Year 1899–1900*, p. 43.
71 BPP 1849, vol. XXXIV, Reports to Secretary of State on the Past and Present State of Her Majesty's Colonial Possessions, 1848, p. 286; *Port of Spain Gazette*, 4 March 1857.
72 *Port of Spain Gazette*, 19 February 1859, 4 February 1863, 4 March 1865.
73 BNA, CO 295/278, fos 144–5, 9 March 1877, Des Voeux to Carnarvon; fos 191–4, 4 April 1877, Des Voeux to Carnarvon; fos 196–8, 4 April, 1877, Crane to Colonial Secretary; fos 200–1, 14 February 1877, Martin to Crane; fos 295–6, note dated 27 April 1877.

Work in British West Indian asylums 161

74 BNA, CO 295/291, fos 426–9, 1 November 1881, Freeling to Kimberley; fos 431–6, 29 October 1881, Crane to Freeling.
75 BNA, CO 295/291, fos 427–8, 1 November 1881, Freeling to Kimberley; fos 707–10, 28 November 1881, Freeling to Kimberley; fos 711–7, 28 November 1881, Crane to Freelling.
76 London Metropolitan Archives, Metropolitan Asylum District: Board Minutes, vol. IX, 1875/6, p. 105; vol. X, 1876/7, Medical Superintendent's Report, 1 October 1876, p. 549; vol. XV, 1881/2, Medical Superintendent's Report, 31 December 1880, p. 88; vol. XVI, 1882/3, Medical Superintendent's Report, 31 December 1881, p. 48; vol. XV, 1883/4, Medical Superintendent's Report, 31 December 1882, p. 390; MAB/0251, Committee Minutes, 16 June 1882. Seccombe's contribution had been well regarded.
77 BNA, CO 298/39, Colonial and Criminal Lunatic Asylum, Trinidad, 1 May 1883, pp. 1–3; *Journal of Mental Science*, 30 (1884), 141–4.
78 BNA, CO 298/39, Colonial and Criminal Lunatic Asylum, 1 May 1883, p. 3; *Journal of Mental Science*, p. 142.
79 BNA, CO 298/40, Colonial and Criminal Lunatic Asylum, Trinidad, 1 May 1884, p. 1.
80 BNA, CO 298/40, Colonial and Criminal Lunatic Asylum, 1 May 1884, pp. 3, 14.
81 BNA, CO 298/41, Colonial and Criminal Lunatic Asylum, 28 February 1885, pp. 1–2, 4, 16–18; CO 298/42, Colonial and Criminal Lunatic Asylum, 31 March 1886, pp. 16–18; CO 298/43, Colonial and Criminal Lunatic Asylum, 31 March 1887, pp. 2, 8–9.
82 *Trinidad: Report of the Surgeon-General for the Year 1887*, pp. 12–13.
83 *Trinidad: Report of the Surgeon-General for 1887*, p. 14.
84 *Trinidad: Surgeon-General's Reports on the Medical Department*, 1889, p. 86; 1890, p. 90; 1893, p. 43; 1895, p. 56.
85 *Trinidad: Surgeon-General's Reports*, 1896, p. 59; 1898, p. 54.
86 *Trinidad: Surgeon-General's Report*, 1900, p. 87.
87 *Trinidad: Annual Report of the Surgeon-General*, 1907/8, pp. 91, 102.
88 *Trinidad: Annual Report of the Surgeon-General*, 1902/3, p. 65.
89 *Trinidad: Annual Reports*, 1903/4, p. 55; 1904/5, p. 52; 1905/6, p. 52.
90 *Trinidad: Annual Report*, 1907/8, p. 91.
91 BNA, CO 295/450, fos 26–43, 4 March 1909.
92 *Trinidad: Annual Report*, 1913/14, pp. 52, 64–5.
93 For fuller consideration of these transfers, see 'Introduction' in Waltraud Ernst and Thomas Mueller (eds), *Transnational Psychiatries: Social and Cultural Histories of Psychiatry in Comparative Perspective, c. 1800–2000* (Newcastle: Cambridge Scholars, 2010), pp. ix–xxiii, and Jacqueline Leckie, 'Islands, communities and entangled madness: Transferring psychiatry to the colonial Pacific, 1884–1964', in the same volume, pp. 24–50.
94 These aspects of patient 'occupation' were particularly well developed at the asylums of Jamaica and British Guiana, during the superintendence of Thomas Allen and Robert Grieve respectively.

95 *The Asylum Journal* (1 April 1881), p. 9.
96 The description 'brown' also comprises people of East Indian origin.
97 The interactions between race and mental disorder are considered more fully in Smith, *Insanity, Race and Colonialism*.

7

Work and activity in mental hospitals in modern Japan, *c.* 1868–2000

Akira Hashimoto

Historians have argued that the modernisation of Japan has not been a simple case of Westernisation, but that in the process of forming a nation state equal to Western countries, modernisation has been intertwined with Japanese nationalism.[1] What is more, the Western concept of modernity itself has been questioned.[2] Yet, broadly speaking, the course of Japanese modernisation can be mapped in terms of two major sociopolitical changes, both of which were influenced by Western powers: the Meiji Era restoration (1868–1912) that led to the rise of modern Japan under the influence of Europe, and the reconstruction that took place after the Second World War led by the United States of America.

The history of work or occupational therapy (OT) and rehabilitation science has followed a similar path. In pre-Second World War Japan, work and activity in a therapeutic context, later understood as OT, developed mainly from three fields: psychiatry, orthopaedics and internal medicine, and was particularly prominent in the treatment of tuberculosis.[3] Within these three fields, work and activity for mental patients has the longest history, being associated with the reform of psychiatric institutions in the early twentieth century, which was initiated by elite psychiatrists who had studied in Europe, especially in Germany and Austria.[4]

This chapter explores the history of work and OT in modern Japan, focusing on the changing context of work and activity in mental hospitals and the professionalisation of occupational therapists during a period when Japan fluctuated between Western and Japanese modernity. It will be shown that during the earlier period work and activity were managed by psychiatrists and later on by specially trained and qualified occupational therapists. Either way, the work regimes remained strongly influenced by Western theories and practices until more recently a new generation of occupational therapists concerned itself with issues pertaining to the specificities of the Japanese cultural context.

Within the context of this chapter, the term 'work therapy' denotes work and activity practised within a therapeutic context before the 1910s and 1920s. Subsequently, the practice of 'occupational therapy', undertaken by specially trained staff, was established in Western countries and referred to as such in Japan, too. The Japanese translation for both 'work therapy' and 'occupational therapy' remained the same, namely *sagyō ryōhō*. However, after the Second World War a different type of *sagyō ryōhō* (commonly translated as 'work therapy' in English) was introduced in Japan within the wider framework of 'life therapy'. Life therapy was inspired by the observed positive effects of habit training in the aftercare of lobotomised patients in psychiatric institutions. This therapy was newly conceptualised against the former 'occupational therapy' as practised in Japan and the United States and embraced habit training, recreational therapy and 'work therapy'. In contrast to its earlier usage, 'work therapy' within the context of 'life therapy' had only a narrow meaning. To follow Western usage of the terms, in this chapter 'work therapy' is used to refer to the earlier type of *sagyō ryōhō* and 'occupational therapy' for the post-Second World War version of *sagyō ryōhō*.

The early stages of occupational therapy: Kure Shūzō and his contemporaries

The idea of work and activity was first introduced into psychiatric institutions by foreign teachers after the Meiji Restoration, which began in 1868. In Kyoto, the first public mental hospital in Japan, Kyoto Tenkyōin, was established in 1875. Work and activities such as sewing, rope and paper-string making were practised under the instruction of the Austrian physician Ferdinand A. Junker von Langegg (1828– ?), who taught medicine in a public hospital in Kyoto from 1872 to 1876. Before his arrival in Japan in 1872, he had graduated from the University of Vienna, obtained British nationality, and worked as a physician in the Samaritan Free Hospital, London. He is considered to have acquired his knowledge of moral treatment and the principle of non-restraint from John Conolly (1794–1866). Kyoto Tenkyōin was closed in 1882 for financial reasons.[5]

Meanwhile, in 1879, the Austrian physician Albrecht von Roretz (1846–84), who taught at various medical schools in Japan, designed a new building for the public mental hospital in Tokyo, Tokyo Fu Tenkyōin, which was established in the same year. He was probably commissioned by Hasegawa Tai (1842–1912), medical director of the public general hospital in Tokyo (Tokyo Fu Byōin). Based on the non-restraint system, Roretz also proposed the introduction of work and activity into the new hospital.[6] But it seems that neither work nor activity were practised before Sakaki Hajime's (1857-97) tenure as medical director of Tokyo Fu Tenkyōin in 1887.[7] In the same year it was decided that the Imperial University in Tokyo should take charge of the treatment of patients in this institution, which at the time was the only public mental hospital in Japan. As there were no psychiatric beds on the university campus, it was difficult to garner patients for clinical lectures other than those from Tokyo Fu Tenkyōin.[8]

In the previous year, 1886, Sakaki had been appointed as the first professor of psychiatry at the university after studying for four years in Germany. In his 1887 article on the treatment of mental patients, Sakaki looked at a psychiatric institution near Leipzig (probably Alt-Scherbitz, mentioned below), where the patients were occupied in farm work.[9] In 1889, Tokyo Fu Tenkyōin changed its name to Tokyo Fu Sugamo Byōin, and Sakaki and his pupils made patients engage in light work such as sewing or knitting. On 18 September 1890, Sakaki wrote in his diary: '[F]rom today we give *shokugyō* (work) to the patients.'[10] But the effect was very limited: the number of patients this applied to and the work to be done was restricted, and the available equipment and the physicians' experience were insufficient.[11]

Work and activity in Tokyo Fu Sugamo Byōin went into full swing under the direction of Sakaki's pupil Kure Shūzō (1865-1932). After Sakaki died young at the age of thirty-nine in 1897, Kure was sent to Europe by the government to study psychiatry for four years (1897-1901). During his stay abroad, Kure visited a number of psychiatric institutions and was particularly inspired by the mental hospital in Alt-Scherbitz near Leipzig, which was well known among psychiatrists worldwide for its agricultural colony where, as part of their treatment, many chronic patients were engaged in agricultural work.[12]

Shortly after his return to Japan in October 1901, Kure was appointed professor of psychiatry at the Tokyo Imperial University and medical director of Tokyo Fu Sugamo Byōin. He at once reorganised the treatment of mental patients in Sugamo Byōin. He prohibited the use of chains and introduced diversions such as musical concerts, garden parties or short-time excursions for the patients. In November 1901, Kure established two rooms for sewing in a female ward. There the female patients made pillows and clothes for the hospital. In December 1901, based on his experiences in Europe, he gave a lecture on work therapy (*sagyō ryōhō*) for the mentally ill at a conference.[13] He complained about what he perceived as backwardness in Japan: 'No work therapy has been practised until today.'[14] From 1902, seventeen male and twenty-five female inmates (out of 400 inmates) were engaged in weeding the grounds. The workers were restricted to public patients, who made up about 80 per cent of all inmates.[15] According to the hospital rules of 1905 wages were to be paid to public patients. Self-funded patients were not expected to work, but encouraged to take part in leisure activities such as theatre performances.

There were different rules regarding outdoor activities for self-funded patients and public patients: the time of day when all patients could exercise was fixed, but self-funded patients could stay outside longer and were attended to by more nurses than public patients. The rules also stipulated the strict separation of male and female patients: they could not approach each other when working, or while outside.[16]

From today's vantage point, Kure's reforms may seem restricted, but the Tokyo prefectural government did not fully condone them. There were safety concerns as the number of patients who escaped from Sugamo Byōin increased with the introduction of work and non-restraint. In 1903 the Tokyo prefectural government complained about Kure's methods, referring to the first national law for mental patients in 1900, the Mental Patients' Custody Act, which stipulated strict guidelines for patients' confinement in psychiatric institutions. In Japan the forty-seven prefectural governments possessed limited powers until 1947, when the Local Autonomy Law came into force. However, even before 1947 each prefecture had a local assembly that had a voting right of local finance and was responsible for local administration such as police, education, health and welfare. Public hospitals in Tokyo, including Sugamo Byōin, were placed directly under the jurisdiction of the Tokyo prefectural government. The authorities claimed that Kure's reforms frightened the nurses, who were prohibited from physically restraining patients, and that imitating foreign countries was bound to fail.[17] Yet later the prefectural government seems to have accepted Kure's reforms, although the reasons for this are unknown. Sugamo Byōin developed more and more lines of work and activities such as farming, dyeing, washing, plastering, painting, and so on. By 1904, a pig farm and two workshops, one each for male and female patients respectively, were completed in the grounds.[18] However, the restricted site at Sugamo Byōin was a barrier to improving work and activity in the hospital on a large scale, and as the surroundings had become increasingly urbanised, the hospital was not suitable for agricultural work. Even so, the agricultural colony of Alt-Scherbitz in Germany was always in Kure's mind.

Kure's reforms were extended after the hospital was moved from Sugamo to Matsuzawa village in the suburbs of Tokyo in 1919. The grounds of Matsuzawa Byōin, or Matsuzawa Mental Hospital, were much larger than those at Sugamo. The new hospital was built in pavilion style: the hospital buildings were decentralised and consisted of numerous pavilions, like in Alt-Scherbitz.[19] According to Katō Fusajirō (1887–1968), it became easier for patients to work and carry out various activities after moving from Sugamo to Matsuzawa because Matsuzawa had sufficient land. Furthermore, the Mental Hospital Act of 1919 enabled patients to have more freedom within the hospital, whereas the previous law, the Mental Patients' Custody Act (1900), had emphasised only the secure confinement of the mentally ill in psychiatric institutions.[20]

Katō Fusajirō and occupational therapy

The psychiatrist Katō Fusajirō was appointed by the director Kure to be in charge of OT from 1919 to 1925 in Matsuzawa Byōin. His work was summarised in his doctoral thesis on OT and published in the medical journal *Shinkeigaku zasshi* in 1925. Katō stated that OT is most effective for schizophrenic and mentally retarded patients, and that they should be taken out of their rooms and outside to accustom them to group activities, and then encouraged to participate in group OT before taking part in individual OT. He also paid attention to trends in OT in the United States, where the National Society for the Promotion of Occupational Therapy was founded in 1917. For instance, he referred to psychiatrist William R. Dunton (1868–1966) of Philadelphia, who has been considered as one of the founding fathers of OT in the United States. However, it is unclear whether Katō's practice in Matsuzawa was directly influenced from overseas. Katō noted that specialist OT staff were required in Japan as much as in the United States, but that it would be impossible to directly apply European and American experiences to mental hospitals in Japan.[21] Meanwhile, Katō's collaborator, Maeda Norizō (1893–1976), who worked as a nurse in Matsuzawa from 1921 to 1933, published an abridged translation of Dunton's 1919 book *Reconstruction Therapy*, which is said to have been highly regarded before the Second World War when no other text on OT existed in Japan.[22]

In February 1921, Maeda visited Matsuzawa for the first time and was introduced to Katō by the director Kure.[23] At that time, eighty out of 600 patients worked in the wards and thirty outside and in the hospital's workshop. They made paper bags, cleaned the corridors, set the tables, worked in the fields, raised pigs, and so on. Shortly after he was employed as a nurse, Maeda was involved in collective outdoor work: he was able to recruit seventeen or eighteen applicants from male public patients who were to improve the arable land within the hospital grounds. The work was safely completed in about a month. He had the impression that the patients probably enjoyed the work, otherwise they would have preferred to spend the time idling in their rooms all day.

After this successful outdoor experience, a remarkable construction project began in July of the same year in the hospital grounds. Katō and Maeda themselves, together with the patients, dug the grounds, made a pond, carried soil in straw baskets, accumulated this soil, and created a mountain, singing songs in turn to encourage one another.[24] The enormous earthquake of September 1923 did some damage to the mountain under construction, but actually ended up giving it a better form. For several months after the earthquake, about half of all patients were mobilised for repair work on the hospital buildings as the number of regular workers was insufficient. The building work was restarted later. The mountain and the pond were finally completed in March

1925 and subsequently developed into a Japanese garden. In the same year Katō resigned and returned to his home town in Aichi to open a clinic, and Kure left the hospital on reaching retirement age.[25]

The construction of the mountain and pond by Katō with his colleague and patients is often retold as the heart-warming story of an anti-authoritarian doctor.[26] But Katō was sometimes seen as a tragic pioneer of OT in the history of Japanese psychiatry, for at that time many colleagues looked down on him as the 'construction doctor'.[27] However, Katō's OT in Matsuzawa might have been overestimated to some extent, as it was realised under select conditions. As Maeda wrote, the collective outdoor work for the improvement of arable land was performed only by public patients – in other words, poor inmates (70 per cent of patients were receiving welfare at the time). All work in Matsuzawa before the Second World War is said to have been done by them.[28] In terms of the relationships between the various social classes of mental patients and work in mental hospitals, what Maeda noted in his summarised translation of Dunton's book might also be applied to the patients of Matsuzawa: the well-to-do and the well-educated tended to dislike work. He referred to the statement by John M. Galt, Superintendent of the Eastern Lunatic Asylum of Virginia at Williamsburg, that: 'No class of patients is so happy as the labourers; no other convalescents recover so rapidly and favourably; many of these would be completely miserable without labour and their recovery retarded.'[29]

Moreover, there was a gender divide in the organisation of work activities. Of the 700 patients (male: 60 per cent; female: 40 per cent) in 1925, 140 men and 90 women worked. While the work in the wards such as cleaning, setting the tables and making paper bags was done by both male and female patients; outdoor work such as construction, cultivation, and horticulture was carried out by male patients only. In contrast, sewing and washing were restricted to female patients.[30]

For psychiatrist Katō, on the other hand, diagnosis was crucial for the selection of patients suitable for work. The kind of patient seen to be most eligible was a chronic schizophrenic who led an idle life in his or her room all day. At the time, more than half the patients were diagnosed as schizophrenic. Katō stated that those patients who were able to walk, eat, and imitate other people were also able to work, even if they suffered from dementia. Unstable patients who talked excessively and had destructive tendencies were taken outdoors to help with weeding. They were encouraged to comply by means of incentives such as rice crackers, cigarettes, or rice balls tinged with soy sauce. Katō emphasised that OT was not suitable for paralytic dementia patients and psychopaths, as they made other patients uneasy.[31]

In the 1930s other mental hospitals introduced OT, but the regime often faced problems. For example, at Nakamiya Byōin in Osaka, established

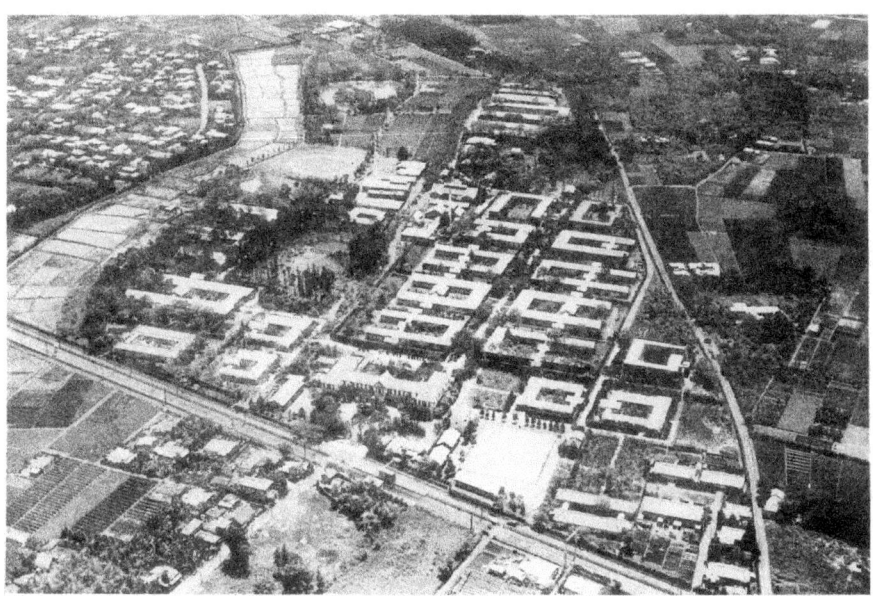

7.1 Aerial photograph of Matsuzawa Byōin, c. 1935.

in 1926 as the second public (prefectural) mental hospital in Japan, OT was begun in 1931 by psychiatrist Nagayama Yasumasa (1893–1986), who studied from 1929 to 1930 in Germany as a promising neuropathologist. He was deeply impressed by Gustav Kolb's (1870–1938) *Außenfürsorge*, or extramural care, and Hermann Simon's (1867–1947) *Arbeitstherapie*, or work therapy, and lost his interest in biological study. After returning to Osaka, he found a job at Nakamiya Byōin as the head doctor. However, doctors in the public mental hospital, who had graduated from elite universities and were more interested in biological studies of mental illness than in the care and cure of mental patients, did not take well to Nagayama's practice. According to Nagayama, they believed that, if work were introduced, patients would escape from the hospital. The nurses, who were entrusted with inmates' safety, felt uneasy about patients' freedom to engage in work outside the wards and feared the possibility that they might escape and staff be required to give a written apology or, at worst, be dismissed by the hospital director.[32]

The Second World War cast a shadow over OT in mental hospitals. While mental patients tended to be treated as a burden on society during wartime, the psychiatrists at Matsuzawa emphasised that the patients were useful even in an emergency situation, stating that their work would help ease food and labour shortages. As the war intensified, patients were engaged in constructing air-raid shelters and digging graves for deceased patients in the grounds, in which they themselves might be buried the next day.[33]

OT, as implemented by prominent psychiatrists such as Kure and Katō, has been well documented by historians.[34] However, the number of hospitalised mental patients who were engaged in work was so small that the influence of OT on psychiatry in pre-war Japan is thought to have been very limited. For the wider acceptance of OT, psychiatry and psychiatric institutions needed to be popularised.

Post-war Japan and the invention of 'life therapy'

The environment for psychiatry in Japan drastically changed after the Second World War. Many new mental hospitals were constructed from the 1950s onwards, and more and more patients were hospitalised all over the country. After 1950, the number of psychiatric beds in Japan continued to increase (1950: 17,686; 1960: 95,067; 1970: 247,265) until the mid-1990s (1993: 363,010), while in other developed countries the de-institutionalisation of mental patients had become a common trend.[35]

In Japan, post-war OT emerged as a form of rehabilitation but also as a tool to control psychiatric patients in crowded hospitals. Above all, a new practice called *seikatsu ryōhō*, or 'life therapy', spread throughout mental hospitals all over the country from the 1950s to the 1970s.[36] The Japanese word *seikatsu* (or *kurashi*, meaning 'life') of *seikatsu ryōhō* was a key word of the time. A variety of phrases that referred to *seikatsu* were coined after the 1950s: *seikatsu tsuzurikata* (writing education), *seikatsu taiiku* (physical education), and *Kurashi no techō* (title of a popular magazine). People tried to take back their own lives and appreciated the positive and creative nuances of the word *seikatsu* during this period.[37]

'Life therapy' was first coined in a 1956 article by Kobayashi Hachirō, a psychiatrist at Kokuritsu Musashi Ryōyōjo (National Musashi Hospital) in the suburbs of Tokyo. According to Kobayashi, the concept of OT used in America, which sometimes even included therapies such as psychodrama, was very broad. In Japan in contrast, *sagyō ryōhō*, or OT, enunciated the narrow meaning of patient work as practised by Kure and Katō before the Second World War. Kobayashi intended to change the old understanding and practice of Japanese OT by using the new phrase 'life therapy'.[38]

Kokuritsu Musashi Ryōyōjo was originally established in 1940 as a sanatorium for disabled veterans suffering from mental illness (Shōigunjin Musashi Ryōyōjo). According to the institution's commemorative publication, from its opening staff found it difficult to deal with inmates' dirty and destructive behaviours. Intensive nursing and care was considered necessary and seen to improve patients' condition. This led later to the idea of *seikatsu shidō*, or 'habit training'. After the war Japan's army was abolished under the new constitution, and in 1946 the hospital came under the jurisdiction of the Ministry of Health and Welfare and changed its name to Kokuritsu Musashi Ryōyōjo.[39]

Psychosurgery had its golden age in Japan around 1950. It may have been stimulated by its founder Egas Moniz's Nobel Prize award in 1949, but the main reason for the positive reception of psychosurgery was that it required less expense and effort than other treatments such as insulin shock therapy. This was an important consideration at a time when food and goods shortages still prevailed throughout the country.[40] Kokuritsu Musashi Ryōyōjo introduced psychosurgery in 1948, but as psychiatrist Sekine Shin'ichi, the first director of this institution (in service 1940–66), pointed out: 'It would be meaningless if we only did lobotomy. Its effect will be produced only after we retrain the lobotomised patients. Even if the condition of the patients did not seem to improve after the surgery, it would be rash to give up their treatment.'[41] During the war Sekine had observed that intensive nursing and care improved patients' condition. So habit training, or *seikatsu shidō*, as Sekine called it, was introduced after psychosurgery, and a special ward for the aftercare of post-operative patients was established in 1951. The implementation of the new regime was facilitated by the institution's head nurse, Hanyū Ritsu. She felt that psychosurgery contributed to the development of psychiatric nursing after the war. Nurses were able to enhance their practices while looking after patients who recovered their communication skills as a result of surgery. Habit training became subsequently more generally applied to chronic patients.[42]

In 1956 Sekine's colleague Kobayashi suggested that 'life therapy' should be composed of habit training, recreational therapy and work therapy. Habit training was recognised as the basis of or pre-treatment for recreational and work therapy. Kobayashi produced detailed guidelines for habit training. They stipulated a range of daily activities: getting up, going to bed, taking a bath, and so on. Each activity was packed tightly into a daily schedule. Ideally, patients' time in hospital had to be entirely devoted to habit training.[43]

'Life therapy' is understood to have its origins in Kobayashi's theory. Its development within psychiatry has been considered as peculiar to post-war Japan.[44] But was this really the case? 'Life therapy' was invented by Kobayashi, but its ideas and practices were strongly inspired by American and British OT in place during the early years of the twentieth century. Kobayashi and his colleagues at Kokuritsu Musashi Ryōyōjo did not, however, comment on this fact. Kobayashi chose the English phrase 'habit training' in his 1956 article to translate the Japanese *seikatsu shidō*.

Habit training is said to have first been attempted at Rochester State Hospital, New York, in 1901 by Eleanor Clarke Slagle (1876–1942), who was deeply influenced by Adolf Meyer (1866–1950), professor of psychiatry at Johns Hopkins University. From his psycho-biological viewpoint Meyer contended that newer conceptions of mental conditions should not frame them as mere diseases of a structural and toxic nature, but as problems of living. He emphasised the benefits of structured use of time and work.[45] Slagle described a typical habit training schedule, which called for mental patients to rise at six o'clock in the morning, wash, go to the toilet, brush their teeth, and air their beds; then have breakfast, return to their wards and make their beds, sweep the floors, and so on. The fundamental plan was to arrange a twenty-four hour schedule in which physicians, nurses, attendants and occupational therapists should play a part.[46]

In Britain, the founder of Dorset House, Elizabeth Casson (1881–1954), imported ideas such as the medical control of OT, standardised education programmes, and habit training from America and used these in the development of British OT.[47] Moreover, the first full-length textbook on OT in mental illness was published in Britain by John Ivison Russell in 1938. He proclaimed that the general principle of any system of occupational treatment might be described as 'habit training' and provided a detailed habit training schedule.[48]

Notwithstanding these earlier developments in America and Britain, criticism of 'life therapy' increased in Japan during the 1970s. For instance, at Karasuyama Byōin in Tokyo, one of the most famous private mental hospitals that employed 'life therapy', promoters and opponents strongly fought each other. Eventually, the hospital administration dismissed the critics, who claimed that 'life therapy' was exploitation of labour, leading to a court battle.[49] When a symposium on 'life therapy' was held in 1972 at the annual meeting of the Japanese Society of Psychiatry and Neurology, some delegates expressed their concerns about the approach, criticising it for oppressing and controlling the details of patients' lives in the name of therapy.[50] In the same year, the birthplace of 'life therapy' in Japan, Kokuritsu Musashi Ryōyōjo, stopped using the term under its director Akimoto Haruo. He noted that 'life therapy' was just a medley of medical and nursing practices. He suggested that habit training should be separated from recreational therapy and work therapy, and positioned within psychiatric nursing, where he thought it belonged.[51] Subsequently, the controversy on 'life therapy' in mental hospitals was gradually replaced by debates on social rehabilitation outside mental hospitals and community mental health.[52]

A new paradigm from the United States

Aside from 'life therapy', which was initially promoted by doctors and nurses in mental hospitals, a new paradigm emerged in the 1960s. This was a 'new' kind of OT, once again influenced by the United States. The American impact on Japan is often connected to the works of occupational therapist Gail S. Fidler (1916–2005), who pursued psychoanalytic theory in OT and:

> [H]oped to present occupational therapy as a psychotherapeutic function rather than as a maintenance function or diversional activity ... based on our definition of occupational therapy as that form of psychiatric or psychologic [sic] treatment which uses constructive activity as the mode of operation.[53]

The 1963 book written by Gail and Jay W. Fidler was translated into Japanese shortly after the profession of occupational therapist received state accreditation in Japan in 1965.[54] The translation is said to have contributed to the spread of psychoanalytic thinking in Japanese OT.[55]

American predominance, goes back to the occupation of post-war Japan and the policies of General Headquarters, the Supreme Commander for the Allied Powers (GHQ/SCAP). The Japanese government's interest in forming a welfare state and improving the social security system was initiated by the 'Report of the Social Security Mission' submitted by William H. Wandel (Social Security Administration of the United States) to GHQ/SCAP in December 1947. The report also contributed to an improvement in education and the social status of doctors, nurses and other medical and welfare professionals, though it did not refer to the profession of occupational therapist directly. On the other hand, in 1951, when the San Francisco Peace Treaty between Japan and the Allied Powers was officially signed, Japan joined the World Health Organization (WHO), which pointed out the backwardness of rehabilitation and the lack of experts in Japan. Rehabilitation was a crucial part of the medical and welfare policies of the post-war era, and this led to the state qualifications of physical therapist and occupational therapist.[56]

The movement to establish these two state qualifications prospered from the early 1960s. The 1962 'Annual Report' by the Ministry of Health and Welfare suggested that a school for physical therapists be established in a tuberculosis sanatorium and a school for occupational therapists in a mental hospital (the above-mentioned Kokuritsu Musashi Ryōyōjo was a candidate). However, this plan was not implemented. Instead, three-year training institution for both professions, Rihabiritēshon Gakuin (The School of Rehabilitation), was established as an annex school of Kokuritsu Ryōyōjo Tokyo Byōin (The National Tokyo Hospital) in 1963.[57]

According to the government official Ōmura Junshirō (1915–87), who was in charge of the establishment of Rihabiritēshon Gakuin, it was initially difficult to find staff for the new school. As there were few Japanese trained professionals education depended on foreign teachers. The chief instructors at the time were American experts who were dispatched through the WHO as consultants: the heads of the physical therapy department were Tali A. Conine (in service 1964–66) and Barbara Nash (1966–69), and the chief of the OT department was Janet M. Hirata (1966–70), a second-generation Japanese American. Conine, the wife of a high official of the US forces stationed in Japan, had already been teaching as a volunteer at the school from the time it opened in 1963. She later became a professor of physical therapy at the University of British Columbia in Canada. When Elizabeth Fuchs, the first chief of the OT department, left the school within a short period of time (probably for mental-health reasons), Hirata succeeded to the post. There were also many other full-time and part-time American teachers.[58]

The curriculum at the school was modelled on the educational philosophy and methods of four-year colleges in the United States.[59] Hirata recalled that the lecturers were very eager to teach OT that was directly imported from America, and although this was difficult as the Japanese pupils had to learn everything in English, they were strongly motivated to absorb state-of-the-art knowledge.[60]

Shortly after the establishment of Rihabiritēshon Gakuin, two other schools for physical therapists and occupational therapists opened in Kitakyūshū (1966) and in Fuchū, Tokyo (1969) respectively. American OT was taught in both of these schools in English, by American teachers. According to a former student of the school in Kitakyūshū, it was difficult for the students to follow the class because they did not understand English well.[61] It seems odd that so many foreigners taught Japanese students in English in educational institutions in the 1960s and the 1970s. This would have been more understandable during the early modernisation period of the late nineteenth century, before the psychiatrists Sakaki and Kure studied in Europe. Praise, however, must be given, as it was epoch-making that such high standards were introduced into medicine-related education in Japan, even if somewhat forced. Some of the graduates went on to study abroad and became leading professionals after returning to Japan.[62]

In 1965 OT entered a new era when the state qualifications of physical therapist (*rigaku ryōhō shi*) and occupational therapist (*sagyō ryōhō shi*) were established. The following year, all the graduates of Rihabiritēshon Gakuin passed the state examination, and fourteen physical therapists and five occupational therapists started work in these fields for the first time in Japan.[63] While the number of state-qualified occupational therapists increased in mental hospitals, it seems that other medical professionals, especially psychiatrists, held older ideas about patient work and did not necessarily welcome OT. When OT for physical and mental disorders began to be covered by the national medical insurance system in 1974, the Japanese Society of Psychiatry and Neurology (JSPN) strongly criticised it. They claimed that at a time when many patients were hospitalised compulsorily and inmates involved in forced labour in the name of therapy, it would be impossible to regard 'occupational therapy' as medical treatment.[64]

There were also some who doubted that this new OT, imported directly from America, would be effective in Japan. Occupational therapists felt concerned about practising and teaching American OT in a Japanese context. A pioneering 'America-oriented' occupational therapist and the first president of the Japanese Association of Occupational Therapists, Suzuki Akiko, who studied at Columbia University in the early 1960s, seems to have felt an invisible barrier, which she thought came from cultural differences between Japan and the United States. She insisted that the philosophy of OT should be based on individual dignity supported by psychological independence, although according to Suzuki this was lacking in Japanese people.[65] Suzuki's view was anchored not only in American psychoanalytic thinking but also popular Japanese cultural theory, such as the 1971 bestseller by psychoanalyst Doi Takeo (1920–2009) who described the Japanese mental structure using the concept of *amae* or dependence, which he thought to be peculiar to Japanese human relations.[66] Suzuki appeared to be dissatisfied with the immaturity of the self in the Japanese to promote OT, while hoping that a Japanese model of OT would appear.[67]

Beyond Western blueprints

The history of Japanese OT can be divided into two distinct phases: work and OT until the 1960s and 1970s, and OT after the establishment of state qualification in 1965. The former has been mapped and shaped by famous psychiatrists such as Kure and Katō in Matsuzawa, and Kobayashi in Kokuritsu Musashi Ryōyōjo. The latter phase, in contrast, has been assessed critically by only a few authors. Tajima Akiko describes the contemporary history of Japanese OT after the introduction of state qualification, arguing that in the early stages occupational therapists struggled to establish their professional identity among other medical professions. From the late 1980s, however, they succeeded by drawing on overseas ideas and practices.[68] Finally, as the pioneering Japanese occupational therapist Suzuki had hoped, occupational therapists focused on developing an approach suited to Japanese conditions.

Around the year 2000 the *kawa* (river) model of Japanese occupational theory appeared in opposition to Western theories. Okuda Mayumi, occupational therapist in Okayama, Japan, wrote:

> Many Japanese clinical occupational therapists experience difficulty when attempting to explain their profession to others. Occupational therapy theories should help alleviate this problem but many conceptual models have been directly imported and developed in different cultural context.[69]

According to other advocates, the theory and model imported from the West and taught at training colleges in Japan, emphasises the primacy of the self and the celebration of independence, which, they argued, did not work well within the Japanese cultural context. In the *kawa* model, the life of a patient is compared to a river. The role of occupational therapists is to help the river flow smoothly, although there may be obstacles such as illness, disorder, and so on.[70]

Michael Iwama, a Canadian professor of OT at Georgia Regents University in Augusta, Georgia, with Japanese connections, played a crucial role in the development and international spread of the *kawa* model. He has become a spokesman for what could be seen as an 'idealised' Japanese tradition and culture. In his doctoral dissertation about OT in Japan, Iwama stated: 'The Japanese person's life being depicted by a metaphor of nature seemed like a natural interpretation for a society whose cosmologies are based on a naturalistic paradigm.'[71] In an article published in 2010, he contended that:

> The *kawa* model is a new conceptual model of practice that heralds an important shift in the discourses of theory and culture in occupational therapy. The profession's first substantial theoretical work to emerge outside of the West impels occupational therapy beyond its familiar bases of individual autonomy and agency, toward collective-oriented, interdependent views of human occupation.[72]

These statements affirm that, while occupational therapists internationally serve an increasingly diverse population, their professional discourse remains culturally biased towards Western sociocultural contexts.[73] However, Iwama's own views encapsulate clichés of Japanese culture (naturalism, groupism, familism) as represented in the West. Tajima, a Japanese occupational therapist, argues that the *kawa* model may succeed in freeing Japanese OT from the predominance of Western paradigms. But at the same time she regards the emphasis on culture in the discourse of the *kawa* model to be questionable. She suggests a modification of the *kawa* model that respects a client as an individual, whose life could be explained by the metaphor of a river, rather than as 'a Japanese', 'an Oriental' or 'a non-Westerner'.[74]

Conclusion

The emergence and further development of the *kawa* model, which attempts to broach the intriguing and contested relationship between culture/tradition and health/rehabilitation, might be described as a new phase of Japanese OT. It might herald the liberation from Western-focused discourses, which has never been experienced before in the one hundred and fifty year history of work and OT in Japan. However, Japanese occupational therapists will need to be aware of the dangers of falling into the trap of narrow Japonism.

Notes

1 Sadami Suzuki, *Nyūmon nihon kingendai bungeishi* (*An Introduction to the History of Art and Literature in Modern Japan*) (Tokyo: Heibonsha, 2013).
2 Ryūichi Narita, *Kingendai nihonshi to rekishigaku* (*Modern History of Japan and History*) (Tokyo: Chūōkōron shinsha, 2012).
3 Akiko Suzuki, *Nihon ni okeru sagyō ryōhō kyōiku no rekishi* (*The History of Occupational Therapy Education in Japan*) (Sapporo: Hokkaido University Press, 1986), pp. 77–84; Hajime Kagaya, 'Tokyo shi ryōyōjo ni okeru sagyō ryōhō seiritsu no haikei to sono igi' ('Background and significance of occupational therapy formation in a sanatorium in Tokyo'), *Sagyō ryōhō*, 19:5 (2000), 445–53.
4 Yasuo Okada, 'Nihon deno seishinka sagyō chiryō narabini seishin shikkan kanja ingai chiryō no rekishi haisen mae' ('The history of psychiatric occupational therapy and extramural treatment for psychiatric patients in pre-war Japan'), in Seishinka iryōshi kenkyūkai (ed.), *Nagayama Yasumasa sensei chosakushū* (Tokyo: Nagayama Yasumasa sensei chosakushū kankōkai, 1994), pp. 341–78.
5 Naoka Ono, 'Kyoto furitsu "Tenkyōin" no setsuritsu to sono keii' ('Kyoto Prefectural Hospital "Tenkyo-in" for the mentally disabled: Its opening, development, and abolition'), *Nihon ishigaku zasshi*, 39:4 (1993), 477–500.
6 Hideo Tanaka, *Oyatoi gaikokujin Rōretsu to igaku kyōiku* (*The Foreign Teacher Roretz and Medical Education*) (Nagoya: Nagoya University Press, 1995).
7 Sakaki was also a professor of psychiatry at the Imperial University, later to become the Tokyo Imperial University and then the University of Tokyo
8 Yasuo Okada, *Shisetsu Matsuzawa Byōin shi* (*The History of Matsuzawa Mental Hospital*) (Tokyo: Iwasaki gakujutsu shuppansha, 1981), pp. 138–41.
9 Hajime Sakaki, 'Tenkyōnin toriatukai hō' ('The treatment of the insane'), *Tokyo igakukai zasshi*, 1:3 (1887), 120–8.
10 Yūshi Uchimura, 'Sakaki Hajime sensei to Tokyo Teikoku Daigaku Igakubu Seishinbyōgaku Kyōshitsu no sōsetsu' ('Professor Sakaki Hajime and the foundation of the Department of Psychiatry at the Faculty of Medicine, Tokyo Imperial University'), *Seishin shinkeigaku zasshi*, 44 (1940), 63–79, 70. Unless otherwise stated, translations from Japanese are the author's own.
11 Osamu Kusakabe, 'Kindai nihon ni okeru seishinka sagyō ryōhō no rekishiteki kōsatsu: Sakaki Hajime wo chūshin ni' ('A historical study of psychiatric occupational therapy in modern Japan: Centred around Hajime Sakaki'), *Nihon ishigaku zasshi*, 59:3 (2013), 365–77.
12 Yasuo Okada, *Kure Shūzō so shōgai to gyōseki* (*The Life and Works of Kure Shūzō*) (Kyoto: Shibunkaku, 1982).
13 Japanese *sagyō ryōhō*, which Kure coined around 1900, still remains today as a translation of English 'occupational therapy'. As a result, *sagyō ryōhō* has a double image of old 'work therapy' of the time of Kure and new 'occupational therapy' developed afterwards in the West. In the process of establishing the state qualification of occupational therapist in 1965, another Japanese term *shokunō ryōhō* was proposed for 'occupational therapy', but it was not adopted. Shōhei Mōri, 'Sagyō ryōhō kara mita seishin igakushi' ('History of mental health from

the viewpoint of occupational therapy'), *Seishin igakushi kenkyū*, 15:1,2 (2011), 132–9.
14 Shūzō Kure, 'Tenkyō mura (seishin byōsha no sagyō ryōhō) ni tsukite' ('On the colony for the insane and work therapy'), *Kokka igakukai zasshi*, 185 (1902), 427–52, 447.
15 Shūzō Kure, *Wagakuni ni okeru seishinbyō ni kansuru saikin no shisetsu* (*Recent Psychiatric Institutions in Japan*) (Tokyo: Tokyo igakukai jimusho, 1912); Okada, *Matsuzawa*, p. 238.
16 Tokyo Fu Sugamo Byōin, *Tokyo Fu Sugamo Byōin kisoku* (*Hospital Rules of Tokyo Fu Sugamo Byōin*) (Tokyo: Tokyo Fu Sugamo Byōin, 1906).
17 Okada, *Matsuzawa*, pp. 264–71.
18 *Ibid.*, pp. 280–3.
19 Akira Hashimoto, 'Matsuzawa to Aruto Sherubittsu: Nichidoku no seishin byōin purojekuto no hikaku kenkyū' ('Matsuzawa and Alt-Scherbitz: A comparative study of mental hospital projects in Japan and Germany'), *Seishin igakushi kenkyū*, 15:1/2 (2011), 81–95.
20 Fusajirō Katō, 'Seishin byōsha ni taisuru sagyō ryōhō narabini kaihō chiryō no seishin byōin ni okeru korega zisshi no igi oyobi hōhō' ('Practice and method of occupational therapy and open medical treatment for the mentally ill in mental hospitals'), *Shinkeigaku zasshi*, 25:7 (1925), 371–403.
21 *Ibid.*
22 William R. Dunton, *Reconstruction Therapy* (Philadelphia, PA, and London: W. B. Saunders, 1919). Norizō Maeda, 'Okyupeishon no hanashi: Dunton shi no shosetsu shōkai' ('On occupation: Introduction to Dunton's work'), in Kyūchikai (ed.), *Seishin byōin ni okeru sagyō ryōhō no riron to jissai* (Tokyo: Kyūchikai, 1932); Yasuo Okada, 'Sagyō ryōhō no sendatsu no shōzō: Maeda Norizō jō' ('The portrait of the pioneer of occupational therapy: Maeda Norizō, Part 1'), *Sagyō ryōhō jānaru*, 36:9 (2002), 1105.
23 Norizō Maeda, 'Ichi joshu no kiroku: Matsuzawa Byōin sagyō jidai no Katō sensei' ('Dr Katō and occupational therapy in Matsuzawa Mental Hospital'), in Gentarō Mori *et al.* (eds), *Hakutenroku* (Tokyo: Katō Kiyomitsu, 1969), pp. 271–9; Norizō Maeda, 'Kure inchō jidai ni sagyō chiryō ni jūjishita ichi kangofu no omoide' ('A nurse recalls the occupational therapy in the time of the director Kure'), in Seishinka iryōshi kenkyūkai (ed.), *Kure Shūzō sensei sono gyōseki* (Tokyo: Seishinka iryōshi kenkyūkai, 1974), pp. 496–500.
24 Maeda, 'Ichi joshu', p. 275.
25 Maeda, 'Ichi joshu'; Maeda, 'Kure inchō'.
26 Suzuki, *Nihon ni okeru*, pp. 78–80.
27 Okada, *Matsuzawa*, p. 467.
28 *Ibid.*, p. 528.
29 Dunton, *Reconstruction Therapy*, p. 22; Maeda, 'Okyupeishon'.
30 Maeda, 'Kure inchō'.
31 Katō, 'Seishin byōsha'.
32 Hideki Moriguchi, 'Nagayama Yasumasa sensei to Osaka Furitsu Nakamiya Byōin' ('Dr Nagayama Yasumasa and Osaka Prefectural Nakamiya Byōin'),

in Seishinka iryōshi kenkyūkai (ed.), *Nagayama Yasumasa sensei chosakushū* (Tokyo: Nagayama Yasumasa sensei chosakushū kankōkai, 1994), pp. 255–89.
33 Okada, 'Nihon deno'.
34 Okada, *Matsuzawa*; Tsuguo Kaneko, *Matsuzawa Byōin gaishi* (*The History of Matsuzawa Mental Hospital*) (Tokyo: Nihonhyōronsha, 1982); Gōhei Yagi and Akira Tanabe, *Nihon seishinbyō chiryōshi* (*The History of Treatment of Mental Illness in Japan*) (Tokyo: Kanehara shuppan, 2002).
35 Yasuo Okada, *Nihon seishinka iryōshi* (*History of Psychiatry in Japan*) (Tokyo: Igakushoin, 2002).
36 Hidema Seki, 'Seishinbunretsubyō no rihabiritēshon to sagyō ryōhō' ('Rehabilitation and occupational therapy in schizophrenia'), *Rigaku ryōhō to sagyō ryōhō*, 15:6 (1981), 547–51.
37 The National Museum of Modern Art, Tokyo, *Bijutsu ni burru!* (*Art Will Thrill You!: The Essence of Modern Japanese Art*) (Tokyo: The National Museum of Modern Art, NHK Promotions Inc., 2012), pp. 202–3.
38 Hachirō Kobayashi and Sugao Kobayashi, 'Rekuriēshon ryōhō' ('Recreation therapy'), *Nihon iji shinpō*, 1662 (1956), 35–41; Hachirō Kobayashi, 'Seishin shikkan no seikatsu ryōhō' ('Life therapy for mental illness'), *Nihon rinshō*, 17:1 (1959), 154–62.
39 Kokuritsu Musashi Ryōyōjo, *Kango no ayumi: shōwa 15 nen – shōwa 55 nen* (*The Development of Nursing from 1940 to 1980 in Kokuritsu Musashi Ryōyōjo*) (Tokyo: Kokuritsu Musashi Ryōyōjo, 1982).
40 Kaneko, *Matsuzawa Byōin gaishi*, p. 257.
41 Shin'ichi Sekine, 'Sagyō ryōhō ni tsuite' ('On occupational therapy'), in Tsutomu Ezoe and Hiroshi Utena (eds), *Sagyō ryōhō ni tsuite* (Tokyo: Dai kyūkai kantō seishin igaku konwakai, 1953), pp. 11–19.
42 Kokuritsu Musashi Ryōyōjo, *Kango no ayumi*, pp. 53–78.
43 Kobayashi and Kobayashi, 'Rekuriēshon ryōhō'; Hachirō Kobayashi, 'Seikatsu ryōhō' ('Life therapy'), in Tsutomu Ezoe (ed.), *Seishinka kango no kenkyū* (Tokyo: Igakushoin, 1965), pp. 174–9.
44 Seki, 'Seishinbunretsubyō'; Hirotake Asano, *Seishin iryō ronsōshi* (*The History of Disputes of Psychiatry in Japan*) (Tokyo: Hihyōsha, 2000).
45 Adolf Meyer, 'The philosophy of occupational therapy', *Archives of Occupational Therapy*, 1:1 (1922), 1–10.
46 Robert K. Bing, 'Occupational therapy revisited: A paraphrastic journey', *American Journal of Occupational Therapy*, 35:8 (1981), 499–518.
47 Ruth Levine Schemm, 'Bridging conflicting ideologies: The origins of American and British occupational therapy', *American Journal of Occupational Therapy*, 48:11 (1994), 1082–8.
48 Ann A. Wilcock, *Occupation for Health* (London: British Association and College of Occupational Therapists, 2002), vol. 2, pp. 153–6; John Ivison Russell, 'The Occupational Treatment of Mental Illness' (MD thesis, University of Glasgow, 1938).
49 Asano, *Seishin iryō ronsōshi*.
50 Toshio Fujisawa, '"Seikatsu ryōhō" wo umidashita mono' ('What produced "life

therapy"'), *Seishin shinkeigaku zasshi*, 75:12 (1973), 1007–13; Isao Ozawa, 'Seikatsu ryōhō' wo koeru mono' ('What goes beyond "life therapy"'), *Seishin shinkeigaku zasshi*, 75:12 (1973), 1013–18.

51 Haruo Akimoto, 'Sagyō ryōhō wo kangaeru' ('Thinking of occupational therapy'), in Haruo Akimoto (ed.), *Sagyō ryōhō no genryū* (Tokyo: Kongō shuppan, 1975), pp. 9–22.

52 Asano, *Seishin iryō ronsōshi*.

53 Gail S. Fidler and Jay W. Fidler, *Introduction to Psychiatric Occupational Therapy* (New York: Macmillan, 1954), p. 178.

54 Gail S. Fidler and Jay W. Fidler, *Seishin igakuteki sagyō ryōhō* (*Psychiatric Occupational Therapy*) (Tokyo: Igakushoin, 1966). (Japanese translation of *A Communication Process in Psychiatry: Occupational Therapy* (New York: Macmillan, 1963).)

55 Mōri, 'Sagyō ryōhō kara mita seishin igakushi'.

56 Suzuki, *Nihon ni okeru*; Rihabiritēshon Gakuin, *Rihabiritēshon Gakuin heikō kinenshi* (*Commemorative Publication of the School Closure*) (Tokyo: Kokuritsu byōin kikō Tokyo Byōin Fuzoku Rihabiritēshon Gakuin, 2008).

57 This hospital had originally been a tuberculosis sanatorium before the Second World War. Rihabiritēshon Gakuin, *Rihabiritēshon Gakuin heikō kinenshi*.

58 Rihabiritēshon Gakuin, *Rihabiritēshon Gakuin heikō kinenshi*.

59 Noriko Tomioka, 'Sagyō ryōhō no 40 nen wo furikaeru: Seishinkei sagyō ryōhō no miryoku to kurō' ('Fascinations and sufferings of 40 years of occupational practice in education and mental health'), *Sagyō ryōhō*, 25 (2006), 409–16.

60 Janet M. Hirata and Noriko Tomioka, 'Janet M. Hirata sensei ni ukagau' ('An interview with Janet M. Hirata'), *Rigaku ryōhō to sagyō ryōhō*, 20:1 (1986), 59–64.

61 Takashi Hashimoto, 'Rigaku ryōhō kyōiku: Gaikokujin kyōin kara nihonjin kyōin no te e' ('Physical therapy education in Japan: Japanese physical therapy teachers inherited the 'education baton' from foreign teachers'), *Rigaku ryōhōgaku*, 38:2 (2011), 154–60.

62 Rihabiritēshon Gakuin, *Dōhyō: Rihabiritēshon Gakuin 10 nen no ayumi* (*The Tenth Anniversary of the School of Rehabilitation*) (Tokyo: Kokuritsu ryōyōjo Tokyo Byōin Fuzoku Rihabiritēshon Gakuin, 1973).

63 As a result of the first state examination in 1966, in addition to five occupational therapists who graduated from Rihabiritēshon Gakuin, fifteen occupational therapists came into being as an interim measure. The latter had been already engaged in OT for a certain period of time, or had acquired a license as occupational therapists in foreign countries. Suzuki, *Nihon ni okeru*.

64 The Japanese Society of Psychiatry and Neurology (JSPN), 'Kaikoku (Notices of the JSPN)', *Seishin shinkeigaku zasshi*, 77:7 (1975), 541.

65 Akiko Suzuki et al., 'Zadankai: OT ni totteno seishin iryō no kabe' ('A round-table talk: The barrier of psychiatry for occupational therapists'), *Rigaku ryōhō to sagyō ryōhō*, 9:12 (1975), 840–8; Suzuki, *Nihon ni okeru*; Keiko Yoshimi and Akiko Suzuki, 'Nihon ni okeru sagyō ryōhō no rekishi' ('History of occupational therapy in Japan'), *Nihon ishigaku zasshi*, 42:2 (1996), 128–9.

66 Takeo Doi, *Amae no kōzō* (*The Anatomy of Dependence*) (Tokyo: Kōbundō, 1971).

67 Suzuki, *Nihon ni okeru*, p. 171.
68 Akiko Tajima, *Nihon ni okeru sagyō ryōhō no gendaishi* (*The Contemporary History of Occupational Therapy in Japan*) (Tokyo: Seikatsu shoin, 2013).
69 Mayumi Okuda *et al.*, '"How does your river flow?": A new conceptual model of occupational therapy developed by Japanese clinical occupational therapists', *Sagyō ryōhō*, 19: Tokubetsugō (special issue) (2000), 517.
70 Naoe Yoshimura *et al.*, 'Wākushoppu "Kawa moderu"' ('Workshop "The Kawa Model"'), *Sagyō ryōhō*, 22 suppl. (2003), 5630; Michael Iwama *et al.*, 'Understanding and applying client centred occupational therapy in Japanese practice settings', *Journal of Japanese Association of Occupational Therapists*, 23 suppl. (2004), 662.
71 Michael K. Iwama, 'A Social Perspective on the Construction of Occupational Therapy in Japan' (PhD dissertation, Kibi International University, Japan, 2001).
72 Michael Iwama, http://individual.utoronto.ca/michaeliwama/ (last updated 4 January 2010; last access date 2 August 2015).
73 Alison J. Gerlach, 'A critical reflection on the concept of cultural safety', *Canadian Journal of Occupational Therapy*, 79:3 (2012), 151–8.
74 Akiko Tajima, '"Kawa moredu" no inpakuto to "bunka" toiu kyōchōten eno gigi' ('The impact of "*kawa*-model" and the doubt of emphasize [sic] the concept of "the culture"'), www5.ocn.ne.jp/~tjmkk/ta5.htm (2005; last access date 15 August 2014).

8

Patient work and family care at Iwakura, Japan, c. 1799–1970

Osamu Nakamura

Iwakura is a village located seven kilometres northeast of Kyoto, the ancient capital of Japan. It has a famous legend. During the reign of Emperor Go-Sanjo (reigned 1068–72), a princess who was afflicted with a mental condition was cured after praying to the image of Buddha at Daiunji-Temple in Iwakura and drinking water from the temple well.[1] This is a well-known story that highlights the connection between Iwakura and mental illness. It was not uncommon for those suffering from a mental condition to be received at temples. Kumogahata Iwayayama Hudoin-Temple, for example, which is located fifteen kilometres north of Kyoto, provided for mentally ill people from 1690.[2] Though Iwakura was not the first place that was sought out by the mentally ill in Kyoto, it became famous for receiving mentally ill patients in home-style Japanese inns in which they were taken care of by their hosts and attendants. These inns appeared from 1717 onwards.[3] As Hashimoto has shown, Iwakura soon developed a reputation as a 'Japanese Gheel', where mentally ill patients were taken care of by host families.[4]

The diseases that visitors to Iwakura suffered from were varied. The first patient reported to have stayed at the temple, in 1697, was afflicted with an eye disease; the image of the Buddha at Daiunji-Temple was seen to be particularly effective in the cure of ophthalmic problems.[5] Mentally ill people seem to have paid visits to, or stayed at, inns near Daiunji-Temple increasingly from around the middle of the eighteenth century.[6] In 1773, a famous haiku poet, Buson Yosa (1716–84), composed a well-known seventeen-syllable poem, which mentioned a mentally ill female patient who confined herself in Daiunji-Temple for prayer.[7] In 1796, a famous doctor, Kinkei Nakagami referred to the way in which mentally ill people were taken care of by host families in Iwakura.[8] By 1875, more than twenty patients were in Iwakura.[9]

How did Iwakura establish its reputation as a place for the mentally ill? One reason was the Daiunji-Temple's efforts to attract patients. For example, the temple made a woodcut print of its Buddha image in 1707 and printed its history for visitors. It also built a waterfall for therapeutic bathing and accommodation consisting of a fifteen-tatami-mat room for patients and attendants in 1709.[10] Since charges for prayers and accommodation together with money offerings from patients and their attendants were Daiunji-Temple's main source of income, it made a consistent effort to attract patients. Another reason for the popularity of Iwakura was that inns in the village provided good accommodation for patients. At first, inns were prohibited from doing so. However, with increased demand for lodging houses from the late eighteenth century, inns such as Ueda, Kimori and Imai (figure 8.1) extended their buildings for the hosting of mentally ill people in 1796, 1815 and 1818, respectively.[11] The occupants as well as the temple's lodging house were transferred to inns between 1818 and 1830, as the service in them was more attractive for the patients.[12] From the beginning of the nineteenth century, inns at Iwakura were the main providers for the reception of mentally ill patients within family-style settings. During the late nineteenth century, patients mainly came from elite families who had left the old capital of Kyoto for the new one in Tokyo during the early 1870s.[13]

One reason why patients and their families were attracted to inns was that from the late eighteenth century they employed attendants (figure 8.2).[14] The

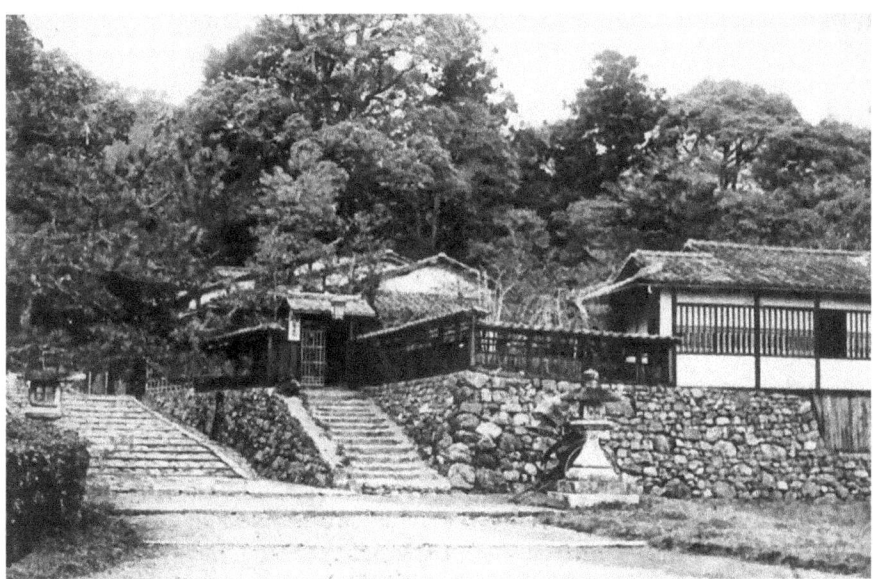

8.1 Imai Inn, *c.* 1905.

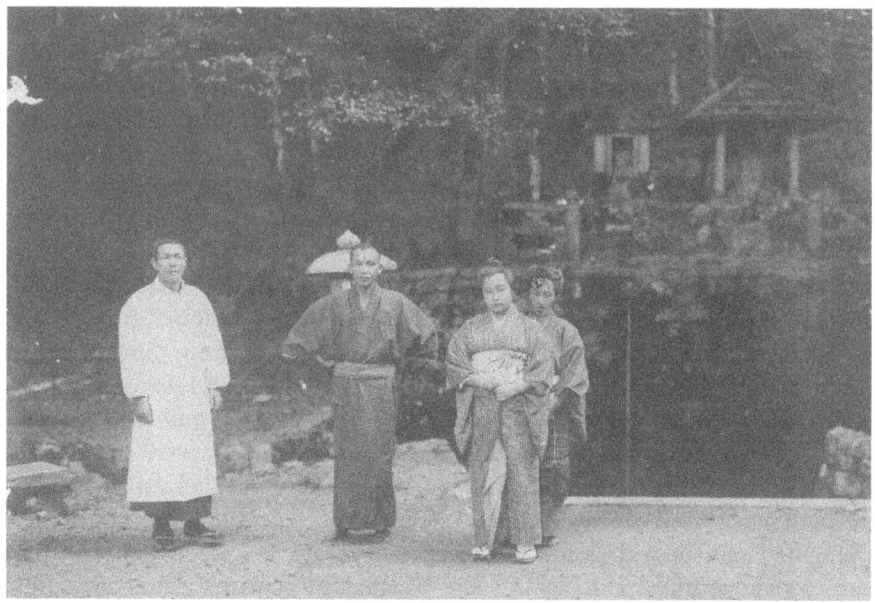

8.2 A patient with two attendants and a cook in front of the waterfall, c. 1910.

care and services offered by family-style inns constituted a welcome opportunity for families to provide for their mentally ill relatives.

Most of the attendants at the inns appear to have been family members and neighbours of the inn owners. An announcement in 1799 by Jissoin temple, which owned Daiunji, declared that innkeepers should not only offer entertainments to patients and induce them to help with household chores, but also make them visit the temple for prayer.[15] Although patients were paying guests and not hired hands, they appear to have been engaged in domestic labour at the inns.

Iwakura and the challenges of Westernisation

After Japan opened its country to foreigners in 1854, Western ways of thinking and Western medical treatments were introduced into the country. Kyoto Prefecture hired an Austrian doctor, Ferdinand Adalbert Junker von Langegg, and founded Kyoto Hospital in 1872. In June 1875, Kyoto Prefecture ordered Nanzenji-Temple, which had more than ten buildings, to vacate one of its buildings (the 'Hojo' or 'abbot's drawing rooms') and make those rooms available for the use of mentally-ill people (figure 8.3). In the same month, Kyoto Prefecture disallowed the inns in Iwakura from receiving patients, noting that they did not provide medical treatment.[16]

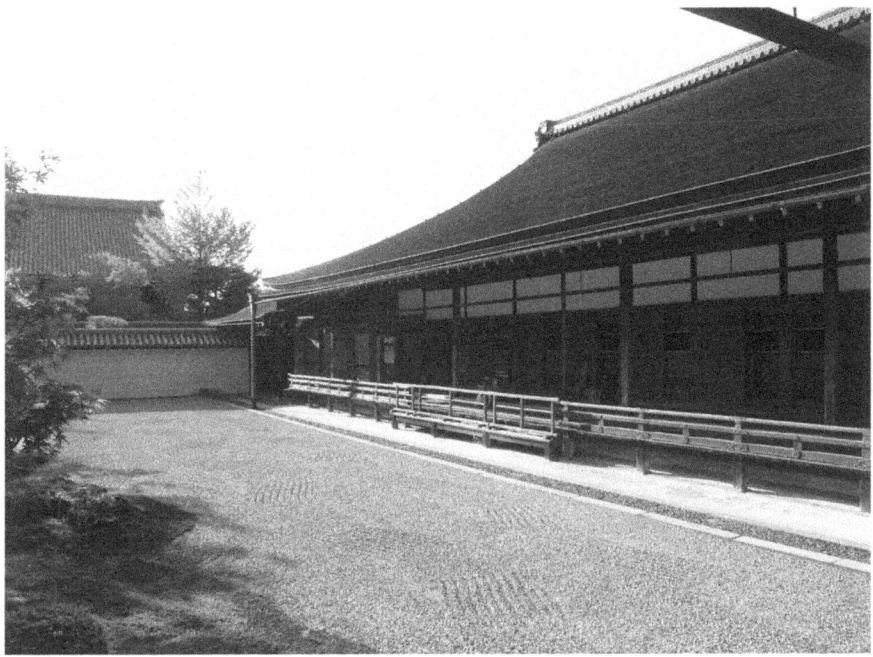

8.3 Hojo, Nanzenji-Temple.

However, Kyoto Mental Hospital was closed in 1882 due to its large deficit.[17] As a result, many patients again returned to the inns in Iwakura, where they were looked after, as before, by attendants, without recourse being had to medical treatment.[18] Kyoto prefecture considered this unsatisfactory and forced some powerful farmers and inns in Iwakura to found a mental hospital.[19] Iwakura Mental Hospital was established in 1884, and it became increasingly difficult for inns to receive mentally ill patients after the Japanese government enforced the Mental Patients' Custody Act in 1900.[20]

A new building was constructed in 1899 and by 1905 forty-three patients were resident in the institution.[21] When the premises were set on fire by a patient in 1907, with seventy-two patients resident at that time,[22] new buildings were constructed in the neighbourhood in 1909 (figure 8.4) and the hospital developed steadily under the leadership of its director, Eikichi Tsuchiya.[23] The number of patients increased from 149 in 1911,[24] to 180 in 1918,[25] 398 in 1930,[26] and 459 in 1935.[27]

Despite the Mental Patient Custody Act of 1900 and the development of Iwakura Mental Hospital, mentally ill patients were still accommodated in inns in Iwakura. One reason was the demand for treatment and scarcity of mental-hospital beds. Although the number of hospital in-patients increased

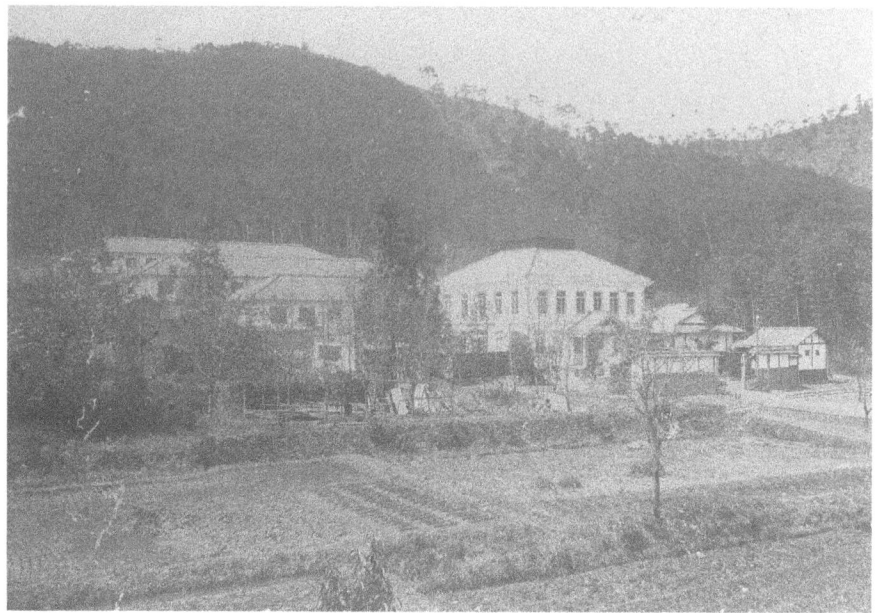

8.4 Iwakura Mental Hospital, 1909.

in Japan from 4,794 in 1924 to 10,602 in 1935, the overall number of mentally ill people in need of care and treatment increased from 32,964 in 1912 to 83,365 in 1935.[28] Iwakura therefore filled a gap in care provision. In addition, in the wake of the Mental Hospital Act of 1919, poor patients were sent to mental hospitals at public expense. Middle- and higher-class patients were expected to pay for mental health services.[29] At Iwakura Mental Hospital, for example, the charges were about ¥100–¥200 per month in 1929, when the monthly salary of a twenty-four-year-old man who worked at the Kyoto Agricultural Association was ¥38. Care expenses at the inns, on the other hand, were ¥36–¥63 per month exclusive of medical expenses and fees for attendants.[30] Hence, families who could afford having a relative taken care of outside their homes, preferred family care at the comparatively cheaper inns to hospital provision.

Another factor in the popularity of inns related to the fact that from around 1923 they began to call themselves 'Hoyojo' (guest house), which means a place where one re-creates oneself.[31] This designation was seen as preferable to the potential stigma of confinement in a mental hospital. New inns that marketed themselves as 'Hoyojo' did particularly well by introducing exercise, walks and work activities into patients' everyday lives.

Finally, the reputation of Gheel in Belgium resonated within the Japanese context. In 1901, Professor Shuzo Kure of Tokyo University visited Gheel and noted that Iwakura had a similar family-care system to that of Gheel.[32] When Dr Wilhelm Stieda of Russia and Professor Frederich Peterson of Columbia University visited Iwakura in 1906 and 1909, respectively, they praised its family-care provision.[33] Moreover, the director of Iwakura Mental Hospital, Eikichi Tsuchiya, proposed a family-care arrangement controlled by Iwakura Mental Hospital in the 1930s, urging families around the hospital to found 'Hoyojos' (guest houses).[34] In contrast to the public mental hospitals, Iwakura Mental Hospital was, like the Hoyojo, privately run. In order to attract patients, Eikichi Tsuchiya began to advertise Iwakura as the 'Japanese Gheel' and a place where occupational therapy was undertaken.[35] Consequently, six new guest houses were founded between 1923 and 1934, in addition to the existing four old inns (guest houses), and by 1935 as many as 320 patients stayed at guest houses in Iwakura. At the guest houses, some mentally ill patients spent their lives helping with carrying water, wood-chopping and farming, as well as going for walks (figures 8.5 to 8.7).

Work and activities at the inn

In 1930, twelve out of sixty-six residents in guest houses engaged in some kind of work. This is a relatively low number, which can be explained by the fact that paying patients and their families were comparatively rich in order to be able to afford the inn charges and hence not overly inclined to engage in physical labour. The director of Iwakura Mental Hospital, Eikichi Tsuchiya, reported:[36]

> *Kimori Guest House*: two male patients engaged in chicken raising and gardening (of a total of twenty male and seven female patients).

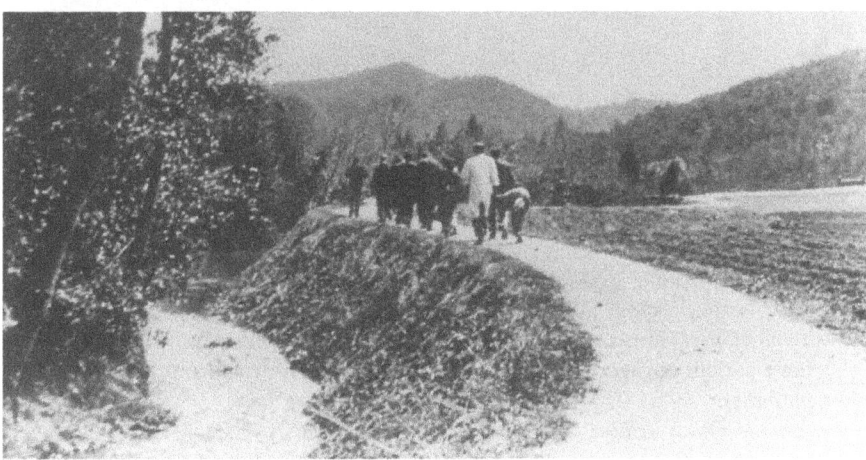

8.5 Patients of Muramatsu Guest House walking around Iwakura, *c*. 1935.

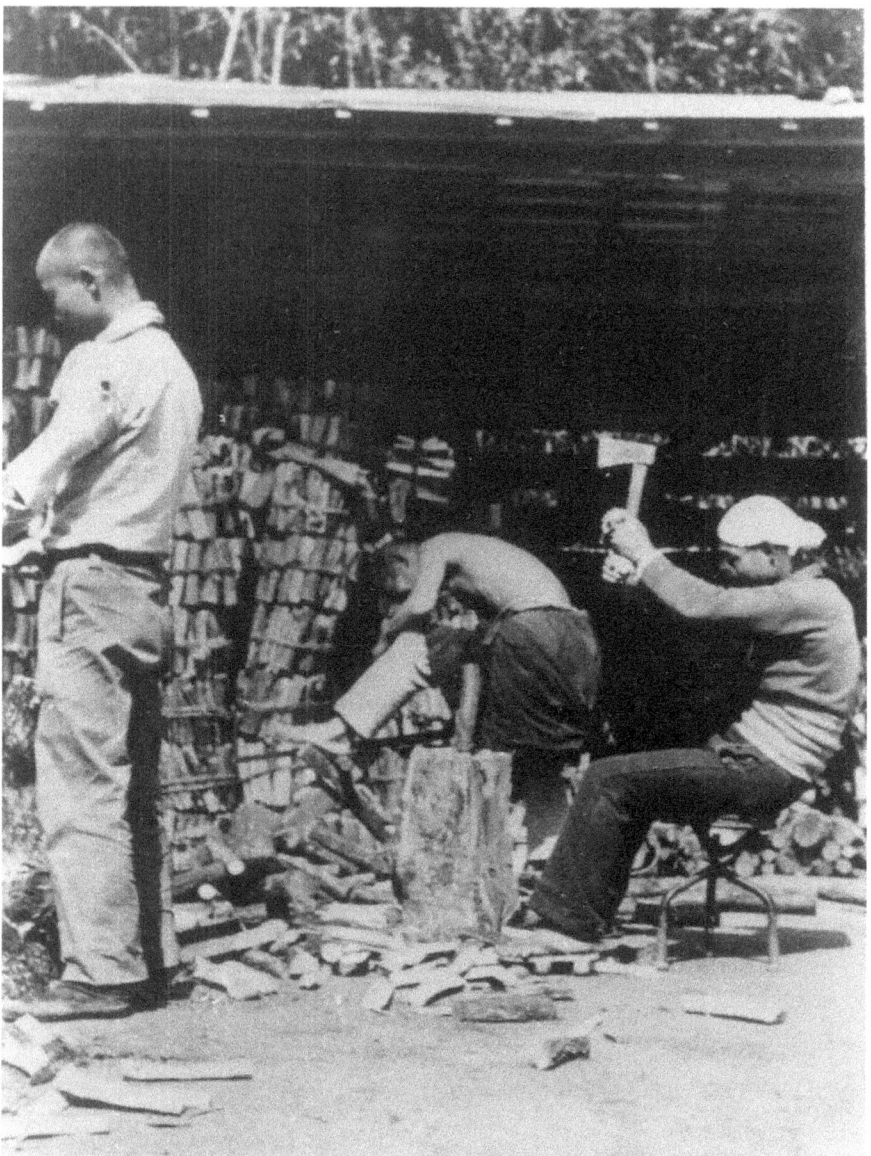

8.6 A patient at Muramatsu Guest House chopping wood, c. 1935.

Okayama Guest House: two female patients performed domestic chores and one male patient engaged in farming (of a total of twelve male and four female patients).

Watanabe Guest House: one male patient engaged in chicken raising, four female patients in sewing and washing, and one female patient in domestic chores (of a total of seven male and twelve female patients).

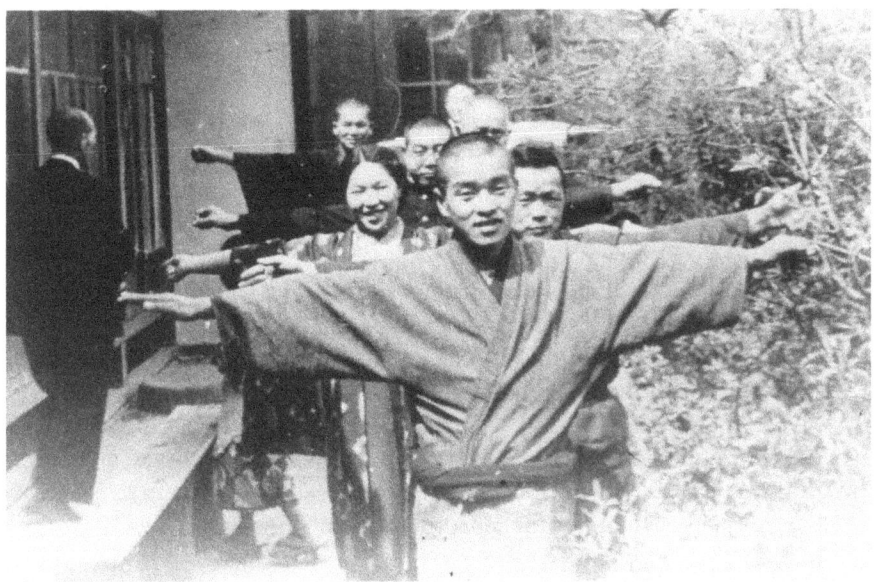

8.7 Patients at Muramatsu Guest House doing exercises, *c*. 1935.

Muramatsu Guest House: one male patient engaged in gardening (of a total of four male patients).
Iwakura Mental Hospital: several male patients engaged in farming and chicken raising (of a total of 274 male and 124 female patients).

Family host care and the local economy

Both the inns and Iwakura Mental Hospital benefitted not only from the fees they charged for accommodation, but local produce such as rice, vegetables and firewood became part of patients' boarding necessities rather than needing to be carried for sale to Kyoto city. Villagers were able to get employment as attendants, washerwomen and cooks. Until 1928, when a railway opened between Kyoto and Iwakura, it had been difficult for inhabitants to make a living in Iwakura unless they inherited some land or were adopted by or married into well-to-do families. The Mental Hospital and the inns therefore contributed to the local economy. From 1928 onwards, villagers' livelihoods depended less on the hospital and guest houses, as they were now able to commute to Kyoto city and make a living that did not involve the hosting of mentally ill patients. Attitudes towards inn keeping changed concomitant on these infrastructural developments.

Other changes in the wider social economy in Japan led to a decreased need for residents in Iwakura to host mentally ill patients and make use of their labour after the Second World War when large-scale farmers had to distribute their land to smallholders, with a limit of one hectare being the norm. While earlier on people in Iwakura had received mentally ill people in order to make a living, they now no longer needed to provide family care because they were able to make a living by other means. This was also true for Gheel, Belgium, where people began to work in factories in the surrounding areas and the number of mentally ill patients declined from 3,736 in 1938 to 1,300 in 1979.[37]

Like other mental institutions during the Second World War, Iwakura Mental Hospital and the guest houses in Iwakura, too, suffered from a shortage of food. No government help was forthcoming. Iwakura Mental Hospital had to vacate its buildings in July 1945 and sent the patients to other hospitals or returned them to their families. After the Second World War the buildings temporarily requisitioned by the army were returned. However, the owners of Iwakura Mental Hospital preferred to sell the buildings to Kyoto Prefecture, which used them as lodgings for repatriates from China and Korea.

The rise of the mental hospital and the decline of family host care

Though a few patients remained in a small number of guest houses in Iwakura, the Japanese government outlawed family care under the Law of Mental Hygiene in 1950, following a Western model of institution-based mental health provision.[38] In response to these developments, the owners of the earlier Okayama guest house founded the new Iwakura Mental Hospital in 1952, and those of the erstwhile Kimori guest house established Kitayama Mental Hospital in 1954.[39] The number of beds for mentally ill patients increased rapidly, as they did all over Japan. Both at Iwakura and Kitayama some patients worked in the fields and helped with the rice harvest. In the 1960s and 1970s, however, mechanisation of farming proceeded and the patients were no longer required to assist in agricultural labour.

After around 1970, Iwakura Mental Hospital actively pursued an open medical care system.[40] However, local residents strongly opposed this for a variety of reasons. Patients were reported to cause trouble in the communities in which they were placed. For instance, it was reported that released patients entered private residences.[41] There had also been concerns in earlier decades about patients living in Iwakura. For example, from around 1925, when Iwakura Mental Hospital rapidly began to increase its number of beds, the volume of sewage pouring into Iwakura River increased and it was reported that the water became so dirty that the residents could no longer use it for washing.[42] There was also a stigma, and Iwakura villagers were mocked by people in surrounding areas such as Kyoto city.[43]

Conclusion

Prior to 1950, mentally ill people from mostly well-to-do families were looked after by host families in privately run guest houses at Iwakura, near Kyoto. Emphasis was on care rather than medical treatment. Patients' relatives who could afford to have family members taken care of outside their own homes preferred host family care at Iwakura to the more costly provision available for paying patients at the mental hospitals founded along Western lines from the late nineteenth century onwards. Only a small number of patients assisted their hosts with domestic chores and agricultural work, but leisure activities commensurate with patients' social backgrounds and their aptitudes were offered by host families.

The family-care provision available at Iwakura contributed to the local economy by providing employment opportunities during a period when villagers could no longer rely on agricultural income alone and infrastructural amenities were still restricted. Following a Western model of institution-based mental health provision, family care was abolished under the Mental Health Act of 1950, putting an end to a practice that had emerged during the eighteenth century to accommodate pilgrims who sought healing and relief at Iwakura's Buddhist Daiujji temple.

Notes

1 Anon., *Eiga Monogatari*, vol. 2 (*Nihon Koten-Bungaku Taikei*, vol. 76) (Tokyo: Iwanami Shoten, 1965), p. 496. The third princess of Emperor Go-Sanjo was afflicted with a disease. It is not certain, however, if she was cured in Iwakura.
2 Anon., *Meisho Miyakodori* (*A Guide to the Main Sights of Kyoto*) (*Shinshu Kyoto Sosho*, vol. 5) (Kyoto: Rinsen, 1968), p. 28.
3 Makoto Atobe, Naoko Iwasaki and Shinji Yoshioka, 'Kinsei Kyoto Iwakura-mura ni okeru "Katei Kango"' ('Family care of mentally ill patients in Iwakura in the Edo period') (1), *Seishin-Igaku* (*Psychiatry*), 37:11 (1995), 1222.
4 Akira Hashimoto, 'The invention of a "Japanese Gheel": Psychiatric family care from a historical and transnational perspective', in Waltraud Ernst and Thomas Mueller (eds), *Transnational Psychiatries* (Newcastle: Cambridge Scholars, 2010), pp. 142–71.
5 Joyu, *Daiunji-Dosha Kyuseki Sannyo* (Summary of History of Daiunji-Temple) (Kyoto: 1699), p. 58. See also the Kyoto guidebook written in 1754: *Yamasiro Meiseki Junko Shi* (Walking Around Kyoto) (Kyoto: Rinsen, 1972), p. 339.
6 It is certain that a mentally ill patient paid a visit to Daiunji-Temple in 1765 based on an official notice of Kyoto, and an earlier document written in 1754 and preserved in Imai Inn indicating that the inn had received a mentally ill patient in 1754. *Kyoto Machibure Shusei* (*Official Notices of Kyoto*), vol. 4 (Tokyo: Iwanami, 1984), p. 380.

7 Buson Yosa, *Buson Kushu* (*Buson's Poetical Works*) in *Buson Shu, Issa Shu* (*Buson's Poetical Works and Issa's Poetical Works*) (*Nihon Koten Bungaku Taikei*, vol. 58) (Tokyo: Iwanami Shoten, 1959), p. 114.
8 Kinkei Nakagami, *Seiseido Itan* (*Medical Advice*) (1796) in *Kinsei Kanpo Igakusho Shusei* (*Medical Books in the Edo Period*) (Tokyo: Meicho Shuppan, 1979), vol. 17, p. 77.
9 Shinkichiro Yamane, 'Kita-Iwakura Daiunji no gi nitsuki Tansakusho' ('Report of Iwakura'), in 'Tenkyoin Ikken' ('Kyoto Mental Hospital') (Seiji-bu Eisei-rui, no. 6 (handwritten booklet), 1875), *Kyoto-Fu Si* (*History of Kyoto Prefecture*), vol. 2.
10 'Jissoin Monjo'('Jissoin-Temple documents'), box 28, doc. 46; Atobe *et al.*, 'Iwakura-mura "Katei Kango"' (1), p. 1224.
11 'Imai-ke Monjo'('Old documents of the Imai family in Iwakura'), 1873.
12 'Imai Hoyojo no Annai' ('A pamphlet of Imai Guest House'), c.1930.
13 Osamu Nakamura, *Rakuhoku Iwakura to Seishin Iryo* (*Iwakura, Kyoto and Care of Mentally Ill Patients*) (Kyoto: Sekai Shisosha, 2013), pp. 28–38.
14 'Jissoin Monjo', box 31, doc. 274; Atobe *et al.*, 'Iwakura-mura "Katei Kango"' (2), *Seishin Igaku* (*Psychiatry*), 37:12 (1995), 1337.
15 'Jissoin-Monjo', box 31, doc. 274; Atobe *et al.*, 'Iwakura-mura "Katei Kango"' (1), p. 1226.
16 Yamane, 'Iwakura Daiunji Tansakusho', in *Kyoto-Fu Si*.
17 Kyoto Furitsu Ika Daigaku Soritsu Hachiju Shunen Kinen Jigyo Iinkai (Kyoto Prefecture Medical School's 80th Anniversary Celebration Executive Committee) (eds), *Kyoto Furitsu Ika Daigaku Hachijunen Shi* (*The Book of Eighty-Year History of Kyoto Prefecture Medical School*) (Kyoto: Kyoto Furitsu Ika Daigaku Soritsu Hachiju Shunen Kinen Jigyo Iinkai, 1955), p. 150.
18 Shuzo Kure, *Wagakuni ni okeru Seishinbyo ni kansuru Saikin no Shisetsu* (*Hospitals and Institutions Receiving Mentally Ill Patients in Japan*) (*Tokyo Igakukai Soritsu 25 Shunen Shukuga Ronbun Dai 2 Shu* (Essays Contributed in Celebration of The 25th Anniversary of the Tokyo Association of Medical Sciences, vol. 2) (Tokyo: Tokyo Igakukai (The Tokyo Association of Medical Sciences) 1912), p. 132.
19 *Ibid.*
20 'Iwakura Byoin Rakusei oyobi Soritsu 25 Shunen Kinen Shiki' ('Twenty-fifth Anniversary of Iwakura Mental Hospital'), *Kyoto Iji Eisei Shi* (*Kyoto Medical Journal*), 180 (1909), 20.
21 *Kyoto Iji Eisei Shi*, 62 (1899), 18; Private collection, Eikichi Tsuchiya, 'Iwakura Byoin Shi Soan' ('A draft history of Iwakura Mental Hospital') (unpublished, 1948), p. 9.
22 *Kyoto Iji Eisei Shi*, 180 (1909), 20; Eikichi Tsuchiya, 'Iwakura Byoin Shi Soan', p. 9.
23 Eikichi Tsuchiya, 'Iwakura Byoin Shi Soan', p. 10.
24 *Kyoto Iji Eisei Shi*, 211 (1911), p. 3.
25 Shuzo Takezaki, 'Honpo Seishinbyosha no Tohkeiteki Kansatsu' ('Statistics of mentally ill patients in Japan'), *Seishin Ijyosha to Shakai Mondai* (*Mentally Ill Patients and Social Problems*) (Tokyo: Chuo Jizen Kyokai, 1918), pp. 153–9.
26 *Kyoto Iji Eisei Shi*, 430 (1930), p. 30.
27 'Kyoto-Shi ni okeru Seishinbyosha oyobi sono Shuyoshisetsu ni kansuru Chosa'

('The survey of mentally ill patients and of institutions for mentally ill patients in Kyoto city'), *Kyoto-Shi Shakaichosa Hokokusho* (Kyoto: Kyoto-Shi, 1935), pp. 45, 49.

28 Yasuo Okada, *Nihon Seishinka Iryoshi* (*History of Japanese Psychiatric Care*) (Tokyo: Igaku Shoin, 2002), p. 181.
29 Mamoru Uchida, *Kumamoto-Ken Shakai Jigyoshi Ko* (*History of Social Works in Kumamoto Prefecture*) (Kumamoto: Kumamoto Shakaifukushi Kenkyujo, 1965), p. 327.
30 'Kyoto-Shi ni okeru Seishinbyosha oyobi sono Shuyoshisetsu ni kansuru Chosa', p. 53.
31 Nakamura, *Rakuhoku Iwakura to Seishin Iryo*, pp. 60–6.
32 Shuzo Kure, 'Tenkyoin no Kazoku Kangoho ni tsuite' ('Family care of mentally ill patients in mental hospitals') (1902), in Yasuo Okada (ed.), *Kure Shuzo Chosaku Shu* (Kyoto: Shibunkaku Shuppan, 1982), p. 72; Shuzo Kure, *Wagakuni ni okeru Seishinbyou ni kansuru Saikin no Shisetsu*, p. 129.
33 Wilhelm Stieda, 'Nihon no Seishinbyogaku' ('Psychiatry in Japan'), *Shinkeigaku Zasshi*, 5:7 (1906), 36–40; Frederick Peterson, 'From Vanves to Iwakura', *The Survey* (The Survey Associates, 5 October 1912), 1–5.
34 Eikichi Tsuchiya, 'Kyoto Fuka Iwakuramura ni okeru Seishinbyousha Ryoyo no Gaikyo' ('Summary of guest houses in Iwakura, Kyoto Prefecture'), *Kyoto Iji Eisei Shi*, 439 (1930), p. 7.
35 For a critical assessment of the myth of the 'Japanese Gheel', see Akira Hashimoto, 'The invention of a "Japanese Gheel"'.
36 Tsuchiya, 'Iwakuramura Ryoyo Gaikyo', pp. 7–8.
37 Eugeen Roosens, *Geel no Machi no Hitobito* (Japanese translation of *Mental Patients in Town Life: Geel – Europe's First Therapeutic Community* (Thousand Oaks, CA: Sage, 1979)) (Tokyo: Seishin Iryo Iinkai, 1981), pp. 3, 11, 70, 73–4.
38 Okada, *Nihon Seishinka Iryoshi*, pp. 197–216.
39 Editorial Board of Iwakura Byoin Shi, 'Iwakura Byoin Shi (1)' ('History of Iwakura Hospital'), *Seishin Iryo*, 4:1 (1974), 57–62.
40 *Ibid.*
41 Akira Nishiura, 'Chiiki no Kaihoiryokan no Henkaku nitsuite' ('Changes of residents' attitude towards the open medical care system in Iwakura'), *Byoin-Chiiki Seishin Igaku* (*Hospital and Community Psychiatry*), 36:3 (1995), 93–4; Takao Kitae, 'Kaiho Iryo niokeru Chiiki Meiwaku to Kango no kakawari nituite' ('Troubles caused by mental patients and the open medical care system in Iwakura'), *ibid.*, pp. 102–4.
42 This is according to interviews with the residents and my own experience. This problem lasted until around 1985 when the public sewage works was improved in Iwakura.
43 Kaichiro Yabuta, 'Iwakura-ko', *Tokyo to Kyoto* (*Tokyo and Kyoto*), no. 5 (Kyoto: Shirakawa Shoin, 1960), p. 51; Tatsusaburo Hayashiya, *Kyoto* (Tokyo: Iwanami, 1962), pp. 92–4; Kaisen Iguchi, 'Iwakura', *Tanko*, 9 (1968), 95.

9

Work and occupation in Romanian psychiatry, c. 1838–1945

Valentin-Veron Toma

Along with other types of occupation, such as reading, writing and sporting activities, work has been used as a form of therapy in Romanian psychiatry from the mid-nineteenth century. For example, the first workshops for mental patients were created at the Mărcuța asylum in Bucharest in 1855, just seventeen years after the institutionalisation of psychiatry in the Romanian principalities. Work and other occupations were considered appropriate mainly in the treatment of long-term, chronically ill patients. From the second half of the nineteenth century, confinement of the insane was initially based on the principles of the French alienist medicine, which recommended the separation of the mentally ill from society. This led to the creation of a 'parallel society', within the psychiatric institutions, where individuals had not only to be physically active, but also productive. Described as a sign of progress in contrast to previous therapeutic practices and other forms of medical care, work and occupational therapy were, time and again, critically examined by leading Romanian psychiatrists by comparing them with equivalent practices – and their economic or social contexts – in other European countries. It will be argued that the controversies as well as models of best practice prevalent in other countries became integral parts of work and occupational therapy in Romanian institutions concomitant with the transfer of particular ideas and practices from abroad, and their adaptation to local circumstances. Although a good range of historical accounts of the development of mental institutions has become available in recent years, to date there are no in-depth appraisals of the role of work in Romania.[1] The aim of this chapter is to explore this issue further. The geographical scope of the research encompasses the United Principalities of Wallachia and Moldavia as well as territories such as the Principality of Transylvania that were under foreign occupation for an extended period (figure 9.1). While overcrowding became

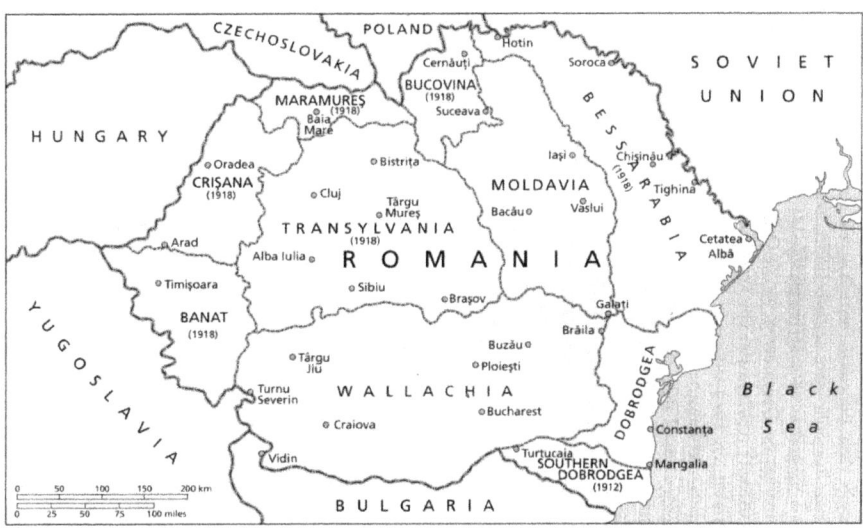

9.1 Map of Romanian territories between the First and Second World Wars.

a problem towards the end of the period, the number of institutions was relatively constant throughout the nineteenth and early twentieth centuries. Most were located near large cities, such as Bucharest (Romania's capital city), Iași, Craiova and Sibiu.

The medicalisation of insanity and the evolution of ideas about mental illness in the Romanian principalities

In the first decades of the nineteenth century, the hospitals in the Romanian principalities (Wallachia and Moldavia) were organised under two separate systems of administration run by previously founded charities. In Wallachia medical establishments were under the supervision of the Ephorate Hospitals (Eforia Spitalelor) formed by a decree issued by the Governor of the Principalities, the Russian general Paul Kiseleff (1788–1872) in 1832. Medical establishments in Moldavia were administered by the trustees (in Romanian: *epitropi*) of the Hospitals of St Spiridon (Epitropia Spitalelor Sf Spiridon), founded as a private charity in the first half of the eighteenth century, transformed into a public institution on 1 January 1757 and then reformed and reorganised by the Law of 1 August 1785 under Prince Alexandru Ion Mavrocordat.[2] From 1864, on the recommendation of Mihail Kogălniceanu, then the Minister of Interior, the two institutions were united under a single public institution called Eforia Spitalelor Civile.[3]

In 1838 it was decreed that insane people ought to be taken care of by medically trained staff within institutional settings (administered by Eforia

Spitalelor). This act, passed under the rule of Alexandru D. Ghica (1796–1862) constituted the first step towards the medicalisation of insanity in the Romanian principalities.[4] Religious hospitals continued to cater for the mentally ill, but from the 1850s, were to be led by a medical doctor. The medical staff was not necessarily specialised in the treatment of mental illness. Nicolae Gănescu (1799–1875), for example, who became the first doctor at Mărcuța in 1840, had been licensed to practise medicine, having obtained the generalist degree of *medicus tertia classis*. We know about the tasks of the different types of medical staff and the internal rules and regulations on patient admissions only from 1861 onwards, when regular reports were published.[5] Prior to 1867, Mărcuța received lunatics alongside people classified as beggars.

Although institutional developments and medical theory lagged behind those in Western European countries, practices became increasingly regulated, with a Romanian tradition of psychiatry emerging from the 1860s onwards, with the appointment of Alexandru Sutzu (1837–1919) at Mărcuța. Sutzu established a new type of specialised, clinical practice.[6] Together with his colleagues and disciples, Sutzu drew on a wide range of French, English and German models of psychological medicine, such as: Pinel and Esquirol's paradigm of mental alienation; Conolly's doctrine of non-restraint; Falret's theory of the clinic; Morel and Magnan's ideas on hereditary degeneracy; Darwin's theory of evolution; and Griesinger's principle of the organic nature of mental illness.

The main figures of Romanian psychological medicine were well attuned to developments in European psychiatric institutions, which they studied with great attention, not only through the specialist literature but also during repeated travels. They were interested in the similarities and differences between the countries they visited and their home country. From the late nineteenth century onwards, they were generally well informed about the latest ideas and practices in the most advanced European countries. A conceptual shift is discernible over the period, from the earlier influence of the French school to new paradigms emanating from Germany. Members of the young generation of psychiatrists, even those who had studied in Paris, became aware of the new trend towards the anatomoclinical model and an international nosology as developed by the German psychiatrist Emil Kraepelin (1856–1926) towards the end of the nineteenth and beginning of the twentieth centuries.[7] As the psychiatrist Ion I. Cantacuzino put it in 1939:

> While creating the Romanian medical psychiatry, Professor Sutzu remained faithful to the views of his time. Back then, the French school considered mental alienation as derived from degeneration, an essentially irreversible phenomenon, which would, therefore, eliminate, in theory, any therapeutic possibility. The German school saw dementia as a complete and global decay of all mental faculties, thus eliminating any therapeutic hope. Under the influence of these

two paradigms, the beginnings of Romanian psychiatry could practically do nothing but tend towards the improvement of the means of assistance while, scientifically, perfecting the spirit of medical observation.[8]

Subsequently, the new stage of Romanian psychiatry was to be dominated by Alexandru Obregia and Alexandru Brăescu in Bucharest and Iași, respectively. Obregia continued Sutzu's work and developed further the clinical teaching of psychiatry and hospital organisation and management, thus making a significant contribution to the field of modern mental healthcare. However, Obregia broke with Sutzu's Francophone theoretic views, which did not employ efficient therapeutic intervention and allow for hope in positive treatment outcomes. At the same time he rejected some of the tenets of the Kraepelinian school and instead mooted new theoretical and therapeutic approaches. Cantacuzino noted:

> By breaking with these directives, Professor Obregia, influenced by Virchow's ideas, guided psychiatry towards the anatomopathological view and, later, in keeping with the progress of science, the Romanian school evolved ceaselessly on its path to new therapy means, introducing the notion of a cure where earlier views were dominated by a belief that degeneracy was irreversible and dementia was imminent.[9]

After Obregia's retirement, in 1934, the Psychiatry Department in Bucharest was led by Petre Tomescu, one of Obregia's former students. He was also Health Minister, for two years (1941–42), in Marshal Ion Antonescu's government.[10] In 1944 he was arrested for his involvement in a far right government and replaced by Constantin I. Parhon (1874–1969), who, although registered as an endocrinology professor, was appointed substitute director of the Psychiatry Department, until the appointment of a new director.[11] Another paradigm shift took place. Through personal research, Parhon contributed to the development of the biological approach in psychiatry, one of his objectives being to establish the role of endocrine factors in psychopathology.[12] Through his political and scientific connections in the academic world of Soviet Russia, Parhon would become a promoter of materialist ideas and Pavlovianism in Romania.[13]

Work and occupation in Romanian psychiatric therapy

Mental institutions in Romania were funded by charities (i.e., Eforia Spitalelor and Epitropia Spitalelor Sf Spiridon) throughout the entire period, with only a small number of private patients contributing to their own upkeep[14] and with the exception of one small private asylum (i.e., Institutul 'Caritatea') founded and run by Sutzu in Bucharest from 1877 onwards.[15] During the late nineteenth century, there existed a relatively small number of public lunatic asylums of which those established in Bucharest, Iași, Craiova and Sibiu will be discussed here.[16]

In the early nineteenth century the Romanian principalities represented a predominantly agrarian country, with a feudal economic system based on private land ownership.[17] Social organisation was characterised by clearly delineated social classes, such as free peasants, peasants with a servile status ('clăcași'), members of the clergy, minor nobles, great boyars and townspeople.[18] In the period 1864–84, however, a process of economic transformation began that led to the gradual transition from feudal structures and manufacturing practices to modern mechanised work, as a result of which Romania gradually entered the industrialisation phase. As pointed out by Victor Axenciuc, after the agrarian reform of 1864 and the adoption of the Constitution of 1866, along with other political, legal and economic measures, the ownership of land became private, being freed from the old feudal rules. In turn, the labour force of peasants was freed from its dependence on landlords and feudal obligations, and it became legally free and a potential commodity on the labour market.[19]

It is not surprising, then, that lunatic asylums in the nineteenth century were mainly populated with peasants and farmhands. Other patients included craftspeople, servants and low-ranking clerks as well as unemployed urban dwellers (vagrants, unemployed townspeople). Asylum doctors were concerned with providing adequate treatment to ease and, if possible, cure the patients. Those considered as incurable performed domestic chores and, depending on their gender, age, education and previous experience, were assigned specific tasks in workshops or on farms. The assignment of work was based on the rationale that chronic patients stayed in the institutions for long periods, which greatly increased the cost of their care. These costs could be reduced if the patients became productive, especially in agricultural work and, albeit less so, workshop activities.

However, work was not considered as a right for the patients who, under contemporary laws, were stripped of their rights and therefore unable to manage their finances and receive income.[20] Work was seen as an obligation that patients had to fulfil during their stay in the asylum. As noted by Pantelimon Miloșescu, in a paper on the history of Mărcuța Lunatic Asylum, article 91 of chapter VI of the Mărcuța rulebook (1864) stipulated that insane people of both sexes 'owed' their work to the institution.[21] At the same time, this owed work was described as 'a means of treatment and pleasure'. Upper-class patients, who constituted a minority, were exempt from work and instead offered intellectually stimulating activities and entertainment.[22] These so-called 'retirees' – patients who paid for their stay at the asylum – were accepted on a voluntary basis.[23] Most asylums, at the end of the nineteenth and the beginning of the twentieth centuries, used the labour power of chronic, intellectually disabled and convalescent patients. The question of patients' choice in this matter was not raised. In fact, financial requirements seem to have been paramount.

Payment for patient work was mentioned at Mărcuța in 1864 in chapter VI of its rulebook entitled 'On various forms of work and leisure'. There were ten hours to a working day. Patients were to receive ten *parale* per day.[24] The accumulated money was paid when the patient left the asylum. Regulations stated that 'the worker could not use the money earned before reaching a capital of 30 lei, a sum that was given to the superintendent for safe keeping'.[25] The rules did not stipulate what happened if a patient died or remained in the asylum. A different model of remuneration called '*pecula*' was introduced by Alexandru Brăescu in 1905, first at the Golia Asylum and then at the newly founded Socola psychiatric hospital in Iași, which he designed and ran for several years, until his untimely death in 1917. The introduction of payment at Mărcuța in 1864 and later by Brăescu in Iași constitutes an important change in the way patients were perceived and treated as human beings and citizens with rights that needed to be respected. In a context where, once admitted into the mental asylum, patients lost all their civil rights, including the right to manage their own affairs or to decide on the use of their own money, such a revision of institutional regulations was revolutionary for the period.

By the early twentieth century, work and occupation held a special role in the therapeutic arsenal of institutional psychiatry. In August 1923 the first section opened in the Central Hospital founded by Alexandru Obregia in Bucharest was the pavilion for 'ergotherapy', as work therapy came to be called in the German tradition. It was run by Dr Mircea Bruteanu (1882–1957). Patients attached to this pavilion contributed directly to the construction and maintenance of the other pavilions.[26] The new hospital's workshops included a smithy, a locksmith, shoemaking facilities and a joinery.[27] They functioned alongside the agricultural farm, which was organised as a colony in an open doors system, until 1945 when all these facilities took on a secondary and negligible role and were gradually abandoned and removed from the medical institution's economic circuit.

Patient work in Bucharest:
The Mărcuța Lunatic Asylum (1839–1923) and the Central Psychiatric Hospital (1923–45)

The first lunatic asylum of the Romanian principalities was launched at Mărcuța, near Bucharest, in 1839. Petre Protici (1822–81) was its head doctor and director between 1854 and 1867. In 1855 he established special workshops for patients: joinery for men and dressmaking for women.[28] Miloșescu notes that by 1864:

Insane people were subject to occupation as a means of treatment, but also as a way to counter the boredom of the time spent in the asylum. These occupations included: participation in orderly service, household tasks (kitchen, laundry, etc.), gardening, agriculture, sewing, joinery, rug making, etc. The occupations were aimed at giving the patients the impression that they are not cut off from society, on the contrary, that they can fit in just like everyone else (sane people), and can be useful to society.[29]

Dr Alexandru Sutzu, who is widely regarded as the founder of Romanian psychiatry, built on Protici's ideas and further developed existing facilities for work, adding new workshops for patients.[30] Sutzu also wrote the first papers theorising the use of work and occupation in psychiatry. The use of work for patients with mental disorders in the principalities was perceived at the time as a sign of progress and a step forward towards more freedom being offered by the asylum doctors to their patients, an example also followed by other mental institutions, for instance those sponsored by monasteries.[31]

Following other European authors, Sutzu grouped the forms of care most appropriate for mental patients into four major types: the lunatic asylum; the so-called cottage system proposed by British authors; villages or colonies for the insane, such as the one in Gheel, Belgium; and agricultural farms within or adjoining the mental asylums.[32] In 1875, Sutzu published in his *Gazette* his reflections on the colony for the insane at Gheel.[33] He had gained direct experience during his visits abroad and, coupled with the evaluation of arguments for and against the use of the various methods, he used this as a basis for the implementation of new forms of care. In contrast to the Belgian system of family care and the British cottage system, Sutzu considered only the agricultural farm model as suitable for Mărcuța and, indeed, Romania as a whole. It was especially the overcrowding at Mărcuța that led Sutzu to propose the open-door system for the practical problems he encountered in his clinical activity.[34] In Sutzu's view, work performed by patients needed to be considered in economic terms and not just from a moral and medical perspective. Patients, as passive consumers of goods and services, could, through the work performed in agricultural farms, contribute actively to a reduction in the costs of their care.[35] The advantages of such a system were also therapeutic, he claimed: 'Thus, the admitted patients will not be subject to the rigorous isolation that is inevitable today; they will perform work that helps convalescence.'[36] Exploitation of patients on the part of farm supervisors would be prevented by farm management being co-ordinated by a doctor.[37] Sutzu referred explicitly to the medical nature of the asylum farm and the central position of the doctor. His model emphasised the position of absolute power held by the medical staff, especially by the chief physician of the asylum. In his view this was not only necessary but also academically and morally justified by the scientific nature of the field he represented.[38]

In his subsequent publications, Sutzu listed the benefits of work, both physical and intellectual, on the mental state of patients. Segregation of the sexes within the asylum was to be enforced not only on the wards and with regard to the opening hours of the hospital garden but also during work activities. Sutzu held that:

> The principles of the general treatment of the mentally ill are: positive regulations, group life, occupation; these are the main influences exercised by the asylum, thus organised, on the admitted patients. ... Occupation is another principle, equally beneficial and powerful, highly recommended by Pinel as well, in several of his writings. In the Mărcuța asylum, occupation, although not sufficiently well organised, although not entirely systemised, exists in some forms; manual work on plantations or in workshops, conferences and readings of historic books in general gatherings, these are the main occupations applied to patients in the asylum. Nobody can doubt that such means produce a powerful repulsion of delirious ideas. Manual work regulates brain excitement; it brings a considerable exhaustion of the nervous force and triggers repose and sleep. Labour and intellectual work replace diseased preoccupations, and they draw the patient's attention towards ideas and notions that are far from delirium, changing the direction of the patient's syllogistic function. Occupation gains ever greater power of action through the influence of example and the stimulation of self-esteem, when it is applied generally for all patients.[39]

Music was another component of what would nowadays be referred to as occupational therapy (OT). Sutzu wrote enthusiastically about its beneficial effects on patients' intellectual and affective faculties.[40] However, the modest financial resources of his institution prevented the further development of music therapy at Mărcuța.[41]

When Sutzu retired in 1909 his position was taken over by Alexandru Obregia (1860–1937), who would lead the Psychiatry Department in the Faculty of Medicine and the Central Psychiatric Hospital, in Bucharest until 1934.[42] At his previous post in the Mărcuța Asylum he had introduced agricultural work in 1899. Large plots of land were purchased to the north of the asylum, where vegetable gardens and farms were set up.[43] In his monograph, published in 1910, Obregia described the institutional structures that were to host therapeutic work within the new hospital that he helped to establish at Bucharest.[44]

Obregia highlighted that work was not only economically essential to the upkeep of a modern mental hospital but also constituted a medical factor for therapy, especially for chronic patients and those in convalescence. He was critical of Kraepelinian therapeutic pessimism, believing that even chronic patients could get better if carefully managed and treated. He therefore considered the advantages of productive activity to be twofold: medical (namely 'progress with a large category of patients') and economic (namely 'monetary savings'). After attending a scientific society exhibition in autumn 1903, where a group of agricultural products from the Mărcuța mental hospital farm 'was well graded and appreciated', Obregia also devised an overall marketing strategy. He argued that if a new location were to be obtained, with larger plots of land: '[T]he product of agricultural work will be so large that it will reduce the costs of hospital maintenance by more than half, as shown in the asylums of Altscherbitz, Dobrzan, Vuhlgarten, Collegne, Grenoble and many others in the West.'[45]

Obregia's vision closely followed Sutzu's ideas. This was also the case with regard to the family colonies for the insane, about which he wrote that:

> This system exists in a well developed state in just one country: at Gheel, in Belgium. It has been the subject of more or less successful experimentation, at Lierneux: then in France at Dun sur Auron and in a few other places. Most of the developed nation states have yet to introduce this system. The system is lauded, indeed, but it is also the subject of controversy. Indeed it is cheaper than the asylums, – but there have also been cases of complications in patients, left untreated, and leading to death or incurability, lack of adequate care, negligence and violence by the caretaker villagers, scenes of cruelty or incest, and a propagation of vices and neuroses, etc.[46]

Obregia's conclusion echoed Sutzu's earlier contention:

> In any case, the following fact is a certainty: family colonies for the insane are only possible in a region where the peasants are highly cultured and accustomed to practising good household hygiene, nutrition and social conduct for themselves and their close ones. These peasants are also required to be open to learning and not to be superstitiously repulsed by the mentally ill, considering that this type of repulsion is widespread in so many countries, including ours.[47]

While Obregia did not consider the Gheel system suitable to the Romanian conditions extant at the beginning of the twentieth century, he believed in future economic and social development that would make the introduction of family care possible. Psychiatric provision was to develop in three stages: first, the establishment of a new asylum; second, adoption of the English open-door system and creation of farming colonies; and, third, introduction of the Gheel system in the vicinity of the newly built institution. Obregia mooted the large-scale application of work therapy to mental patients. In his report sent to the interior minister in 1905, he argued:

> Once the hospital is set up on the new grounds, we will immediately bring great development of manual and agricultural work, which will reduce the costs of maintenance to a minimum. We can see that in Altscherbitz (Saxony) and Ilten costs were reduced by 350 lei per patient per year, and at Ellen the cost is even lower. We will introduce *open door* agricultural colonies and we will gradually

organise the system of treatment in colonies for the insane (*patronnage familial Gheel*), all of which will bring further decreases in the cost of maintenance.[48]

Colonies for the insane and work colonies were also suggested in the Health Act of 1930.[49]

Patient work in Iași:[50]
The Golia Asylum (1858–1905) and the Socola Psychiatric Hospital (1905–45)

Obregia came to hold important government positions, such as director general of the country's health service. He introduced new hospitals, some of them in rural areas others near large cities. Obregia lent his support also to Alexandru Brăescu (1860–1917) in his endeavour to set up a modern psychiatric hospital in Iași. In 1892, the legislative bodies of the Romanian Kingdom had recommended the construction of two new institutions for the care of the mentally ill, one in Bucharest and the other in Iași.[51] Brăescu devoted his full energy to implementing the latter project and, supported by Obregia, he managed to draw a subsidy worth 350,000 lei for the construction of the new institution. Work began in 1897, on the site of the former Socola theological seminary, in a hilly area of the city. The plans used by Brăescu, influenced by his studies in the European countries he had visited, were conceived as a system of pavilions considered most suitable for a psychiatric hospital. The new building, designed to replace the old mental asylum at the Golia monastery, had a capacity of 400 beds and was finished in 1899. The official inauguration could only be organised several years later, in 1905, because of lack of funding.[52] During the construction period, Brăescu continued to act as consultant to the Golia Lunatic Asylum.[53] He subsequently was director of the new institution until 1912.

During his time at the old Golia Asylum, one of his first initiatives was to introduce, for the first time in Iași, a method of remuneration for those among the eighty or so patients who were active in the ergotherapy workshops. He called his payment regime '*pecula*', a term derived from the Latin word *peculium*.[54] It was considered 'as a means for the motivation of patients, with an active contribution to the therapeutic process'.[55] In his text, *Cum sunt considerați și asistați alienații în România* (1903), Brăescu recommended a series of measures that needed to be taken to improve the treatment given to mental patients. Among these was the organisation of 'farm-colonies' using the German system, 'which will host the incurable and harmless chronic patients, epileptics, idiots and some of the patients found in convalescence'.[56] Close to the asylum, workshops for men and women were to be established where 'chronic patients and some of the patients in convalescence will perform work'.[57] Work was recommended especially for chronic and convalescing patients, but was considered contraindicated in the case of acute patients, who needed to remain in the asylum under the observation of the medical staff. Brăescu noted:

> These colonies will be similar to those near the Altscherbitz asylum in Germany and they will be placed under the authority and control of the asylum's head doctor; the colonies need to host approximately the same number of chronic patients we have in our care at the moment.[58]

He considered it vital that chronic and acute patients were segregated from each other:

> These asylums and the ones already in existence will need to host 1,500–1,600 patients, namely the number of acute patients registered; asylums will almost exclusively host acute patients, susceptible to cure, who require close and constant medical care. These asylums will be organised in the system used by the closed asylums in Germany, using the Altscherbitz asylum as a model, or the system used by asylums in Scotland, such as Gartloch, Larbert, etc.[59]

The rationale underlying segregation appears at first sight to have been economic, as is evidenced in Brăescu's explanation:

> These colonies are of extreme importance for us: indeed, since we do not have many asylums in which to place patients and we lack the money to build as many asylums as we need, the placement of patients in colonies is the only way to assist as many mentally ill people as possible in the cheapest way possible. Thus, we will have colonies similar to those in civilised countries, where doctors have long struggled with the need to prevent the overpopulation of asylums with chronic patients.[60]

However, there were also medical in addition to financial reasons for segregation on the basis of envisaged curability and chronicity:

> The removal of chronic patients from asylums and their placement in colonies comes with serious medical and economic advantages. Medical benefits consist of the fact that acute patients, susceptible to cure, remain alone in asylums and will be subject to closer care from doctors who previously lacked sufficient time for the care of chronic and acute patients alike; as a consequence, the chances for a cure will be greater, for the benefit of the patients. Economic benefits will be twofold: (1) the care for patients in colonies costs half as much as care in asylums – which is an important aspect as far as budget is concerned; (2) patients in colonies are working and, through their work, performed in various ways, they cover a large part of the expenditure they cause. There are colonies (Vuhlgarten near Berlin, Altscherbitz, etc.) that cover most of their costs through the work performed by their patients.[61]

A major paradigm shift occurred in Iași in 1912, when Constantin I. Parhon took up the chair in psychiatry and became the new director of Socola

Hospital. He had scientific interests very different from Brăescu, being oriented toward the pathophysiology of nervous processes and the endocrine substrate of mental illness, and particularly of affective psychoses.[62] This does not mean, though, that he completely ignored therapeutic work or denied its importance. On the contrary, Parhon repeatedly referred to this topic. For example, in an article for the newspaper *Adevărul* in September 1925, Parhon evoked, in appreciative terms, the contribution of Brăescu to the development of work therapy at Socola:

> This doctor has made sacrifices of time and work to equip the hospital with all the necessities for the treatment of patients and did not forget, among other things, to use their work for therapeutic purposes, by creating various workshops and also by putting them in the cultivation of land on the plots owned by the Socola Hospital.[63]

In another article, published in the same newspaper, in September 1925, Parhon mentioned that at Socola, because 'animal fodder can be grown on its land, we have been able to breed laboratory animals (rabbits, guinea pigs) whose number now reaches several hundred'.[64] In that year, the number of patients admitted to Socola reached a high level of nearly 600. However, the national authorities, in their efforts to reduce the healthcare costs, considered its dissolution, which probably justified the intense media campaign fought by Parhon in favour of the psychiatry hospital he was leading. Parhon's direction, in terms of scientific research, was continued by Leon Baliff (1892–1967), who added new areas of biomedical research, both fundamental and applied (i.e., studies on the pathology of neurosyphilis, the application of malaria therapy by using the method proposed by W. von Jauregg). In 1924–25, Baliff was awarded a fellowship by the Rockefeller Foundation and went to study neuro-physiology at Oxford and Cambridge. He became professor of mental and nervous diseases at the Medical School of Iași in December 1933. Baliff also held the position of director of the Socola Psychiatric Hospital between 1928 and 1936.[65] He was subsequently appointed director at Socola, being replaced in 1966 by his successor Dr Petre P. Brânzei (1916–85).[66]

Patient work in Craiova:
The Madona-Dudu Asylum (1860–91, 1891–1922)

Since the eighteenth century, the provision of care for the mentally ill in Craiova has been linked to a settlement between the community and a local church known as Madona-Dudu. Rebuilt in 1760 by two wealthy locals this church received an inheritance from them in order to maintain a place of Orthodox worship. In 1860, a medical institution – funded by the church – was established on the lands owned by the Madona-Dudu church, when the

Austrian military doctor Nicolae Hanselman (1826–65) came from Salzburg. As the primary doctor of Craiova, he was the first physician of the asylum for the mentally ill located in the churchyard. He worked there until 1865 when he died from a typhus infection.[67] In the two rooms of this small asylum, six to eight patients were permanently boarded, but their number would sometimes increase to fifteen or sixteen.[68] Dr Hanselman, although not trained as a psychiatrist, banned physical punishments, which were extensively used as a therapeutic method. Instead he relied on a number of alkaloid drugs such as opium, morphine, atropine, etc. Hanselman also recommended some forms of work. The creation of crafts workshops was considered, but it is not known if they were established. What is known is that Dr Hanselman proposed the setting up of a new hospital for the insane to provide better conditions than those prevalent at the time. However, it took thirty years for this to happen. In 1890 the new hospital was completed and, after being provided with the necessary utilities, it was inaugurated in 1891 and the patients were transferred from the old asylum.[69]

Developments at the new Madona-Dudu Asylum, which has been considered by many authors as the first modern psychiatric hospital in Romania, were strongly influenced by Sutzu's ideas. One of his students, George Mileticiu (1853–1917), had been at medical school in Bucharest and had pursued doctoral studies in 1881 under his guidance. Influenced by his mentor, Mileticiu went on to develop in Craiova the knowledge gained in Bucharest. Mileticiu ran the new asylum from 1888 to 1917. The institution was:

> [M]ade up of pavilions with rooms for acute afflictions, with separate pavilions for men and women, divided into sections for calm patients, with eight rooms, and also rooms for epileptics and paralytics, while agitated patients were placed in isolation. There were spacious salons for men and women, 'workshops for physical work and entertainment', areas for interns, and staff, and utilities. In total there were 88 beds (35 government funded beds, 30 private beds in the common area and 6 reserved beds, with an additional 17 beds in the isolation rooms, for agitated patients with contagious diseases). The entire asylum was surrounded by gardens, orchards and fir trees, as well as an agricultural plot spanning 8 hectares, where patients would undergo ergotherapy.[70] Doctor Mileticiu also set up the first bowling alley seen in mental asylums across the nation, for the entertainment of the patients.[71]

In 1895, Mileticiu reflected on the work regime and the activities pursued at Madona-Dudu:

> During the summer, able-bodied patients are tasked with gardening, watering the flowers and trees, cleaning the grass pathways in the garden and park, in a regulated fashion at fixed times. For the entertainment of the convalescing patients, the asylum offers a small library, chess, backgammon, domino, playing

cards, etc.; able-bodied women help the seamstress, the cook, water the flowers, embroider, knit and perform other such feminine arts, all decided in accordance with the social status of the patient. During the winter, mechanical activities for the patients come with greater difficulty. Given the social status of each patient, they cannot all be tasked with pumping water, sawing wood, removing the snow and other such works performed outdoors; there is a lack of indoor mechanical occupations within the asylum.[72]

Another project was planned:

> Personally I plan and hope to succeed, with the help of the Madona-Dudu church administration, in creating a cardboard shop (production of cardboard boxes and paper bags) under the co-ordination of a special foreman. This harmless and uncomplicated craft will keep the patients busy and entertained, which are two factors required by rational treatment.[73]

In his chapter on the history of mental hospitals, Mileticiu engaged in a comparative analysis of the varied types of institutions in Europe and the United States of America. Like Sutzu and Obregia, he argued that colonies for the insane, such as the one in Gheel, were not suitable for the conditions in Romania, and that the open-door hospital designed on the pavilion model was the only viable option.[74] There were two lines of argument against the Belgian family colony system of Gheel. First, Mileticiu referred to the difficulties of controlling such permanent establishments where abuse and exploitation of the labour of the mentally ill could occur. Second, he considered living standards and the culture in Romania unsuited for a colony where the mentally ill would live together with simple rural folk. Considering the social conditions prevalent in Romania he suggested:

> [A]n asylum built in the open pavilion system, on the outskirts of a big city, surrounded by parks and gardens and lucrative land; conducted by able physicians; administered conscientiously; endowed with small workshops to mechanically occupy the sick; a rigorous application of the method of non-restraint, and the results would be very satisfactory.[75]

Similar to Mărcuța, at Madona-Dudu poor patients required a 'pauper's certificate' in order to receive free care. Those who were able to afford the standard 45 lei per month were placed in a separate section. Private patients, who wished to benefit from the services of a personal attendant and have their own room, were charged 150 lei per month.[76] Like at all institutions in Romania, the national guidelines for the treatment of mental hospital patients were applied from 1867.[77] In 1908, the designation was changed from '*ospiciu*' to '*sanatoriu*' and regulations on how patient work and recreational activities had to be managed were devised.[78] Mileticiu was replaced at the helm of the asylum by his intern, Dr George Constantinescu (1881–1962), who had been his deputy between 1910 and 1919. As shown by Olaru et al. (1989), the Madona-Dudu church transferred the Mental Hospital and its entire estate to the Ministry of Public Health, Work and Social Protection in 1922.[79] Alas, the Ministry was not interested in this endowment and transferred the building, with its annexes, on to the Ministry of Education, which turned the premises into a Normal School for girls. All patients were sent to the Socola Mental Hospital in Iași and the Costiugeni Mental Hospital in Chisinau.[80] This ended, for a while, the history of psychiatric assistance in Craiova.[81]

Although during its entire existence the new insane asylum at Craiova – founded in 1891 – was, like the previous one, funded and led by the church trustees from Madona-Dudu, and not by the state, the medical activity followed the model championed by Mileticiu. He drew on the experience he had acquired during his internship in Bucharest, on literature published abroad by renowned psychiatrists, and his observations during many regular visits to the most advanced institutions for the mentally ill in Europe.[82] This resulted in the use of work and leisure activities, along with other forms of therapy, based on the principles of modern psychiatry. Therefore there was no major difference between the work regimes pursued in Mărcuța, for example, and at the Madona-Dudu asylum.

Patient work in Sibiu Mental Hospital (1863–1945)

Sibiu was first mentioned in documents in 1191, under the name of Cibinium. In 1223 it was known under the name of Vila Hermanni and from 1366 as Hermannstadt. In the fifteenth century it became one of the best defended fortresses in Transylvania and between 1692 and 1791 and from 1849 to 1865, under Austrian rule, it was the capital of the Principality of Transylvania.

As Munteanu and Cruceanu have noted:

> Discussions on the establishment of a lunatic asylum in Transylvania date back to the year 1830, when a special fund was created in Vienna, called '*Fondus mente captorum*', in support of construction works. The initial plan was for the new hospital to be constructed in Cluj, but Sibiu was eventually chosen, and a special commission for the management of the project was appointed.[83]

Sibiu asylum possessed a plot of land for an agricultural farm. During the planning stage in 1856, it was suggested that: 'Aside from the greenhouse and garden there needs to be an agricultural plot organised as a model household, serving as a training area for the patients.'[84] Under Dr Ștefan Szabo patients were engaged in work from 1872 onwards. Munteanu and Cruceanu note:

> Work colonies were created for gardening, bee keeping, sericulture, swine and poultry farming, and later cattle and horse farming. In the year 1880, the occupational therapy programme was added, including group hikes and trips around

the city and in neighbouring towns, performed under the supervision of teachers, especially the physical education teacher.[85]

Towards the end of the nineteenth century, greater emphasis was placed on leisure activities, such as reading, writing, sports and gymnastics, dancing, and music, and in 1891 a patients' library was established.[86] In contrast to Bucharest, Sibiu set up an agricultural work system that made use of family care under the supervision of hospital doctors. Family care was introduced in 1906 by Dr M. Epsthein and, as Munteanu and Cruceanu have shown, it was:

> [A]pplied to chronic patients, stabilised and partially recovered socially, who were not taken home by their families. The patients were moved to the towns around Sibiu, especially Cisnădie and Gușterița, to private homes, with the purpose of helping out with various activities in exchange for lodging and meals provided by the families in question. The hospital provided clothing and medical assistance consisting of weekly check-ups. In the year 1914 there were 210 patients under family care. This arrangement lasted until 1925.[87]

Why was family care, which had been rejected by psychiatrists in Wallachia and Moldavia, adopted in Sibiu? A possible answer is that in Transylvania, especially in the region around Sibiu, the ethnic composition of the population – dominated by Germans – and religious affiliation were very different from Moldavia and Wallachia. The villages of ethnic Germans were well developed economically and educational levels were considered high enough to allow mental patients to be included in a family care system similar to that of Gheel. The system involved financial savings as it implied a reduction in the number of patients admitted to the more cost-intensive asylum, and it increased patients' economic utility within rural households in Transylvania.

Between 1911 and 1919, the Hungarian-born psychiatrist Pándy Kálmán (1868–1945) led the hospital in Sibiu, being the sixth director of the institution and the last before the unification of Transylvania with Romania in 1918. He continued the family-care set-up, introduced the open-door system, and developed work therapy and leisure activities (i.e., films and music). In the first three years after his arrival at Sibiu, the hospital leased six hectares of agricultural land where patients cultivated potatoes, cabbages, and other vegetables, both for the needs of the institution and for sale. Some of the profit was distributed to patients, while the rest contributed to the upkeep of the hospital.[88] In the hospital farm, chickens, rabbits and pigs were raised for consumption and horses were bred to be used for carts and carriages.[89]

In 1919, after the union between Transylvania and Romania, the hospital's management was restructured. Dr Gheorghe Preda, a Romanian psychiatrist with an interest in scientific research and preventative psychiatry, was appointed as hospital director. Educated in Bucharest, in the tradition of Sutzu, Obregia and Marinescu, and a collaborator of Parhon, Dr Preda was interested not only in psychiatry but also in neurology. This might explain why in 1919 he changed the old name of the institution from insane asylum to hospital for mental and nervous diseases.[90] In 1921 Preda established the 'Society for the Protection of the Mentally Ill', which aimed at the reintegration of former patients into the labour market. To avoid relapses, free home consultations were provided as part of a prophylactic healthcare initiative. From 1921 to 1937, 770 psychiatric home consultations took place throughout the province of Sibiu.[91]

In 1933, with the support of Dr Liviu Ionașiu, then director of the hospital, Preda introduced so-called 'scientific ergotherapy'. Patients were tasked with specific activities, depending on their mental state. As noted by Munteanu and Cruceanu, the patients' occupation:

> [W]ould be changed, whenever the case required it, and it would be replaced with another activity more suitable to the patients' work capacity, throughout their hospitalisation. A series of workshops was created: knitting, carpet and rug making, basket making, broom and brush making, etc. All workshops were provided with materials and ... staffed with specialised personnel.[92]

Preda also wrote a monograph on patient work entitled '*Ergoterapia*', which was published in 1939.[93] Ergotherapy was used for chronic and convalescent patients alongside the 'old' regime of patient work that focused on domestic work, agricultural work and small production workshops.[94] During the Second World War, the psychiatry and neurology clinics in Cluj-Napoca – one of the most important cities in Transylvania – were temporarily moved to Sibiu, as they were forced to seek refuge on account of the Vienna Dictate.[95] No records on the fate of ergotherapy workshops during this period are currently available.

Conclusion

Work in psychiatric institutions was not seen as a right but a social obligation on the part of the patients, especially those from poor backgrounds. Nevertheless, remuneration for work performed was considered as a patient's right. The recommended type of work was, in most cases, physical labour, which was seen to be most appropriate for the majority of patients who came from farming backgrounds. Patients who had benefitted from some kind of education were tasked with activities seen as more suited to their intellectual abilities. Self-funded middle- and upper-class patients, who were referred to as 'retired patients', were not expected to engage in agricultural or workshop activities, but encouraged to occupy themselves with leisure pursuits. Patients' previous professions and social status were key factors in the therapeutic use of labour in nineteenth-century Romanian asylums.

The first workshops for mental patients were created only two decades after the institutionalisation of psychiatry in the Romanian principalities. The head of the Mărcuța Institute, Dr Petre Protici, introduced the first dressmaking workshops for women and joinery workshops for men, respectively. His initiative was continued by his successor, Dr Alexandru Sutzu, who wrote the first scientific papers in Romanian on the use of work in psychiatry. Sutzu assessed the suitability of different European models of patient work for the Romanian context and recommended agricultural farms in preference to the British cottage system and the Belgian family-care system. From 1899, Dr Alexandru Obregia emphasised that patient work was not only essential for the cost-effective upkeep of a modern asylum, but also part of therapy, especially for chronic patients and those in convalescence. Large plots of land were purchased to the north of the Mărcuța hospital, where vegetable gardens and agricultural farms were set up. Like Sutzu before him, Obregia was not convinced by the adequacy of family colonies in villages distant from the asylum, where supervision was difficult and productivity might be jeopardised on account of host families' prejudice.[96]

The main proponents of Romanian psychological medicine had a profound professional interest in the ways in which other European psychiatric institutions developed. They studied them with great attention, not only through the specialist literature but also by repeated visits. They observed the advantages and disadvantages of different models, their similarities and differences and their applicability to their home region. They were well informed about the latest ideas and practices in the most advanced European countries, and were aware of economic aspects, as well as the principles, of psychiatric care. When Sutzu discussed the colony system, he based his arguments on what he had observed in a number of countries and at international conferences, such as those organised by the Austrian philanthropist Baron Mundy.[97] When Obregia reflected on the type of agricultural farm suitable for patients in Romania, he did so after several visits to asylums in Germany, France and Belgium. Brăescu decided the structure of the hospital he founded in Iași after returning from studies at Salpêtrière. Afterwards, he repeatedly went on research trips to Scotland, England, Belgium, Switzerland, France, Germany and Austria. This recourse to fact-finding trips abroad enabled Romanian psychiatrists to create a solid foundation for the therapeutic and organisational decisions they made in the institutions they led. From a transnational standpoint, we can say that cross-fertilisation of ideas and practices and transfers of knowledge were characteristic of psychiatry in European countries. In Romania's case, such transfers were not merely mechanical, for the sake of keeping up with the most progressive paradigms in European psychiatry, but part of a process of critical reflection and adaptation to conditions existing in different regions of Romania at the time. The varied conditions in the three main provinces led to diversity in the application of particular models.

Before 1944/45, ideas and practices of patient work and OT in Romania moved at the same pace as those in Western Europe. A rupture occurred with the installation of a totalitarian political regime, which imposed a Soviet-type of healthcare structure. Following this rupture, the discrepancy between Romanian and Western psychiatry widened quickly and for at least twenty years the desperate efforts of professionals who were not ideologically locked into the system were unable to bring any significant improvement.

Acknowledgement

I would like to thank Dr Marius Turda (Oxford Brookes University) for his advice on an earlier version of this chapter.

Notes

1 For references on relevant authors and medical institutions designed for the care of mental patients, see Alexandru Olaru, Stela Arsene and Maria Cernătescu, 'Asistența psihiatrică în Oltenia', *Neurologie, Psihiatrie, Neurochirurgie*, 3 (1989), 206–9; Ioan Munteanu and Florin Cruceanu, 'Evoluția asistenței psihiatrice în județul Sibiu (1863–1988)', *Neurologie, Psihiatrie, Neurochirurgie*, 3 (1989), 211–15; Nicolae C. Marcu and Nicolae N. Marcu, 'Spitalul Clinic de Psihiatrie "Prof. Dr. Al. Obregia"', *Revista Română de Sănătate Mintală*, 5:2(10) (1998), 7–11; Constantin Dimoftache Zeletin, *Doctorul Alexandru Brăescu. Contribuții documentare* (Bacău: Editura Corgal Press, 2009); Pantelimon Miloșescu, *Mărcuța – de la ospiciul smintiților la institutul de alienați* (Oltenița: Editura Tridona, 2010).

2 *Epitropi* comes from the Greek ἐπίτροπος (= *epitropos*): an administrator (one having authority), a steward or manager of a household, or of lands; an overseer. The foundation and evolution of the Hospitals of St Spiridon has been discussed by Băileanu in several publications, for example: Gheorghe Băileanu, *Fondarea Epitropiei Sf Spiridon și crearea persoanelor juridice în vechiul drept privat. Partea I – Contribuțiuni la Studiul Fondațiilor* (Iași: Viața Românească, 1929), pp. 8–14; Băileanu, *Evoluția juridică a Epitropiei Sf. Spiridon dela 1757 la 1800. Partea II și III – Contribuțiuni la studiul persoanelor morale* (Iași: Institutul de Arte Grafice 'Presa Bună', 1929), pp. 3–9. The 1785 Law has been published under the title 'Hrisovul lui Alexandru Ion Mavrocordat din 1 August 1785 orânduind administrația spitalului' in Băileanu, *Evoluția juridică a Epitropiei Sf Spiridon*, pp. 46–58.

3 Alexandru G. Găleșescu, *Eforia Spitalelor Civile din Bucuresci* (Bucuresci: Tipografia G. A. Lăzăreanu, 1900), p. 473. The law of 16 October 1864, stating this reorganisation, stipulated that its budget would be submitted to the vote by the House of Representatives (Camera Deputaților), as well as that the budget and administration of its property would be subject to the same rules as those for the state budget, the management control being transferred to the Court of Accounts. From this

point on, all subsequent sanitary laws of Romania maintained and strengthened these operating principles. Eforia Spitalelor Civile was abolished by the communist authorities in 1948 and all its property confiscated.

4 The official document was signed by Prince Alexandru D. Ghica on 1 December 1838.
5 See, for instance, Gheorghe Barbu, 'Nicolae Gănescu, un medic progresist', in Valeriu L. Bologa (ed.), *Din istoria medicinii românești și universale* (București: Editura Academiei, 1962), pp. 309–24; Petre Protici, 'Rapportu medicalu cu tabele de mișcarea bolnaviloru din Institutulu Mărcuța, din ambele despărțiri, pe anulu 1862', *Monitorul Medical*, 2:17 (1863), 133–5.
6 This development of psychiatry as a discipline in Bucharest was built on the previous creation of a legal framework through the law of 1838 and an institutional infrastructure through the creation, in 1839, of the first asylum in the Romanian principalities.
7 See Alexandru Al. Sutzu-son and S. Marbe-Cohen, 'Psihiatria modernă și principalele ei entități morbide', *Spitalul*, Februarie (București: Tipografia Eminescu, 1905); Alexandru Al. Sutzu-son, 'La psychiatrie moderne et l'oeuvre du Professeur Kraepelin. Suite et fin', *Annales Médico-Psychologiques*, 3 (1906), 402–20; Sutzu-son, 'La psychiatrie moderne et l'oeuvre du Professeur Kraepelin', *Annales Médico-Psychologiques*, 4 (1906), 243–57; Sutzu-son, 'Encore la question de la démence précoce', *Annales Médico-Psychologiques*, 5 (1907), 243–64.
8 Ion I. Cantacuzino, 'Centenarul psihiatriei românești', *Revista Fundațiilor Regale*, VI:3 (1939), 697–706, reprinted in Valentin-Veron Toma and Adrian Majuru (eds), *Nebunia. O antropologie istorică românească* (București: Editura 'Paralela 45', 2006), pp. 376–84, 381.
9 Cantacuzino, 'Centenarul psihiatriei românești', p. 382.
10 See Petre Tomescu, *Doi ani de activitate la Ministerul Sănătății* (București: Institutul de Arte Grafice 'Tiparul Românesc', 1942).
11 In 1946, Professor Constantin I. Urechia was transferred from Cluj and took the lead in the Psychiatry Department at the Medical Faculty in Bucharest until 1949 when he was replaced by Dr Constanța Parhon-Ștefănescu. She became a professor, and head of the department, in 1962. Teodor Ilea, Iuliu Ghelerter and Benone Duțescu (eds), *Învățămîntul Medical și Farmaceutic din București. De la începuturi pînă în prezent* (București: Institutul de Medicină și Farmacie, 1963), pp. 361–2.
12 Ștefan M. Milcu, 'Coup d'oeil sur l'oeuvre scientifique du professeur C. I. Parhon', in Ștefan M. Milcu (ed.), *Omagiu lui C. I. Parhon, Președinte de Onoare al Academiei Republicii Socialiste România cu prilejul împlinrii a 90 de ani* (București: Editura Academiei Republicii Socialiste România, 1966), pp. 65–80, 72.
13 Ilea et al., *Învățămîntul Medical și Farmaceutic din București*, p. 95.
14 See art. 21, Secțiunea III – The revenues and expenditure of the service for the mentally ill, from the Mental Health Act (*Legea asupra alienaților*), document enacted through the High Royal Decree, no. 4090 from 10 December 1894, published in *Monitorul Oficial*, no. 203 on 15 December 1894.
15 Although a private property, this institution was subsidised by the State, as it served

not only for internment and treatment but also as a temporary shelter for the mentally ill during their move to Mărcuța.
16 According to Felix, in 1892 three public asylums existed in Wallachia and Moldavia, one church-sponsored (i.e., Madona-Dudu) and only one private hospital owned by Professor Alexandru Sutzu. See Iacob Felix, *Raport General despre igiena publică și despre Serviciul Sanitar ale Regatului României pe anul 1892* (București: Tipografia Statului, 1893), pp. 134–5, reprinted in Toma and Majuru (eds), *Nebunia*, pp. 159–60. By the year 1907 yet another asylum with forty beds had been built at Coșula (Moldavia) for the insane and pellagra patients. Alexandru Obregia, *Raport general asupra Igienei Publice și asupra Serviciului Sanitar al Regatului României pe anii 1898–1904* (București: Institutul de Arte Grafice și Editura 'Minerva', 1907), pp. 259–61. In Transylvania there was only one public asylum at Sibiu, the former capital city of the Principality of Transylvania.
17 See Victor Axenciuc, *Avuția națională a României. Cercetări istorice comparate, 1860–1939* (București: Editura Expert, 2000), pp. 16, 22; Daniel Chirot, *Schimbarea socială într-o societate periferică. Formarea unei colonii balcanice*, trans. Victor Rizescu (București: Editura Corint, 2002), p. 197.
18 Chirot, *Schimbarea socială într-o societate periferică*, pp. 162, 187.
19 Axenciuc, *Avuția națională a României*, p. 53.
20 See Sutzu's texts in which he analyses current legislation on the civil capacity of mental patients and their right to leave accumulated wealth as inheritance. Alexandru Sutzu, *Alienatulu în fața societății și a scienței, Colecția Studii Medico-Psychologice* (Bucuresci: Noua Typographie a Laboratorilor Români, 1877), pp. 7–12, 21–7.
21 Miloșescu, *Mărcuța*, p. 86.
22 On this category of patients, Miloșescu notes that in chapter VI of the rulebook *Regulamentul serviciului Ospiciului Mărcuța* from 1864 the following is stated: 'Those with better education could take up reading and writing. There were also fitness exercises, gymnastics, various games, walks around the asylum etc.' Miloșescu, *Mărcuța*, p. 63. Regarding the benefits of intellectual activity as an occupation with effects on mental protection and the reduction of the risk of dementia, Sutzu notes: 'Such intellectual activity, whatever the consensus may be, does not lead to dementia, unless it is accompanied by emotions and unease. A cultivated and healthy spirit, on the contrary, finds intellectual occupation as a means to distance itself from the cause of grief and suffering that obsesses it, and focuses on an object that is healthy and useful.' Sutzu, *Alienatulu în fața societății și a scienței*, p. 232.
23 Alexandru Sutzu, 'Regulamentul de admissiunea bolnavilor pensionari în Ospiciul Mărcuța și tratamentul lor', *Gazetta Medico-Chirurgicală a Spitalelor*, 4:1 (1873), 63–4, and 4:18 (1873), 192.
24 '*Para, parale*' is a coin division equal to one hundredth of an old leu; also a small Turkish coin made of silver that circulated in the Romanian principalities (DEX, see http://dexonline.ro/definitie/para). According to Axenciuc, until the introduction of the new 'leu' as the official national monetary unit in 1867, the nominal value of the coins in circulation in the Romanian principalities had different and

variable levels. For example, a Napoleon – the equivalent of twenty francs – was worth 54 lei, while the pound sterling was equivalent to 25.20 French francs or 68 lei. In 1867 the new national monetary system was adopted in Romania. The standard new leu (bi-metal coins that were made of gold or silver) was fixed at 0.3226 grams of gold or 5 grams of silver. The Romanian new coins were identical to the standard of the Latin Monetary Union (1865), i.e., the French and Swiss francs. Therefore, at the time, the validation was undertaken as follows: 100 new lei = 270 old lei; 1 new leu = 1 French franc, 1 pound sterling = 25.25 lei; 1 US dollar = 5.18 lei. Axenciuc, *Avuția națională a României*, p. 19.

25 Miloșescu, *Mărcuța*, p. 63. The sum of 10 *parale* a day (i.e., the equivalent of 0.10 Romanian lei) for the work of a mentally ill patient is, in this context, an extremely small income when the sum of about 30 lei could be earned in only 7–8 days by a healthy worker with an average salary of 4 lei per day in the 1860s. Axenciuc, *Avuția națională a României*, p. 43; Sabin Drăgulin, 'Fenomenul migrator în România. Studiu de caz: italienii (1868–2010)', *Sfera Politicii*, 158 (2011), 15.

26 See Marcu and Marcu, 'Spitalul Clinic de Psihiatrie "Prof. Dr. Al. Obregia"', p. 9; Sorin Riga and Dan Riga, 'Restituția Prof. Dr. Alexandru Obregia', in Gavril Cornuțiu (ed.), *Prima Consfătuire Națională de Istoria Psihiatriei Românești. Lucrările Consfătuirii – Vol. I [Proceedings of the First National Conference on the History of Romanian Psychiatry]*, published in *Analele Universității din Oradea. Fascicula Medicală [Annals of the University of Oradea]*, 3:1 (2009), 53–93, 60.

27 Alexandru Obregia, *Noul ospiciu de alienați lângă București. Cu un plan și 6 tabele anexate* (București: Institutul de Arte Grafice 'Carol Göbl', 1910), p. 30.

28 Alexandru Olaru, 'Tradiții și orientări în psihiatria românească', in George Brătescu (ed.), *Trecut și viitor în medicină. Studii și note* (București: Editura Medicală, 1981), pp. 511–25; Miloșescu, *Mărcuța*, p. 86.

29 Miloșescu, *Mărcuța*, p. 63.

30 George Brătescu, 'Contribuția doctorului Al. Sutzu la pătrunderea spiritului filozofic în știința noastră medicală', *Cercetări Filozofice*, 6:3 (1959), 93–101, 101.

31 Miloșescu notes that: 'We can also find a system of ergotherapy in 1869 at the lunatic asylum affiliated to the Adam convent, where female patients, 20–30 in number, were involved in orderly work on the food block, which prepared meals for all patients (80), performing intense household activities, in line with the doctor's orders.' Miloșescu, *Mărcuța*, p. 86.

32 In his monograph, published in 1869, entitled *The Mărcuța Asylum: Clinical and Medico-legal Relations*. Alexandru Sutzu, *Ospiciulu Mărcuța: Relațiuni clinice și medico-legale* (Bucuresci: Noua Tipografie a Laboratorilor Români, 1869), pp. 15–20.

33 Alexandru Sutzu, 'Colonia de alienați din Gheel (I)', *Gazetta Medico-Chirurgicală a Spitalelor*, 6:12 (1875), 316–19.

34 See, for example, Alexandru Sutzu, *Despre mersul alienațiunei mintale în România* (Bucuresci: Tipografia Academiei Române/Laboratorii Români, 1884), pp. 13–15.

35 Sutzu, *Ospiciulu Mărcuța*, p. 19.

36 Ibid., p. 18.

37 Ibid., p. 19.
38 Valentin-Veron Toma, *Alexandru Sutzu: Începuturile psihiatriei științifice în România secolului al XIX-lea* (București: Editura Dominor, 2008), p. 181.
39 Alexandru Sutzu, 'Câteva cuvinte despre tratamentul general din Ospiciul Mărcuța', *Gazetta Medico-Chirurgicală a Spitalelor*, 3:19 (1872), 327–31, 330.
40 Sutzu, 'Influența musicii asupra morbelor nervoase și mintale', *Gazetta Medico-Chirurgicală a Spitalelor*, 3:19 (1872), 299–300.
41 Ibid.
42 Cantacuzino, 'Centenarul psihiatriei românești', in Toma and Majuru (eds), *Nebunia*, p. 381.
43 Obregia, *Noul ospiciu de alienați lângă București*, p. 12.
44 Ibid., pp. 13, 15, 24, 27, 35.
45 Ibid., p. 13.
46 Ibid., p. 13.
47 Ibid., p. 14.
48 Alexandru Obregia's 1905 report to the interior minister was published in 1910. Obregia, 'Raport adresat Domnului Ministru de Interne de către Medicul Director al Ospiciului Mărcuța, relativ la necesitatea urgentă a Clădirii unui Ospiciu Central de Alienați lângă București', in Obregia, *Noul ospiciu de alienați lângă București*, p. 15.
49 'Legea sanitară și de ocrotire', *Monitorul Oficial*, part I, no. 154, (14 July 1930), arts 451 and 454.
50 Psychiatric assistance in Iași dates back to the year 1858 when the management of the Hospitals of St Spiridon (*Epitropia Spitalelor Sf Spiridon*) took over the care of mental patients from the Golia monastery and created the first asylum, in Moldavia, with forty beds. The psychiatrist Julian Lukaszewski was appointed to lead the asylum. He graduated from the medical school of Berlin. Several years later, he published a monograph called *Soarta nebunilor*. Tadeusz Pirozynski, 'Semnal evocator: școala de psihiatrie de la Socola', *Neurologie, Psihiatrie, Neurochirurgie*, 3 (1889), 194–6, 194.
51 Pirozynski, 'Semnal evocator', p. 195.
52 Zeletin, *Doctorul Alexandru Brăescu*, p. 232.
53 Ibid., p. 86.
54 *Peculium* (Civil Law): Some places, such as Rome, allowed slaves to accumulate, manage, and use property in a *peculium* that was legally revocable but could be used to purchase their freedom. This provision gave slaves an incentive to work as well as the hope of eventual manumission. See *Encyclopædia Britannica* online: www.britannica.com/EBchecked/topic/448405/peculium.
55 Zeletin, *Doctorul Alexandru Brăescu*, pp. 83, 261.
56 It is not known why Brăescu suggested adoption of German model of a *farm colony* adjoined to the mental asylum. In the quoted paper, in a footnote, we learn that the author intended to explain in a later work the reasons why Romania needed to apply the German system and reject the systems used in Scotland, Belgium and France: 'For reasons to be discussed, on a later occasion, we are not pleased with the system of placing patients in families, like in Scotland, or in autonomous colonies,

like in Belgium and France.' Alexandru Brăescu, *Cum sunt considerați și asistați alienații în România* (Iași: Tipografia 'Dacia', 1903), pp. 3–14, 12.
57 Brăescu, *Cum sunt considerați și asistați alienații în România*, p. 12.
58 *Ibid.*
59 *Ibid.*
60 *Ibid.*
61 *Ibid.*
62 Radu Iftimovici, *Istoria universală a medicinei și farmaciei* (București: Editura Academiei Române, 2008), p. 712.
63 Constantin I. Parhon, 'Spitalul Socola din Iași. Însemnătatea lui ca centru pentru tratamentul boalelor nervoase și mintale', *Adevărul* (11 September 1925).
64 Constantin I. Parhon, 'Însemnătatea organisației spitalului Socola. Sediu al clinicii boalelor nervoase și mentale', *Adevărul* (12 September 1925).
65 Traian Bratu, *Anuarul Universității Mihăilene din Iași, 1930–1935* (Iași: Editura Universității Mihăilene, 1936), p. 202.
66 A second major paradigm shift occurred in the period when the department of psychiatry was headed by Petre P. Brânzei. He was one of the promoters, at a European level, of the three-dimensional constructivist model of mental illness, a concept called bio-psycho-social determinism. Petre Brânzei, *Itinerar psihiatric* (Iași: Editura Junimea, 1974). The clinical application of the constructivist bio-psycho-social concept significantly changed the orientation of psychiatry at the Socola Psychiatric Hospital. Vasile Chirita and Roxana Chirita, 'The bio-psycho-social concept in the tradition of the "Socola" school of psychiatry', *Bridging Eastern and Western Psychiatry*, 7:1 (2006), 18–22. Due to the importance of the social side of his theoretical model, Brânzei considered integrative psychotherapy (including both ergotherapy and sociotherapy) and vocational rehabilitation as useful tools in the recovery of the mentally ill. Petre Brânzei and Aurelia Sîrbu, *Psihiatrie* (București: Editura Didactică și Pedagogică, 1981), p. 330. But all this happened, much later, in the late 1960s and early 1970s. Petre Brânzei and Iosif N. Nathanson, 'Le constructivisme tridimensionnel bio-psycho-social de l'école de Socola dans la perspective de la psychiatrie contemporaine', *Acta Psychiatrica Belgica*, 81:5 (1981), 425–36.
67 Olaru *et al.*, 'Asistența psihiatrică în Oltenia', p. 207.
68 George Mileticiu, *Studii psihiatrice. Cu trei planuri* (Craiova: Tipo-litografia Naționale Ralian & Ignat Samitca, 1895), p. 98.
69 *Ibid.*, p. 109.
70 According to Mileticiu: '[T]he foundation of the therapy provided for the mentally ill is occupation which distracts them, and causes them to be distracted from their morbid musings, in a word, it transfers them from the imaginary into the real world. And, of all mechanical activities, the first place is occupied by work in the fields and gardening.' Mileticiu, *Studii psihiatrice*, p. 81.
71 Olaru *et al.*, 'Asistența psihiatrică în Oltenia', p. 208.
72 Mileticiu, *Studii psihiatrice*, p. 112.
73 *Ibid.*, p. 113.
74 *Ibid.*, p. 86.

75　*Ibid.*, p. 86.
76　*Ibid.*, p. 112.
77　*Regulamentul pentru primirea bolnavilor în ospiciile de alienați*, published in the official gazette (*Monitorul Oficial*) on 15 July 1867.
78　*Regulamentul Sanatoriului Madona Dudu din Craiova*, published in 1908, included regulations regarding 'the work and recreational activities of patients'. Olaru *et al.*, 'Asistența psihiatrică în Oltenia', p. 208.
79　Olaru *et al.*, 'Asistența psihiatrică în Oltenia', p. 209.
80　*Ibid.*
81　It was not until 1971 that a general hospital was established in Craiova, offering psychiatric consultations in the out-patient department.
82　George Mileticiu, *Dare de seamă despre o călătorie științifică in Austria și Germania adresată D-lor General G. Anghelescu și Petre Chițu, Epitropii așezămintelor bisericei Madona-Dudu din Craiova* (Craiova: Inst. grafic Samitca, I. Samitca & D. Baraș, 1907).
83　Munteanu and Cruceanu, 'Evoluția asistenței psihiatrice în județul Sibiu', p. 211.
84　Patients were trained there in order to perform a variety of agricultural tasks. Munteanu and Cruceanu, 'Evoluția asistenței psihiatrice în județul Sibiu', p. 212.
85　Munteanu and Cruceanu, 'Evoluția asistenței psihiatrice în județul Sibiu', p. 212.
86　Teodor Stoenescu, Inocențiu Micu, Cornel Lungu and Romulus Simu, 'Cîteva date privind evoluția științifică și organizatorică a Spitalului de Neuropsihiatrie din Sibiu', in Gavril Cornuțiu (ed.), *Prima Consfătuire Națională de Istoria Psihiatriei Românești. Lucrările Consfătuirii – Vol. II* [*Proceedings of the First National Conference on the History of Romanian Psychiatry*], published in *Analele Universității din Oradea. Fascicula Medicală* [*Annals of the University of Oradea*], 4–5 (2010), 224–9, 225.
87　Munteanu and Cruceanu, 'Evoluția asistenței psihiatrice în județul Sibiu', p. 212.
88　Albert Veress, 'Activitatea lui Pandy Kalman în Transilvania', in Cornuțiu (ed.), *Prima Consfătuire Națională de Istoria Psihiatriei Românești. Lucrările Consfătuirii – Vol. II*, published in *Analele Universității din Oradea. Fascicula Medicală*, 4–5 (2010), 38–9, 39.
89　Veress, 'Activitatea lui Pandy Kalman în Transilvania', p. 39.
90　Stoenescu *et al.*, 'Cîteva date privind evoluția științifică și organizatorică a Spitalului de Neuropsihiatrie din Sibiu', in Cornuțiu (ed.), *Prima Consfătuire Națională de Istoria Psihiatriei Românești. Lucrările Consfătuirii – Vol. II*, published in *Analele Universității din Oradea. Fascicula Medicală*, 4–5 (2010), 226.
91　*Ibid.*, p. 227.
92　Munteanu and Cruceanu, 'Evoluția asistenței psihiatrice în județul Sibiu', p. 213.
93　Vasile Predescu, 'O sută cincizeci de ani de asistență psihiatrică în România', *Neurologie, Psihiatrie, Neurochirurgie*, 3 (1989), 163–70, 168.
94　A paradigm shift in the Romanian psychiatry only occurred in the late 1960s, at the Central Hospital in Bucharest, when Dr Aurel Romila outlined the principles of his theory of the resocialisation of mentally ill. Romila became very critical of the use of OT, as the last resort, in the case of the chronically ill – and those with disabilities – and recommended instead the application of OT and a resocialisa-

tion programme from the early stages of developing mental illness, i.e., in the acute phase of the disease.
95 The Vienna Dictate, also known as the Second Vienna Award, was the second of two Vienna Awards arbitrated by Nazi Germany and Fascist Italy. As Béni L. Balogh explains it: 'On 30 August 1940, the ministers of foreign affairs of Germany and Italy, Joachim von Ribbentrop and Galeazzo Ciano, proclaimed the Second Vienna Award in the golden chamber of the Belvedere Palace in Vienna. Under the terms of the Award, 43,104 square kilometres of the 103,093 square kilometres of territory ceded to Romania under the Treaty of Trianon were returned to Hungary. With a population of two and a half million, the territory regained by Hungary became known as Northern Transylvania. Southern Transylvania, comprising around 60,000 square kilometres, remained a part of Romania. The Award represents a crucial development in the twentieth-century history of Hungarian–Romanian relations. It continues to influence – to a different extent and in a contrary manner – the collective memory in the two nations.' Béni L. Balogh, *The Second Vienna Award and the Hungarian-Romanian Relations 1940–1944*, Social Science Monographs, Boulder, CO, Atlantic Studies on Society in Change no. 139, trans. Andrew Gane (Highland Lakes, NJ: Atlantic Research and Publications, Inc., 2011). The Second Vienna Award was voided by the Allied Commission through the Armistice Agreement with Romania (12 September 1944). The Soviet Union agreed to return Northern Transylvania to Romania, provided that a pro-Communist government should be established in Bucharest. The Romanian civil administration did not return to Transylvania until March 1945, after the formation of the government led by Petru Groza. The 1947 Treaty of Paris reaffirmed the borders between Romania and Hungary, as originally defined in the Treaty of Trianon, twenty-seven years earlier.
96 According to Obregia, Romanian villagers of Moldavia and Wallachia in the late nineteenth century were not prepared to receive in custody, in their homes, for family care, patients coming from the asylums. The population of these pauper villages was quite backward at the time, with a low level of civilisation, with many preconceptions and superstitions about the causes of mental illness. In this context, fear of insanity and rejection of the patients were quite undisguised, and the possibility of abuses and violence could easily be assessed as being high enough to disquiet the psychiatrist. Under these conditions, the productive work of the mentally ill would have been of low quality and produced very little or no economic return.
97 Alexandru Sutzu, 'Asistanța publică a alienaților și baronul Mundy', *Gazetta Medico-Chirurgicală a Spitalelor*, 9 (1878), 57–62.

10

Between therapeutic instrument and exploitation of labour force: Patient work in rural asylums in Württemberg, c. 1810–1945

Thomas Müller

Labour has begun to figure prominently in recent historical research. It has been scrutinised especially with respect to its organisation in different socio-political systems,[1] in agrarian[2] and industrial societies,[3] for example, and also with respect to 'race'.[4] A frequent focus has been the interaction between global processes and local conditions,[5] and definitions of 'non-work'.[6] In the field of the history of medicine, and especially in the history of psychiatry, the meaning of work performed by patients caught in the crossfire between therapy and economic benefit has only recently been considered.[7] This chapter focuses on work performed by psychiatric patients in rural mental hospitals in Württemberg, in the south-west of Germany. It maps the development from early understandings of work as part of therapeutic regimes to work therapy bound up with humanist and medical ideas around 1900, and ends with National Socialist health policies and the association with the ability to work, thus perverting the idea of therapy. I will argue, first, that the development of work regimes and their value as therapeutic interventions were linked up with changes in the institutions' designs and functions as *Heilanstalten* (institutions intended to provide therapy for 'curable' patients) and *Pflegeanstalten* (homes for the care of the chronically ill) respectively. Second, it will be shown that patients' ability to work and contribute to the economic upkeep of the asylum had a bearing on their personal status and feelings of wellbeing. Both dynamics were heavily influenced by global and national developments, with the two world wars having particularly adverse effects on patients' life and work in the institutions.

The characteristic forms, opportunities and structures of work performed by patients as well as its organisational set-up will be discussed. Emphasis will be on the oldest institution in Württemberg: Zwiefalten asylum. The intention is to identify work and its management inside institutions, its day-to-day organisation and the therapeutic objectives underlying it. It will be important to differentiate between work performed by patients within psychiatric institutions (such as agricultural colonies and workshops) and outside institutions (such as family care). Within the wider German context, when compared to other German states, Württemberg's *Innenministerium* or Ministry for Home Affairs was ahead of its time during the early nineteenth century with regard to the care of the mentally ill. Earlier than in other regions, former monasteries were converted into asylums, as was the case at Zwiefalten (1812), Schussenried (1875), and Weissenau (1892) near Ravensburg, in the southern parts of Württemberg. Former estates of noblemen met with a similar fate, for example at Winnenthal near Stuttgart, where psychiatric services were begun in 1834. Weinsberg, near Heilbronn, which opened in 1903, was the first purpose-built hospital in the Kingdom of Württemberg.

In contrast to other German states, for example neighbouring Baden and especially Prussia, while the first half of the nineteenth century was characterised by engaged and forward-looking policies of healthcare, developments in Württemberg slowed down towards the turn of the nineteenth to the twentieth century. From about 1800 to 1914, Württemberg's mental hospitals diverged in terms of their institutional and administrative trajectories from those of other regions of the German Reich.

Zwiefalten is a case in point for the history of patient work in Württemberg. In 1812 the first forty-six patients were relocated in oxcarts from a madhouse in Ludwigsburg, near Stuttgart, to the new Royal Württemberg State Asylum in Zwiefalten.[8] To King Fredrick I, as well as his ministers of internal affairs and finance in the Württembergian capital of Stuttgart, Zwiefalten's secluded location in this thinly settled region seemed ideal for the permanent housing of mentally ill persons.[9] This view was in line with contemporary considerations on the types of environments supposed to have a healing effect on patients as well as with economic considerations.[10] Zwiefalten is the oldest psychiatric institution in Württemberg. The small, rural community housed this asylum within the walls of a former Benedictine monastery.[11] The opening of the asylum in Zwiefalten in 1812 ended the era of the so-called madhouses, which were built under the ordinance of Duke Carl of Württemberg beginning in 1746.[12] Zwiefalten was established when in other regions in Germany, too, institutions for the confinement of the mentally ill were first established towards the beginning of the nineteenth century.[13]

Work and occupation, therapy and treatment

The principle that physical work has a positive impact on health and therefore lends itself to the treatment of patients, with the goal of recovery or improvement of health, has been known as 'dietetics' since antiquity.[14] At Zwiefalten,

Narciß Schreiber (1774–1817),[15] who was the first medical director, regularly employed individual patients with so-called 'adequate aptitude' in household chores and in the courtyard.[16] Under his successors, Andreas Elser (1773–1837),[17] and Carl von Schäffer (1808–88),[18] occupational opportunities for patients continued to evolve.[19] During von Schäffer's directorship patients were employed for the first time outside the asylum's premises, for instance in road and house building, and as assistants to local craftspersons.[20] Under the medical direction of Julius L. A. Koch (1841–1908)[21] a number of architectural improvements were undertaken that aimed at enlarging the premises and improving conditions inside the asylum.[22] Agricultural productivity flourished and, as was the case also with husbandry, expanded continuously.[23]

Given the large-scale occupation of psychiatric patients, the question arises whether there was a conflict between the actual therapeutic benefits of work for the individual patient and the economic benefit reaped by the asylum through patient labour. Advocates of patient work cited the positive effects of physical activity on promoting a good night's sleep and on the 'ordering of thoughts', which implied medical-psychiatric support and a healthy structure of daily activities,[24] as German historians of psychiatry Schott and Tölle put it in their authoritative 2006 work. Medical director Carl von Schäffer considered the benefits of garden and field work in particular to be that the patients learned to co-operate and live with others as a result of the intellectually non-demanding work conducted in the fresh air and in the company of others. He emphasised the socially reintegrative aspect of work.[25]

If their health allowed, patients were occupied in a variety of different types of work: women for instance were busy with housework and men with field and garden work, cobbling and carpentry (see figures 1 and 2), as well as cutting and sawing wood. Since the asylum was heated with stoves, there was a need for wood year-round.

For women there were additional opportunities for work at the spinning wheel. Knitting tools were available and patients were also employed in the picking of horse hair and in the laundry. Later on, Rudolf Camerer and Emil Krimmel, psychiatrists with directorial charge at Zwiefalten, reported: 'Individual male patients were able to leave the grounds and work for a regular day's wage for local Zwiefalten citizens'.[26] Following an official decree in 1816, the ministry granted a small wage to those patients employed in work that benefitted the institution.[27] This wage enabled them to purchase refreshments, small items or luxuries such as tobacco, scarfs and neckerchiefs, and to supplement their diet.[28]

When Dr Carl von Schäffer took over as director of the asylum from his predecessor the physician Andreas Elser, he announced in his first financial report for the year 1839 that an asylum should try to aim for the 'total recovery of patients in their care'.[29] The task of the asylum was to keep

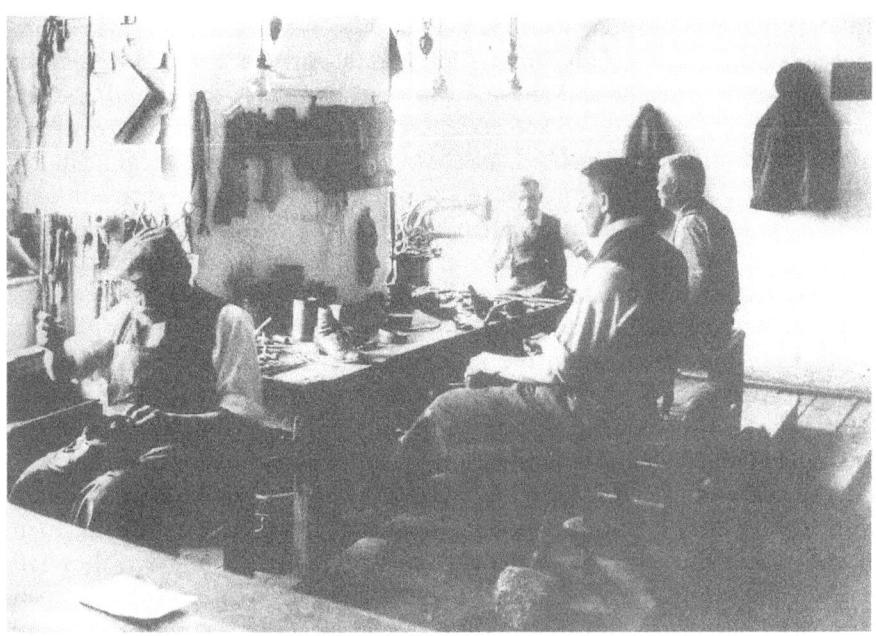

10.1 Zwiefalten Asylum, cobbler's workshop, 1912.

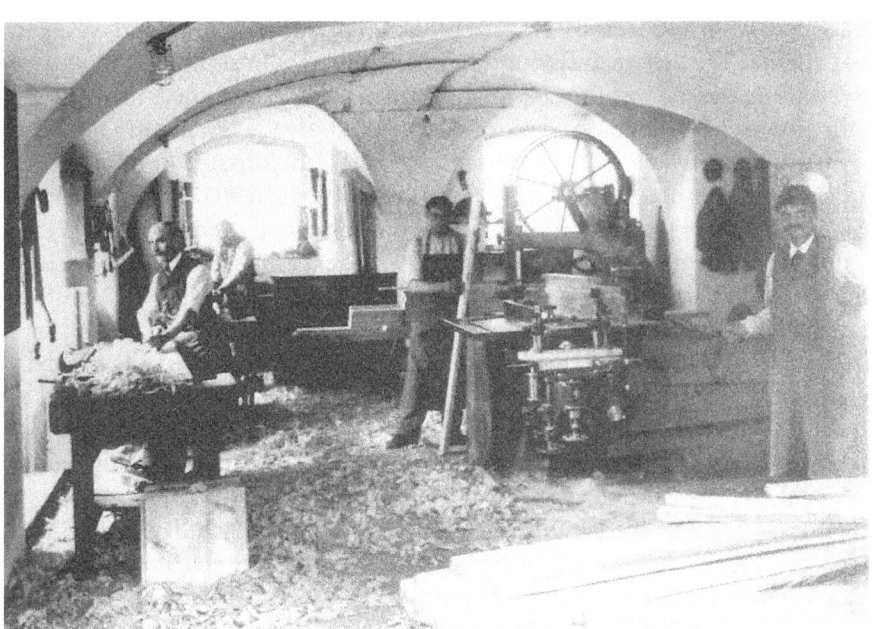

10.2 Zwiefalten Asylum, carpenter's workshop, 1912.

'idiotic' ('*blödsinnig*') patients from sinking deeper, the 'crazy and mad' from exercising their 'crazy and criminal intentions' and the 'deluded of reason' from 'mockery, ridicule and abuse'.[30] However, whatever their condition, all patients needed 'to be forced and accustomed to submit to the house order'.[31] An 'adequate and individualised, psychological-somatic dietary regime in the broadest meaning of the word' was to be implemented and physical ailments were to be treated. In general, patients had to be monitored, with improvement of their health and even recovery being always kept in mind, and be looked after with the greatest care and utilising all possible means.[32]

By the end of Schäffer's first year in office, almost two-thirds of the patients worked on a daily basis and the range of activities was expanded further. Women were employed in the garden and on what were considered typical female chores like knitting, sewing, patching, spinning, fixing laundry, cleaning vegetables, dishwashing, and cleaning windows and floors. Weather permitting, all work was performed outside in the courtyard. This is also where women had their lunch and dinner. In spring, summer and autumn, men carried out field and garden work, while in winter and on rainy days they had to chop and saw wood.[33] The former monastery garden was newly landscaped and paths were laid. Fruit trees were planted and more beautiful and useful gardens created.[34] Schaeffer also started to assign patients for work outside the asylum's premises.[35] He explicitly commented on this innovation in the annual report of 1838/9.[36] Nearly all the wood required by officers, bureaucrats ('*Beamte*') and well-off citizens of the town was now sawn and chopped by patients. The cellars and foundations of newly built houses were dug by asylum inmates, as was the soil for a street construction project through the entire town of Zwiefalten, and more than 4,000 sheaves of grain were threshed in one year for several citizens of both Zwiefalten and the surrounding area.[37] As can be discerned from Schäffer's reports, one particular patient worked as an assistant in the registry of the forestry, foreign and post office ('*Forst-, Kameral- und Postamt*') and as an insurance expert ('*Verwaltungsaktuar*') almost continuously, to the 'complete satisfaction of these officials'. Another patient tended the garden of the brewery opposite the asylum, which had existed since monastery days. In the evenings he even served the resident head-brewer's guests. What is more, although this man had been classified as incurably mentally ill, he was on several occasions put in charge of supervising the waiters at the brewery. Yet another patient worked as a handyman to the local master-workman ('*Werkmeister*') for many months.

Patients were paid for the work they performed outside the asylum and a 'contract was made for the entire work period', to prevent the institution from suddenly withdrawing their patients when the workers were needed in the asylum itself. The salary was paid weekly, but it was small, amounting in 1838, for example, to 10 to 12 *kreuzer*. Bonuses for the guards who worked alongside patients were subtracted from patients' salaries. It was argued that 'the success of the entire thing was dependent on the initiative of the [guards] and also their clothes suffered in the process'. A further portion of the salary went towards the repair and purchase of equipment needed to carry out the work.[38] The senior guard made the calculations under the control of the director. Without authorisation, which had to be obtained in advance, no patient was allowed to work off premises. Schäffer emphasised that there was no obligation whatsoever for the patients to work and that 'the patients know that they could stop working any time if they are willing to put up with the resulting deprivations'. This, he noted, was 'one of the main differences between an asylum and a forced labour facility'.[39]

As a patient's refusal to work implied a loss of privileges and rewards, however small, some critical questions arise regarding the allegedly 'voluntary' nature of patient work and the assurance that 'no force' was applied. Patients had to choose between losing privileges and work. Psychological and social pressure may have been exerted by fellow patients in a work team and by staff keen to earn a bonus. The boundaries between well-intentioned and therapeutically meaningful occupation and economic exploitation of vulnerable, mentally ill persons may have been fluid.

As suggested by Camerer and Krimmel in 1912, Schäffer's financial and annual reports suggest that patients' health, as well as the asylum facilities at Zwiefalten, improved around the time that the director introduced the new work regime between 1838 and 1874.[40] However, both sources map only coincidence, rather than providing clear evidence for a clear causative relationship between the apparent improvements and the modified work regime. According to Camerer and Krimmel, sporadic increases in voluntary admissions during this period were due to the wider public having become aware of the favourable developments and living conditions inside the institution.[41] As a result, it did not take long for the available capacity at Zwiefalten to reach its limits.[42]

Increasing involvement in agriculture

In order to increase the economic viability of the asylum at Zwiefalten, animal husbandry was extended and six cows were purchased during the 1840s. This meant that more work opportunities were created for patients and greater independence from the previous milk delivery service was possible. Waste from the kitchen and garden was used as animal feed and mulch, and the cows' manure was used on the vegetable plots.[43] In 1851 the number of cows was increased, and in the following year 6.5 acres of fields and gardens were added.[44] In addition, ten acres of meadow land in the vicinity of the asylum were rented.

The medical directors did however experience drastic setbacks in their efforts to modernise the institution and the care of patients. In January 1849, for instance, the cellars, ground floors and the courtyards of the buildings were flooded.[45] Inmates also suffered from contagious disease, when an epidemic of cholera spread though the asylum in 1854; 40 out of 164 contracted the disease and 14 died.[46] In 1878 and 1881–82 several patients and staff became ill with typhus, and in the winter of 1889–90 an influenza epidemic caused up to 200 to be bedridden for an extended period.[47] In 1853 and 1863 storms and hail badly damaged the buildings, undoing many years of hard work devoted to the construction and maintenance of the premises.[48] What is more, it became increasingly difficult to find staff to maintain the buildings, as skilled and able workers preferred employment with the railway, in forestry, or as *gendarmes* (policemen) and tax inspectors to the 'uncomfortable duty in an asylum'.[49] The problem became even more acute during and following the Franco-Prussian war of 1870–71 due to the introduction of conscription and of a new law on marriage ('*Verehelichungsgesetz*'). These measures enabled men to make a reasonable living, albeit on a 'rather insignificant little plot of land', and it became increasingly unattractive to take up a salaried position in the asylum.[50]

When Dr Julius Ludwig August Koch became Schäffer's successor in 1874, he tried to adjust the internal management of the asylum to match his own convictions.[51] This meant that he not only closed up the institution towards the outside world, but also instigated a much stricter regime inside the asylum itself. This led to a wave of staff leaving their positions and hence high staff turnover rates, which in turn had a negative impact on the quality of care in general.

Family care and agricultural colonies

In 1896 family care was introduced at Zwiefalten.[52] The impetus for this apparently came from a foundation established by the widow of the renowned Württemberg psychiatrist Wilhelm Griesinger. By the end of 1897, twenty-four patients from Zwiefalten (or about 5 per cent of the asylum population) were transferred to family care, primarily to families of former asylum staff.[53] The care places were distributed over a number of towns, villages and farms in the vicinity of Zwiefalten. Both patients and families were selected with great care; 'care parents' or 'foster families' were even contractually obliged to treat the patients well. The asylum closely monitored the arrangement. Weekly visits by nursing staff from the asylum were routine. In many cases patients seem to have preferred care in even modest family care facilities to life in the asylum. It became apparent that they appreciated the increased independence, the more personal surroundings, and the proximity to real family life.[54]

In 1897 this form of care was also introduced at Weissenau asylum, near Ravensburg, about seventy-five kilometres away from Zwiefalten.[55] In 1902, sixty to seventy patients from Zwiefalten and Weissenau lived in psychiatric family care, i.e., in private families outside the premises of the asylums.[56] In 1904, Schussenried asylum, located just thirty kilometres from Zwiefalten, followed suit, and of an annual mean of 470 patients, fifteen were placed with, mainly, farmers' families. Most of these patients were capable of work. It was reported by the medical director of Zwiefalten, Dr Robert Gross, that in the early 1920s, 'the care placements are all good, thanks to the circumstance that – as a result of the vibrant demand – we were able to become gradually more selective.'[57] As even during the First World War food provision was better in care families than in the asylums, which were 'put on rations', patients were attracted to non-institutional care.[58]

Another form of care provision was in agricultural colonies, a system that was introduced at Zwiefalten from 1897. The picturesque Loretto property was purchased to house twelve male patients, a guard and a cook.[59] It had thirty-three acres of land and was only a short distance from the asylum. Both family care and agricultural colony schemes seem to have worked well in a number of asylums in Württemberg. Care facilities provided outside the asylums were not only convenient and comfortable for the patients, but also cheaper than in-patient care and hence involved considerable cost savings.[60] Agricultural colonies were particularly popular, as they provided patients with a degree of freedom of movement in a more or less comfortable home and they had the opportunity to occupy themselves according to their own choosing.

The positive experiences with the male colony made a similar set-up desirable for the female section at Zwiefalten asylum. A small property was therefore purchased in 1903 in a neighbouring village (Gossenzugen), just twenty minutes on foot from Zwiefalten, and turned into a female colony: 'The female colony is located on a prominent hill in the valley and thanks to its commanding location offers a charming view of the valley and of a regional hill in the background.'[61] Six patients and a guard moved into this new agricultural colony. Three goats and chickens were cared for in a barn. Both the patients and their guard were 'very comfortable in their new home' and they 'did not want to consider returning to the asylum'.[62] When, during the second year of the war in 1915, 'electric lighting was introduced … this improvement was welcomed with great joy since there was almost no petroleum available anymore and the little that was available was of low quality'.[63]

Due to continued overcrowding at Zwiefalten only severely ill patients were admitted into the asylum, while patients suitable for family care were admitted more rarely.[64] In the years between 1910 until 1912, the small number of Zwiefalten patients in family care (in comparison to national numbers) continued to decrease. Notwithstanding the low numbers, family care continued to be an alternative to institutional provision. In contrast to large parts of the German *Reich*, family care continued at Zwiefalten even during the Second World War and long after.[65] The demand for family-care patients on the farms around Zwiefalten was strong at any time, as they constituted cheap labour. As the medical director explained in the annual report of 1927, 'for the farmers the work performance of the patient was considered a primary consideration'.[66] However, the same source pointed out that in some cases 'host families continued to keep patients on account of their affection and devotion until they were in need of nursing care'.[67]

Zwiefalten provided alternative solutions to the confinement of the mentally ill as in-patients on psychiatric wards by establishing agricultural colonies and making use of psychiatric family care. This affected a broadening of the range of work therapy options. However, the therapeutic mind sets and practices of senior staff proved a limiting factor in this process. Economic factors, too, had a bearing on the extent to which improvements in patient care could be implemented. Notwithstanding these challenges, medical directors and other senior staff at Zwiefalten managed to achieve a reorganisation of the institutional care and work structures. It is particularly noteworthy that they successfully implemented the family care and agricultural colonies structures, which required a higher degree of managerial skills and awareness of and dedication to the needs of the various stakeholders than was the case in the running of a mental hospital. The following section explores the eminent role of political ideology in the design and evaluation of patient work.

The First World War

The war years saw far-reaching changes for asylums in Württemberg. In particular these affected the organisation of work regimes and associated tasks. First of all, the mobilisation for war led to dramatic shortages in asylum staff. Within a month of the outbreak of war, in August 1914, there was a staff shortage, leaving just '[75 per cent] of all guards ... as a result of which service provision especially on the wards for restless patients was compromised to the highest degree'.[68] Even though recruitment officers at the asylum were no longer 'very selective' when they hired temporary guards and attendants, it became necessary to cancel patients' walks and outings, and to considerably decrease patient work 'due to a lack of suitable supervisory staff'.[69] In consequence, the work regime for male inmates was restructured. In contrast, there were plenty of female staff members, since women who had a well-paid position did not wish to lose it while their husbands, brothers or fathers were in the war and unable to contribute to their families' incomes. The authorities considered it inappropriate for women to supervise male patients, and hence garden and field work at the asylum were in danger of being neglected and of impacting on food supply.

The general food shortage, which became increasingly acute during the course of the war, led to an increase in patient mortality in southern German asylums. The consequences of the hyperinflations of 1919 and 1923, followed by the national currency reform of 1923, manifested themselves in the years following the war and, to a certain degree, replicated the economic emergency situation of the war. The exact causes of death during this period and the numbers of those dying from starvation-related diseases has to date been only partially verified. Many asylum inmates died of lung and gastro-intestinal tuberculosis, the common cold, and typhus.[70] As a result of the typhus epidemic in 1918, lack of fuel and hence of warm water, and a considerable shortage of bed linen, garments and underwear[71] made it practically impossible to maintain healthy hygiene standards. In order to confront this state of emergency, it was decided to cultivate flax on the land attached to the asylum in order to produce linen.[72] To secure the supply of elementary needs such as food, heating, light, and warm water, asylum authorities considered the purchase of an additional land domain and the construction of its own water-treatment plant.[73] It is very likely that these circumstances led to a deterioration of the conditions and therapeutic effects of patient work in the asylum and inmates were no longer free to choose engagement in particular tasks. Given the general crisis situation during and after the war, it is important to assess to what extent patient work became solely subject to economic considerations, with therapeutic considerations being sidelined if not absolutely abandoned.[74]

The years of the Weimar Republic

In 1924, the Annual Report emphasised that even pensive and tranquil Zwiefalten was affected by the political currents and upheavals of the Weimar period. The economic crisis of the post-war era, social problems, and the resulting insecurity and dissatisfaction of the population were not limited to political centres and large cities. People in asylums also vented their resentment. 'Due to strikes and threats of strikes', there were disputes between the senior medical officer, two party secretaries and subordinate staff. These had effects on work in the asylum, including patient work. Staff and party secretaries were confronted with the management's insistence 'that it was not possible to continue to cut working hours'.[75] Towards the end of the 1920s, there was a precarious shortage of physicians and medical interns, with detrimental effects on therapies such as bed rest or bed treatment, continuous baths, and, later, sedative medication. By the beginning of the 1930s, large numbers of patients were still not able to pursue any work. What is more, in order to focus on their 'curable' patients, psychiatric clinics attached to German universities transferred chronically ill patients to the asylums, where limited economic and staff resources did not allow doctors to conduct research on how to improve the medical therapies and work regimes. This became all too obvious in Zwiefalten.

Psychiatry during National Socialism

National Socialist health doctrine was based on a preventive notion of racial hygiene and sterilisation and, from 1939, mooted even to murder those 'unworthy of living'. It put labour and the ability to work in the centre of decision making. Together with a reinterpreted notion of work therapy or *Aktivere Krankenbehandlung*, the shock therapies, established and developed during the 1930s, supported German psychiatrists' self-perception of being members of a therapeutically active discipline that aimed at cure.[76] Given this perspective, patients whose therapy did not prove successful were considered to be incurable, hopeless cases. In those situations where patients' conditions prevented them from engaging in regular work their lives were in danger from those among the medical staff who were responsible for the selection of victims for euthanasia. This horrifying scenario existed at Zwiefalten asylum from the late 1930s to the end of the Second World War.[77]

Due to its geographically secluded location, which was nonetheless useful for the purposes of the *Reich*, the asylum – in line with Nazi health policy – took on a central role in the decline of psychiatry during this period. The asylum of Zwiefalten became the last regional station for many patients on their way to death by gassing in Grafeneck, a mere twenty minutes by car from Zwiefalten. As alleged hopeless cases, chronically ill patients received attention from the regime and from local representatives of racial hygiene, who were trying to promote a 'hereditarily healthy body of people'.[78] Almost 500 of the patients who had received long-term treatment in Zwiefalten were murdered. They were deported in buses, with the windows painted in grey to prevent the passengers from looking out and outsiders from looking in. Most of these victims were murdered during campaign 'central euthanasia' ('T4') at Grafeneck, others at Hadamar in Hesse. A total of more than 1,500 persons, who were admitted to Zwiefalten during the war years, perished as a result of malnutrition, inadequate care and infectious disease or were victims of secret killing by means of 'decentralised euthanasia'. During the National Socialist era, or at least from 1939 onwards, the inability to work became the decisive criterion for being selected for systematic mass murder.

Conclusion

During the second half of the nineteenth century, the majority of patients at Zwiefalten asylum were regularly engaged in work inside and outside the asylum.[79] As a *Pflegeanstalt* this institution was dedicated to the care of incurables or chronic patients.[80] Patients were either looked after in the asylum until they died or worked and were cared for within family care and agricultural colony settings. The lack of detailed medical documentation can be accounted for by the care and work focus of the institution and the relative absence of therapeutic intervention. In many cases, merely one case-book entry per patient per calendar year was provided and a break of several years between entries was not unusual. Therapeutic considerations with regard to work can therefore be reconstructed only with difficulty. In the majority of cases recovery and discharge were rare, and cures unlikely.

A large number of patients at Zwiefalten had been ill for years, if not decades, prior to admission. On entering the institution, many were in a desperate situation in which they themselves, as well as their families, were overwhelmed by the social and personal demands required in the care and treatment of mentally ill people. Some patients endangered themselves, with self-destructive behaviour, and others during violent outbursts. For the families, the asylum could be considered as a relief. Ideally, the institution was supposed to provide patients with an environment in which they could live a life of dignity and without fear, and where they could, to a modest degree, develop individually. Work served as a measure to structure the day and relieve the maintenance costs for the institution. A wage, which allowed working patients to purchase small items functioned as an incentive.

However, the 1890s brought significant changes, when Zwiefalten asylum became a '*Heil- und Pflegeanstalt*', namely a place for both the care and cure of chronically ill as well as curable patients, respectively. Work practices became diversified, and patients worked in the asylum, in agricultural colonies, and within family care settings. As conditions deteriorated due to overcrowding and, during and following the First World War, on account of staff and food shortages, therapeutic measures and the principle of inmates' freedom to choose their chores became restricted. Global and national events and developments had local repercussions.

Patients who engaged in work within family care and agricultural colony settings appear to have enjoyed their relative independence and during the interwar years in particular might have experienced better living conditions than inmates left to work within the asylum itself. Work opportunities for those confined in the asylum itself became increasingly scarce on account of the lack of suitable supervisory staff on the male wards in particular. Epidemic diseases as well as food shortages had a fatal impact on those who were not involved in family care or agricultural colonies.

The end of the First World War and the early Weimar years did not lead to improvements in conditions inside the asylum, nor did political changes effect the re-establishment of work therapy. Strikes and social upheaval affected rural Swabia, impacting on medical and care regimes during the interwar period. The continued shortage of trained nursing staff, as one among other consequences of the war, as well as the general lack of physicians, which hit psychiatry particularly badly in the late 1920s, constituted structural barriers to therapeutic practice. New treatments such as the rest cure distracted staff attention away from work and occupational therapy. In contrast to the period prior to the First World War, a large number of asylum patients were no longer actively engaged in work by the 1930s. Finally, from the 1930s onwards, the inability to work (rather than diagnostic considerations or the alleged heredity of mental illness, as has so often been suggested by historians) became the decisive criterion for numerous patients' extermination by means of central or decentralised euthanasia.

Notes

1 See, among other recent publications, Jürgen Kocka (ed.), *Work in a Modern Society. The German Historical Experience in Comparative Perspective* (Oxford: Berghahn Books, 2013).
2 For example, Global History of Agrarian Labor Regimes, 1750–2000, organised by the Weatherhead Initiative on Global History, Harvard University, Cambridge, MA. See www.hsozkult.gschichte.hu-berlin.de/termine/id=21607 (accessed 6 March 2015).
3 See Sabine Lichtenberger and Günter Müller (eds), *'Arbeit ist das halbe Leben … .' Erzählungen vom Wandel der Arbeitswelten seit 1945* (Vienna: Böhlau, 2012). The Vienna International Conference of Labour and Social History (ITH) in 2014 focused on 'Work and compulsion: Coerced labour in domestic, service, agricultural, factory and sex work, c. 1850–2000', and put emphasis on the exploitative aspects of labour, also touching on matters of slavery. See www.hsozkult. geschichte.hu-berlin.de/termine/id=22839 (accessed 6 March 2015).
4 See the collaborative research project of Birkbeck, University of London, The Pears Institute for the Study of Anti-Semitism and the Wiener Library, London, seeking to explore the interaction between 'labour' and 'race' especially in modern German history, www.hsozkult.geschichte.hu-berlin.de/termine/id=22407 (accessed 6 March 2015).
5 See the Swiss research programme (*Schweizerisches Sozialarchiv*) in transnational perspective, initiated by Zürich historian Jakob Tanner, www.h-sozkult.geschichte. hu-berlin.de/termine/id=21632 (accessed 6 March 2015).
6 See the 2013 contributions of Eastern European and South-Eastern European histo-

rians to the conference 'Nicht-Arbeit': multidisziplinäre Auseinandersetzungen mit einer analytischen Kategorie, organised by Stefano Petrungaro in Regensburg, www.hsozkult.geschichte.hu-berlin.de/tagungsberichte/id=5103 (accessed 6 March 2015).

7 Martina Huber and Thomas Müller, 'Patientenarbeit in Zwiefalten. Institutionelle Arbeitsformen des ausgehenden 19. Jahrhunderts zwischen therapeutischem Anspruch und ökonomischem Interesse', in Thomas Müller, Bernd Reichelt and Uta Kanis-Seyfried (eds), *Nach dem Tollhaus. Zur Geschichte der ersten Königlich-Württembergischen Staatsirrenanstalt Zwiefalten. Vol. 1 Psychiatrie, Kultur und Gesellschaft in historischer Perspektive* (Zwiefalten: Verlag Psychiatrie und Geschichte, 2012), pp. 71–84; Thomas Müller and Uta Kanis-Seyfried, 'Eine kurze Geschichte der Psychiatrie Württembergs am Beispiel der Anstalt Zwiefalten', in Müller *et al.* (eds), *Nach dem Tollhaus*, pp. 9–56. The current chapter is an extended version of an earlier publication: Thomas Müller, 'Patienten-Arbeit in ländlichen psychiatrischen Anstalten im Spannungsfeld zwischen therapeutischem Zweck und ökonomischem Nutzen', in Monika Ankele and Eva Brinkschulte (eds), *Arbeitsrhythmus und Anstaltsalltag*, (Stuttgart: Steiner Verlag, 2015), pp. 51–70. On this subject see also Thomas Beddies, '"Aktivere Krankenbehandlung" und "Arbeitstherapie". Anwendungsformen und Begründungszusammenhänge bei Hermann Simon und Carl Schneider', in Hans-Walther Schmuehl and Volker Roelcke (eds), *'Heroische Therapien'. Die deutsche Psychiatrie im internationalen Vergleich, 1918–1945* (Göttingen: Wallstein, 2013), pp. 268–86.

8 Rescript by King Friedrich I of Württemberg on the transmittance of patients from the Ludwigsburg 'madhouse' ('*Tollhaus*') to Zwiefalten, 10 May 1811. Hauptstaatsarchiv at Stuttgart (hereafter HStA), E 31, BÜ 1080, 'Verzeichnis der nach Zwiefalten zu transportierenden Irren, und der zweckmäßigsten Art ihres Transports', 3 March 1812. Zwiefalten Library, 'Dokumente zur Gründung der königlichen Irrenanstalt Zwiefalten 1812–1817'. See also Staatsarchiv Ludwigsburg (hereafter StA LB), under E 163, BÜ 674, 675, 714.

9 On the history of psychiatry, both in general as well as concerning the specific case of Zwiefalten, see the series of publications by Renate Wittern, 'Vom Tollhaus zur psychiatrischen Klinik – Zur staatlichen Irrenpflege im Württemberg des 19. Jahrhunderts', in Hans Schadewaldt and Jörn Henning Wolf (eds), *Krankenhausmedizin im 19. Jahrhundert*, Schriftenreihe der Münchner Vereinigung für Geschichte der Medizin (München: Demeter, 1983), pp. 112–27; Wittern, 'Zur Geschichte der psychiatrischen Versorgung in Deutschland im 19. Jahrhundert', in Deutscher Paritätischer Wohlfahrtsverband (ed.), *Zur Rehabilitation in der Psychiatrie* (München: München-Germering: Braun, 1988), par. 3.1.1.

10 Rudolf Camerer and Emil Krimmel, *Geschichte der Königl. württembergischen Heilanstalt Zwiefalten 1812–1912* (Stuttgart: Greinr und Pfeiffer, Königl. Hofdrucker, 1912), pp. 79–80. An archive series called 'Etatberichte Zwiefalten' has been a main source for this chapter. So-called 'Etatberichte' represented a kind of further annual report by the medical director. Although they focused on financial data, medical information was still included. Etatbericht Zwiefalten (hereafter Etatbericht), 1838/39, sect. I, pp. 24–5. See also the report of a visiting

commission ('Bericht Kommission Besichtigung Kloster Zwiefalten') of 18 May 1811 at StA LB, D 39, BÜ 804 ('Genehmigung mit K. Dekret 5 July 1811'). This source has also been studied by Isabel Hegenbarth, 'Von der Verwahrung zur Behandlung. Die Anfänge des "Königlichen Irrenhauses Zwiefalten", betrachtet vor dem Hintergrund der entstehenden Psychiatrie des frühen 19. Jahrhunderts' (MA dissertation, University of Tübingen, 1994), p. 50.

11 See the earlier publication in German, Huber and Müller, 'Patientenarbeit in Zwiefalten', in Müller et al. (eds), Nach dem Tollhaus, pp. 71–84.

12 Müller and Kanis-Seyfried, 'Eine kurze Geschichte', in Müller et al. (eds), Nach dem Tollhaus, pp. 9–56.

13 For example at Bayreuth where Johann Gottfried Langermann reconstructed the madhouse in 1805 into a medical institution for the mentally ill. Also in the Saxonian town of Pirna-Sonnenstein in 1811, or in Schleswig, Northern Germany, at Stadtfeld, in 1820, as well as the renowned 'Sachsenberg' close to the city of Schwerin on the Baltic in 1830. Compare with Wittern, 'Zur Geschichte der psychiatrischen Versorgung', in Deutscher Paritätischer Wohlfahrtsverband (ed.), Zur Rehabilitation, par. 3.1.1. See also Asmus Finzen, Das Pinelsche Pendel. Die Dimension des Sozialen im Zeitalter der biologischen Psychiatrie, in Sozialpsychiatrische Texte series (Bonn: Psychiatrie-Verlag, 1998), pp. 10–39, 10–13.

14 Heinz Schott and Rainer Tölle (eds), Geschichte der Psychiatrie (München: Beck, 2006), p. 436; Roy Porter, Wahnsinn. Eine kleine Kulturgeschichte (Zürich: Dörlemann, 2005).

15 Dr Narciß Schreiber, Medical Director of Zwiefalten asylum 1812–17.

16 Camerer and Krimmel, Geschichte, pp. 29, 79.

17 Dr Andreas Elser, Medical Director of Zwiefalten asylum 1817–37.

18 Dr Carl von Schäffer, Medical Director of Zwiefaltern asylum 1838–74. Various versions of the name were in use: in the birth register Karl Schaeffer; in publications Karl Schäffer, Carl Schaeffer, or Carl Schäffer. In this chapter the form Carl Schäffer has been used throughout.

19 Camerer and Krimmel, Geschichte, p. 34.

20 Ibid., pp. 79–81.

21 Dr Julius Koch, Medical Director of Zwiefalten asylum 1874–98.

22 Camerer and Krimmel, Geschichte, p. 117. Patients were also involved in house construction, ibid., p. 119.

23 Ibid., pp. 101, 130.

24 Schott and Tölle, Geschichte, p. 436, and the following paragraphs.

25 Camerer and Krimmel, Geschichte, p. 101.

26 Ibid., p. 29. See also StA LB, E 163, BÜ 766 ('Visitationsbericht Zwiefalten' of 30 August 1816).

27 See Camerer and Krimmel, Geschichte, p. 25.

28 The source lacks clear information on the precise amount of money offered. In 1817, however, the maximum tariff per person per day had been fixed ('jeder Person, die arbeite, täglich 8 Kreuzer gegeben werden dürften'). See Camerer and Krimmel, Geschichte, p. 29. About the refreshments see Etatbericht, 1838/39, sect. I, p. 30.

29 Etatbericht, 1838/39, sect. I, p. 13.
30 Etatbericht, 1838/39, sect. I, p. 14.
31 Etatbericht, 1838/39, sect. I, p. 14.
32 Camerer and Krimmel, *Geschichte*, p. 79; Etatbericht, 1838/39, sect. I, pp. 16–17.
33 Camerer and Krimmel, *Geschichte*, pp. 79–80; Etatbericht, 1838/39, sect. I, pp. 24–5.
34 Etatbericht, 1838/39, sect. I, pp. 125–6. For further sources see also Müller and Kanis-Seyfried, 'Eine kurze Geschichte', in Müller *et al.* (eds), *Nach dem Tollhaus*, p. 24.
35 Camerer and Krimmel, *Geschichte*, pp. 79–80.
36 Etatbericht, 1838/39, sect. I, pp. 1–41, especially pp. 8–16 and 20–34.
37 Here and in the following paragraph quotations relate to Etatbericht, 1838/39, sect. I, pp. 27, 29 and 30.
38 Etatbericht, 1838/39, sect. I, p. 30.
39 Camerer and Krimmel, *Geschichte*, pp. 76–7; Etatbericht, 1838/39, sect. I, pp. 20–34, 32–3 ('Der Unterzeichnete legt hier auf die Worte "ohne allen anderen Zwang" ein besonderes Gewicht … daß die Kranken wissen, daß sie aufhören können zu arbeiten, wenn sie sich nur die damit verbundenen Entbehrungen gefallen lassen wollen, einer der Hauptunterschiede einer solchen Pflegeanstalt von einem Zwangsarbeitshause ausgedrückt ist und braucht … einem bald mehr freundlichen, bald mehr ernsten, ermunternden Zuspruch … keine Art von Strafe oder Zwang gegen irgend einen Kranken angewandt worden, um ihn zur Arbeit zu nöthigen.').
40 Camerer and Krimmel, *Geschichte*, p. 85.
41 *Ibid.*
42 Despite this 'Oberregierungsrat Geßler', as reporting agent to the ministry ('*Referent des Ministeriums*'), reported only positively on the asylum after his visit in 1851. See Camerer and Krimmel, *Geschichte*, p. 100. This pertains to the years 1812 to 1834, during which Zwiefalten had the status of an asylum for the curable ('*Heilanstalt*'). It was referred to as an asylum for the curable again in 1899.
43 Camerer and Krimmel, *Geschichte*, p. 98.
44 *Ibid.*, p. 101.
45 Etatbericht, 1848/49, no. XI, pp. 14–15. Most probably Schäffer is here referring to 'democratic ideas' related to the proponents of the 1848 Revolution in German Lands.
46 Etatbericht, 1854/55, no. XVII, pp. 10–11.
47 Camerer und Krimmel, *Geschichte*, pp. 100, 133; HstA, E 151/53, *Annual Report of the Medical Director* (hereafter *Ärztlicher Jahresbericht*) for the year 1890, p. 10.
48 Etatbericht, 1863/64, sect. XXVI, p. 16.
49 Camerer and Krimmel, *Geschichte*, p. 109.
50 *Ibid.*, p. 112.
51 *Ibid.*, p. 114.
52 On the history of psychiatric family care in the German Reich (of 1871) see, for example, Paul-Otto Schmidt, *Asylierung oder familiale Versorgung. Die Vorträge auf der Sektion Psychiatrie der Gesellschaft deutscher Naturforscher und Ärzte bis 1885*

(Husum: Matthiesen, 1982); Michael Konrad and Paul-Otto Schmidt-Michel (eds), *Die zweite Familie. Psychiatrische Familienpflege – Geschichte, Praxis, Forschung* (Bonn: Psychiatrie Verlag, 1993); Thomas Müller, e.g. 'Community spaces and psychiatric family care in Belgium, France and Germany. A comparative study', in Leslie Topp, James Moran and Jonathan Andrews (eds), *Madness, Architecture and the Built Environment: Psychiatric Spaces in Historical Context* (London: Routledge, 2007), pp. 171–89; or Thomas Müller, 'Re-opening a closed file of the history of psychiatry: Open care and its historiography in Belgium, France and Germany, c. 1880–1980', in Waltraud Ernst and Thomas Müller (eds), *Transnational Psychiatries: Social and Cultural Histories of Psychiatry in Comparative Perspective, c. 1800–2000* (Newcastle: Cambridge Scholars, 2010), pp. 172–99.
53   Konrad Alt, *Die familiäre Verpflegung der Kranksinnigen in Deutschland* (Halle a.d. Saale: Carl Marhold, 1903), p. 17.
54   *Ibid.*, p. 42.
55   *Ibid.*, p. 17.
56   Robert Groß, 'Landes-Heilanstalt Schussenried', *Psychiatrisch-Neurologische Wochenschrift*, 22 (1921), 32–3.
57   *Ibid.*
58   *Ibid.*
59   HstA, E 151/53, BÜ 537, 'Pflegeanstalt Zwiefalten', *Ärztlicher Jahresbericht 1897*, p. 19, 'An agricultural farm, the "Lorettohof", as well as farming land at the "Bronnstaigäcker", had been bought by the asylum itself and included into its financial administration.'
60   Camerer and Krimmel, *Geschichte*, pp. 142, 168.
61   HstA, E 151/53, Ärztlicher Jahresbericht 1904, p. 29.
62   Both quotations are from HstA, E 151/53, Ärztlicher Jahresbericht 1904, p. 29.
63   HstA, E 151/53, Ärztlicher Jahresbericht 1915, p. 31.
64   Camerer and Krimmel, *Geschichte*, p. 168.
65   HstA, E 151/53, Ärztlicher Jahresbericht. See especially the reports for: *1941 p. 8; 1944, p. 6; 1946, p. 6; 1948, p. 7; 1858, p. 10; and 1959, p. 13. For an early historiographical description of these facts see* Reinhold Eisenhut, 'Familienpflege in Zwiefalten während des Nationalsozialismus', in Hermann J. Pretsch (ed.), *Euthanasie. Krankenmorde in Südwestdeutschland* (Zwiefalten: Psychiatrie und Geschichte, 1996), pp. 47–50.
66   HstA, E 151/53, Ärztlicher Jahresbericht. See the reports for 1927, p. 25; 1941, p. 8; and 1944, p. 6.
67   HstA, E 151/53, Ärztlicher Jahresbericht 1927, p. 25.
68   HstA, E 151/53, Ärztlicher Jahresbericht 1914, p. 27.
69   *Ibid.*, for both quotes.
70   HstA, E 151/53, Ärztlicher Jahresbericht 1917, p. 21.
71   HstA, E 151/53, Ärztlicher Jahresbericht 1920, p. 37.
72   HstA, E 151/53, Ärztlicher Jahresbericht 1918, p. 21.
73   HstA, E 151/53, Ärztlicher Jahresbericht 1920, p. 38.
74   In contrast to Zwiefalten, neighbouring asylums like Weissenau near Ravensburg met conditions of restructuring in that they were involved in military planning

during both world wars. Weissenau was transformed into a military hospital ('*Militärlazarett*'), mainly though not exclusively for the care of soldiers with traumatic neuroses ('*Traumatische Neurosen*') or 'war neuroses' ('*Kriegsneurosen*'), what, in retrospect to us, seems to meet current diagnostic criteria for post-traumatic stress disorders (PTSD).

75 HstA, E 151/53, Ärztlicher Jahresbericht 1924, p. 10.
76 See, for example, Gerrit Hohendorf, 'Therapieunfähigkeit als Selektionskriterium. Die "Schocktherapieverfahren" und die Organisationszentrale der nationalsozialistischen "Euthanasie" in der Berliner Tiergartenstraße 4, 1939–1945', in Hans-Walther Schmuehl and Volker Roelcke (eds), *'Heroische Therapien'. Die deutsche Psychiatrie im internationalen Vergleich, 1918–1945* (Göttingen: Wallstein Verlag, 2013), pp. 287–307.
77 Iris Pollmann and Thomas Müller, 'Dr Martha Fauser – eine württembergische Psychiaterin in der NS-Zeit', in Bernd Holdorff (ed.), *Schriftenreihe der Deutschen Gesellschaft für die Geschichte der Nervenheilkunde* (Würzburg: Königshausen and Neumann, 2011), vol. 17, pp. 63–76.
78 Thomas Müller and Thomas Beddies, 'Psychiatrie und Psychotherapie im nationalsozialistischen Deutschland. Teil I: Die Psychiatrie', *Psychologische Medizin. Österreichische Fachzeitschrift für medizinische Psychologie, Psychosomatik und Psychotherapie*, 15 (2004), 16–23; Thomas Müller and Thomas Beddies, 'Life unworthy of living'. Psychiatry in National Socialist Germany', *International Journal for Mental Health*, 35:3 (2006), 94–104.
79 Huber and Müller, 'Patientenarbeit in Zwiefalten', in Müller *et al.* (eds), *Nach dem Tollhaus*, pp. 71–84, and the examples of patients provided in this publication.
80 Camerer and Krimmel, *Geschichte*, p. 120.

11

The patient's view of work therapy: The mental hospital Hamburg-Langenhorn during the Weimar Republic

Monika Ankele

This chapter focuses on the Weimar period (1919–33) and the German mental hospital (*Staatskrankenanstalt*) Hamburg-Langenhorn. It examines the wider political and social factors that impacted on work therapy. My emphasis will be on how patients perceived their role as inmates, how they reacted to work therapy and how they dealt with an uncertain future on their discharge from the institution. I will argue that work therapy meant different things to different people at different times. Looking at the practice of work therapy provides an insight into its manifold effects. Thus I am going to show that work therapy opened up new possibilities for those patients who were capable of working, but that it had devastating consequences during the Nazi era for those unable to work. Case records as well as documents written by the patients themselves will be used to engage with several questions concerning the role of patient work during the 1920s.

The Hamburg-Langenhorn asylum

The end of the First World War marked the end of the German *Kaiserreich* (1871–1918), and the revolution of 1918 led to the proclamation of the Republic and a new democratic constitution in 1919. The Weimar period was shaped by civil-war-like conditions in the first years of the Republic and by hyperinflation, followed by poverty and high unemployment, and by a short period of economic expansion and political stability (the so called 'golden age'), with conditions starting to deteriorate during the Great Depression of 1929 and leading to the transition to the Nazi era in 1933. In German history the Weimar period still stands for (failed) democratisation, for the implementation and development of the welfare system, for social reforms as well as for the strengthening of organised labour.

The *Irren-Colonie* at Langenhorn was founded in 1893 on the outskirts of the city of Hamburg. Hamburg was a city-state of the *Kaiserreich* as well as the Weimar Republic, governed by the Senate. At the turn of the twentieth century, Hamburg had a population of 706,000.[1] It was already the second largest industrial city in Germany (after Berlin) and due to the large port an important commercial and trade city.[2] There was no uniform law in either the *Kaiserreich* or the Weimar Republic to govern the institutionalisation, accommodation and discharge of the mentally ill. As a city-state, Hamburg deployed its own law in this regard, as was the case in all other German territories.

The *Irren-Colonie* at Langenhorn was conceived as a subsidiary of the institution at Friedrichsberg, founded in 1864 as the first asylum in Hamburg. Only a few years after its opening, Friedrichsberg had become overcrowded and a new asylum was urgently needed. Langenhorn was founded as an agricultural colony – combining the care of the mentally ill with work on the land. The colony was supposed to admit only those male and female patients from Friedrichsberg who were calm, chronically ill and able to work. Patients were to be occupied on the basis of their abilities and in accordance with medical considerations.[3] Gender relations at the time dictated that men should work in agriculture and in workshops, and women in the kitchen, garden, laundry and sewing rooms. From the beginning, work therapy was a central part of the treatment regime at Langenhorn, as it had been in many other asylums since the beginning of the nineteenth century. In the 1920s, when Hermann Simon's (1867–1947) 'more active therapy' became prominent in Germany, Langenhorn referred proudly to its long history of work therapy.[4]

The significance of work, especially of physical labour, in the recovery of the mentally ill had one of its origins in 'dietetics', which had been an important aspect of medicine from antiquity to the nineteenth century and also had an impact on alienists' ideas about the treatment of the insane.[5] 'Dietetics' can be explained as a set of principles for the appropriate management of life in both a medical and ethical sense. Dietetics prescribed a balance between eating and drinking (*cibus et potus*), sleep and waking (*somus et vigilia*), light and air (*aer*), secretion and excretion (*repletio et evacutio*), the affects (*accidentia*) as well as between physical labour and rest (*motus et quies*). Any disturbance of balance could lead to a disease. Commitment to an asylum as well as the institutional conditions – the daily routines, the change between work and recreation, the chosen location – were supposed to be arranged on the basis of dietetic principles. Work was a pivotal element of the treatment of the insane in German asylums, and location as well as architecture played an important role in the provision of a variety of work opportunities, especially in the open air.[6]

The eminent German psychiatrist Christian Friedrich Wilhelm Roller (1802–78) in his book *Die Irrenanstalt nach allen ihren Beziehungen* of 1831 outlined the knowledge of his time; placing emphasis on occupations in the fresh air like gardening and field work.[7] A central idea was to keep the hands of the patients occupied with some useful work in order to divert their thoughts from focusing on delusions or fantasies and bring them back to the material world. By citing famous psychiatrists like Jean-Étienne Dominique Esquirol (1772–1840), Philippe Pinel (1745–1826) and Maximilian Jacobi (1775–1858), Roller claimed that every asylum should offer their patients manifold possibilities to work and that the chosen activities should be adapted to the patients' conditions and abilities.[8] The attendants should provide instruction for the inmates and hard-working patients should be recompensed. The aim of this method of treatment was not only to relax and tire the patients, as Roller emphasised, but also to enable them to realise the usefulness of their work as well as its value for the asylum.[9] Very similar arguments concerning the intent of work therapy can be found in the 1920s, albeit in a completely different historical setting.

Langenhorn, conceived as an agricultural colony for the mentally ill (*Irren-Colonie*), was located on the outskirts of Hamburg, fifteen kilometres from the city, in a nearly uninhabited area surrounded by woods, moors and heath.[10] The village of Langenhorn was at a distance of three kilometres from the asylum and could only be reached by a horse bus.[11] The *Irren-Colonie* was built in the pavilion style with an open-plan system that was very popular in the construction of hospitals and asylums at the end of the nineteenth century. The different buildings were spread across the grounds, divided by a main axis to separate men and women. The agricultural buildings were located on the eastern side and the area was bounded by woods, fields, and gardens. There was no wall or fence until the end of the 1920s to separate the hospital from the adjacent grounds. This layout was supposed to offer patients a maximum of individual freedom and create a village-like atmosphere (*dorfartiges Gepräge*)[12] rather than a prison-like surrounding. Initially the *Irren-Colonie* was projected to house 200 patients, but over the years it was extended steadily, so that by 1914, before the outbreak of the First World War, beds for almost 2,000 patients were available.[13] The asylum (now called *Irrenanstalt*) was then open for all kinds of patients, not only for those who were diagnosed as 'chronic' yet able to work. At that time Langenhorn ranked among the largest *Irrenanstalten* of the German *Kaiserreich*.

Bed rest and prolonged bath treatment, the consequences of the First World War on the concept of 'healing', and Hermann Simon's 'more active therapy'

At the beginning of the twentieth century new methods of treatment entered the stage in German asylums and put work therapy (temporarily) in the background. The so-called 'bed rest' (*Bettbehandlung*) and 'prolonged bath' treatments (*Dauerbad*) were introduced as a combined therapy especially for restless patients by well-known psychiatrists like Emil Kraepelin (1856–1926) and Clemens Neisser (1861–1940).[14] Patients were put to bed or in the bathtub for days and weeks and even months, as reported by Kraepelin and his colleagues.[15] Following psychiatrist Wilhelm Griesinger's (1817–68) famous statement of 1845 that mental diseases were brain diseases,[16] the new treatments were aimed at bringing relaxation to the affected brain (*Gehirnruhe*) and were therefore seen as somatic therapies based on their physiological impact on the brain.[17] Furthermore, these treatments heightened patients' realisation and acknowledgment that they suffered from mental illness (*Krankheitseinsicht*), which was considered as an important step on the road to recovery. Lying in bed, especially by day, was associated with being physically ill and therefore helped to make patients realise that they were indeed suffering from some kind of affliction. These new methods were rapidly spreading at the beginning of the twentieth century, leading to the temporary decline of work therapy, until its revival during the Weimar period.[18]

The First World War constituted a break regarding psychiatric practice. Soldiers who suffered from war neuroses were, among other forms of treatment,[19] successfully treated by means of work therapy. Success was defined in relation to the restored employability of men needed as workers in war industries, given that it was considered inappropriate to send them back to the trenches.[20] Within this context the idea of treating the somatic cause of a mental disease receded in favour of an approach that was intended to induce the remission of the symptoms and hence the recovery of employability. The parameters of an achievement-oriented society, based on the worth of labour, were gradually adopted as therapeutic aims. This paved the way, as suggested by Hans-Ludwig Siemen, for psychiatric reforms in the Weimar Republic.[21] These reforms can be described as the 'opening-up' of the care of the mentally ill in two respects, first, the introduction of 'open care' (*offene Fürsorge*)[22] and provision for patients outside the asylum, and, second, the reintegration of patients into the process of production in line with the needs of the welfare state and the wider economy.

Another factor that led to changes in institutional practice related to the experiences and needs of mental hospital doctors. German psychiatrist Hermann Simon, whose name is strongly linked to the boost of work therapy in the 1920s, is a case in point. His concept of a 'more active therapy' (*aktivere Krankenbehandlung*) was based on the belief that 'the root of all evil' is idleness: 'Idleness is the beginning not only of all vice – or antisocial tendencies, as we call it in our patients – but also of impending idiocy.'[23] He strongly criticised what he perceived as the excessive application of bed rest and prolonged bathing, and described the surveillance wards (*Wachsäle*)[24] for chronically ill and quiet patients as a 'cemetery of ghosts' (*Friedhof der Geister*),[25] where patients vegetated bodily and mentally, became increasingly apathetic and lost their social abilities.[26] While the body seemed to repose, the mind stayed restless. Simon advocated 'more activity', not only on the part of the patients but also in relation to the attendants and doctors.

Simon was director at the asylum in Warstein, where he developed his ideas at the beginning of the twentieth century. As this new institution was still under construction after its inauguration in 1905, Simon set patients to work. At the beginning he selected only those inmates who were fit to work, but soon also those who were laid up or in a state of agitation. He noticed that the atmosphere in the mental hospital became less violent, calmer and more orderly than it had been before, and sedative drugs and isolation had to be used less frequently. When Simon published his experiences in the *Allgemeine Zeitschrift für Psychiatrie* in 1927, he was director at the mental hospital at Gütersloh, where he had begun to work in 1919.[27] Gütersloh became a model institution for his method of treatment and psychiatrists from all over Germany and other countries came here to get an idea of its application and effects. The innovative part of Simon's ideas was that unlike in earlier applications of work therapy, when treatment was only to be applied to convalescent patients, the 'more active therapy' was intended for all kinds of patients and at any stage of their illness. According to Simon, every mental patient should be set to work immediately after admission to an institution, being initially assigned a simple task, to be followed by activities that required autonomy and responsibility.[28] Patients should no longer be perceived as 'children', irresponsible for their actions, as had been common in the nineteenth century. Work therapy as a form of psychotherapy was supposed to be anchored in an orderly community and adapted to its needs, with patients taking responsibility for themselves as well as for others. Education was the keyword in this regard.[29]

During the Weimar period, work became the essence of the psychiatric institution, the centre of its organisation. In this respect, mental hospitals came to resemble other welfare institutions such as alms-houses, youth centres, correctional facilities, inebriate asylums, but also prisons, where the work of the inmates was pivotal and described as a substantial means of education. Work was also useful to offset the cost of patients' maintenance in these institutions.[30] From 1930, with the opening of the department for work and welfare (*Arbeitsfürsorge*), employability became the criterion for welfare benefits in Hamburg.[31]

It was not until the 1920s that Simon's approach achieved wider attention among psychiatrists. This was for two reasons. First, biological and social Darwinist ideas, on which Simon's ideas were based, explicitly formulated in the second part of his book of 1929,[32] began to be received more widely among psychiatrists. Second, due to the economic crisis during this period, psychiatrists were forced to focus on cost savings and cheaper forms of institutional care. It was economically and socially important to decrease the number of inmates in costly institutions, and work therapy was presented as one way to achieve this. The aims of work therapy resonated strongly with social and political mores that lay beyond the realm of the merely medical. They were directly connected with the interests of the state. No longer was the cure of patients the primary ambition. Rather it was their reintegration into the labour market and process of production. Cure and 'healing' were therefore no longer primarily directed at a somatic disorder and its possible causes.

Employment constituted one of the cornerstones of the Weimar Republic. Historic developments, such as inflation, high unemployment, the Great Depression, as well as internal conflicts and near civil-war-like conditions in the years immediately after the First World War, posed major challenges to the young Republic. Within this context work became an important factor. It drove the implementation of the welfare state and the social security system, and enabled the realisation of new democratic structures. Resonating with the meaning of 'national work' (*nationale Arbeit*),[33] it was essential for overcoming the defeat of the war, expressive of the collective belief in a resurgent and aspiring nation, and it had in this respect also an ideational significance for the self-conception of the young democracy of Weimar and its people. The sociopolitical dimension of work was written into the Weimar Constitution from 1918:

> Every German shall, without prejudice to his personal freedom, be under the moral duty to use his intellectual and physical capacity as may be demanded by the general welfare. Every German shall be given an opportunity to gain a living by productive work.[34]

Work became a right and a duty; a (moral) duty to the nation and a right for one's own protection and wellbeing. This raises questions about the effects these developments had on the asylums and their patients, which will be discussed now with reference to three examples.

Work therapy in practice[35]

Before the outbreak of the First World War, on average only 35 per cent of inmates at Langenhorn worked regularly.[36] In the 1920s work therapy was extended, as was the case in many other German mental hospitals at that time, following the example of Hermann Simon. By 1926, 56 per cent of the patients were occupied in activities ranging from heavy physical labour to minor tasks.[37] This was seen as a satisfactory development in view of the fact that most patients who had been transferred from Friedrichsberg were restless and incurable. The patients were working about five hours a day and, as was noted, some worked efficiently. At that time most of the male patients were employed outdoors in work teams (*Kolonnenarbeiter*); the rest performed household tasks in the wards (*Hausarbeiter*). Female patients mainly worked indoors as knitters or peeled potatoes in the kitchen. Towards the end of the 1920s work therapy was further extended. In 1930 the staff representative at Langenhorn proudly proclaimed that 65 to 70 per cent of patients were employed every day.[38]

The patients' work had a number of effects on the asylum. First of all it had economic advantages. Many products for daily use – such as food and basic articles like shoes, trousers, mattresses, jackets and baskets – were produced with the help of patients. They also carried out maintenance and repairs; the women knitted and stitched; men and women helped in the kitchen, in the household, in agriculture and in the gardens as well as in the offices and library, and in the private households of the medical staff. Workshops for shoemaking, printing, basket weaving, tailoring, and cap making were situated in the wards, most of them in the forensic department, where the 'antisocial' and criminal inmates were accommodated – most of them diagnosed as 'not mentally ill'. This group's labour seems to have made a significant contribution to the institution's economy.[39] When in 1928 the health authority inquired about the expenses for and income from work therapy at Langenhorn, the superintendent reported 46,591 *Reichsmark* (RM) for the former and 78,891 RM for the latter. The highest contribution to the earnings was made by inmates on the forensic wards employed in shoemaking (20,161 RM) and tailoring (19,326 RM).[40]

Although these figures show that the economic output of work therapy was not insignificant, the asylum's director repeatedly emphasised that financial factors did not have priority and that work therapy should primarily be motivated by therapeutic or, more precisely, educational motives. Above all, patients' work was supposed to be meaningful and purpose-orientated, and this meant, as the director pointed out, that the institution or greater good should benefit from the work not merely in an economic sense. Only useful or purpose-orientated work (*nutzbringende Arbeit*) rather than merely playful or leisurely occupation (*spielerische Beschäftigung*) had a wholesome and educational effect (*heil-erzieherische Wirkung*) on patients.[41] But what was the benchmark for the terms 'useful', 'purpose-orientated' and 'meaningful' – was it again the economic output or could it be measured in other ways? Especially from the city authorities' perspective, the effectiveness of work therapy was indicated by its economic benefits for the institution (and consequently the public purse), even though hospital staff avoided putting too much stress on this aspect.[42]

The description of work therapy in the annual reports shows that therapy and economy were dependent on each other, even though not only the director of Langenhorn but many psychiatrists at that period pointed out that work therapy was not primarily motivated by economic benefits, but that these were mere, albeit welcome, side effects. Psychiatrists, especially during times of inflation and depression, feared that mental hospitals would be placed on the same funding level as workhouses or other social welfare institutions, with severe consequences for their medical status.[43]

The products manufactured by the inmates at Langenhorn were solely intended for use within the institution. This was important as commercial enterprises and professional interest groups saw patient labour as potential competition. Tensions increased especially in the wake of the Great Depression, when there was unemployment and a lack of demand for goods and services.[44] This raises the question of whether competition was one of the reasons why patient work at Langenhorn was restricted to handicraft and did not extend to manufacture.[45] Admittedly, the latter may not have been acceptable to the doctors' understanding of work therapy as an activity that focused on the activation of mind and body through appropriate (physical and mental) exercises rather than potentially alienating occupations.[46]

Another aspect of patients' work highlighted in the annual reports from Langenhorn related to its therapeutic effects, namely daily life in the institution and patients' mental and physical condition. Work was seen to distract from delusions and make patients forget about their complaints by channelling their urge for movement and activity.[47] However, it was not considered as a cure for mental illness.[48] Rather, it was intended to shift patients' focus away from internal to external occupation, to prevent self-absorption and encourage participation in the institution's communal life, and help them become once again 'useful' members of society.

Work and wages

In the case files of a female patient three pieces of fabric embroidered mainly in red and made to look like bank notes can be found (figure 11.1). They are representative of a period of high inflation as well as fictional ideas on currency: '*900 Dollar Mark Schein*' (900 dollar mark note), '*500 Tausend Mark Schein*' (500,000 mark note), and '*500 Mark Schein*' (500 mark note). The embroideries are undated, but they were most probably made in the early 1930s as a comment inserted in the record suggests.[49] The woman who did the embroidery was born in Doernitz in 1868 and had worked as a seamstress before she came to Langenhorn, where she died in 1940. We do not know much about her life prior to and during admission to the mental hospital at Langenhorn, far away from her home town. We can glean from

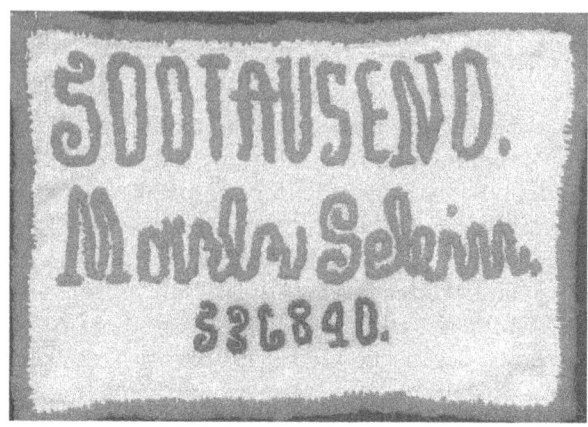

11.1 Piece of fabric, embroidered by a female patient in the Staatskrankenanstalt Hamburg-Langenhorn, 1930s.

the record that she did house- and needlework in the institution and that she collected bread, yarn and bits of fabric. The usefulness of work was seen as crucial to work therapy; staff therefore would not have considered the woman's embroideries as particularly useful. The doctors described her as wilful and grumpy. She argued that she did not come to the mental hospital in order to work. This was a point that was often made by patients. Although she spent many years at Langenhorn, there are just a few entries in her files, as was common in the case of female patients. Their lives, views, thoughts and actions seem to have been less noteworthy to the doctors than those of the male and especially the criminal inmates. Most of the female patients at Langenhorn were diagnosed as chronically ill and they were unlikely to ever be released.

The embroideries are one of few details known about the woman from Doernitz. They look like imitation banknotes. Despite the large sums embroidered in red colour, they are worthless in an economic sense, as nearly were the real notes during times of inflation. Nothing could be bought with them. The fake notes, so plainly and simply crafted, were nothing more than numbers stitched on a piece of cotton. These material objects as well as the patient's statement that she had not come to the hospital to work raise the question of the relationship between work and wages, a relationship that exists so intimately in a capitalist society, based on the exchange of money and labour, where money is seen to mean freedom and self-determination and a motivator to seek out work. How was this relationship and its meaning handled in a mental hospital? And how did patients react to the separation of money and work, as was common in most mental hospitals, in favour of a connection between work and recovery from illness? And how could work be defined as therapy and not perceived as a form of punishment, as was the case in workhouses?

Patients frequently questioned why they were supposed to work without getting paid proper wages. They associated being ill with repose and lying in bed and not primarily with work activities. But work therapy turned this principle upside down. During this period being mentally ill was linked to working without remuneration. This caused discontent among patients. Some refused to work. Others asked why they were not yet released, given that if they were supposed to work in the hospital, they could also work outside.[50] From the patients' viewpoint work was not primarily seen or accepted as a form of therapy or as a therapeutic measure. In a society that was based on the idea of work as a means for personal freedom, work and therapy (with its coercive elements) could not easily be aligned with one another.

Generally, working patients got no wages at Langenhorn during the Weimar period, although a very few, who held a position of trust, received pocket money for their 'extraordinary accomplishments'. This was mentioned in a note in 1931 from the asylum's director, in response to a request from the institution's engineering department to raise the pocket money of patients employed there.[51] The director refused the request, referring to the severe austerity measures and explaining that most of the patients who worked regularly hardly ever got pocket money although they too would deserve it.

A statement from 1925, which was overwritten with the word 'confidential', reveals that patients got more or less food dependent on what work they did.[52] Patients who worked as craftsmen, seamstresses, tailors and in the garden, in agriculture or in the laundry were supposed to get more food. Those who mended clothes, worked in the house or peeled potatoes got less to eat. Dietary requirements were assessed in relation to different types of work. In the view of psychiatrists this was justified by the fact that hard-working men and women needed more energy to find the physical strength that their work required. In addition, the work of craftsmen and tailors was perceived as more valuable for the hospital and its economy than kitchen and house work. This was to become horrifically apparent in the selection criteria employed within the national-socialist 'T4 Euthanasia Programme', when more than 70,000 mentally ill or disabled people were gassed between 1940 and 1941. Patients' ability to work decided life or death, and those whose work was perceived as more valuable had a higher chance of survival.[53]

In addition to food rationing, there was also the practice of recompense in kind for working patients. Tobacco, especially, was in great demand. This is illustrated by a male patient who asked in a letter to the superintendent to be given work because he wanted to smoke and tobacco was only given to workers.[54] Staff occasionally consented to requests for such things as painting implements and sheet music for those who were diligent and hard working.[55] And some of the female patients employed indoors were granted the wish to be allowed to go for a walk in the garden and enjoy fresh air after work.[56]

Beyond the walls of the asylum unpaid labour at Langenhorn provided a target for communist agitation.[57] During the 1920s, a number of articles relating to work therapy as a system of exploitation, based on the coercion to work, were published in communist newspapers in Hamburg by patients from Langenhorn.[58] The names of the authors are not known but it is likely that most of them were accommodated on the forensic ward. The patients referred in the articles to political achievements such as the eight-hour working day, instituted by law in 1918 and softened in 1923. One referred to the law, reporting that he had first worked as a shoemaker in the mental hospital and had felt imprisoned and exploited.[59] Subsequently, he worked in the private household of a doctor, where he was not paid for work lasting more than ten and a half hours a day. He highlighted the apparent contradiction that on the one hand he was considered a lunatic and on the other normal. He called for action by the communist party to bring an end to the existing political system and, by implication, to the psychiatric institutions and their employment of work therapy. His article was noted by the city's health authorities and the mental hospital's director was asked to respond to the allegations.[60] In his letter the superintendent admitted that it was not only for therapeutic reasons that patients were occupied in the households of the medical staff, but also to be of help to the staff.[61] This example shows that the line between occupation for therapeutic reasons and occupation that suited the staff's private needs was permeable. But this example also tells us that the patient's grievances were not ignored but taken seriously by the authorities, if only for economic reasons: If patients worked in private households, medical staff had to pay for their services.

Questions concerning work therapy, including accident insurance for patients and attendants, were also discussed in the *Reichstag*.[62] The initiator of the debate was the *Reichssektion Gesundheitswesen im Verband der Gemeinde- und Staatsarbeiter*, a union with links to the Social Democratic Party. After years of discussions attendants at mental hospitals were finally accepted into insurance schemes in 1928, but patients were excluded.[63] Remuneration was a central criterion for somebody's status as a worker and for insurance purposes, as it was stated in the *Reichsversicherungsordnung*. So as long as patients were not officially paid for their work, they were not perceived as workers in the eyes of the law, and would therefore not qualify for insurance cover. In order to exclude patients suffering from mental illness from any future claims, a section was added to the *Reichsversicherungsordnung* to the effect that mentally ill people could not be considered as workers in the legal sense because of their mental and physical deficiencies (*Mängel*).[64]

Work therapy and working life

In January 1921, a 29-year-old woman was admitted from the Friedrichsberg mental hospital to Langenhorn. Years after her admission she wrote a *curriculum vitae* that the doctors kept in her record.[65] The document was handwritten on plain white paper and consists of four pages. It was not uncommon for doctors to urge patients to write down their life story. As noted in her account, the woman had worked as a maid. During her time at the hospital, she engaged in ironing and darning, but she always had to be tightly supervised to keep her focused on her tasks. Several times she tried to escape to the city of Hamburg. According to the case files, she refused to work in 1930 and she often had to be fed. In 1939, after eighteen years at Langenhorn, she was transferred to Ricklingen with other patients. Ricklingen was a welfare institution in Schleswig-Holstein led by the Inner Mission, where inmates were poorly cared for and the diet was bad, as was commonly the case in most of these institutions during the Second World War. A large number of women and men transferred from Langenhorn to Ricklingen died there.[66]

In her *curriculum vitae* the woman had listed the names of her previous employers, one below the other, the length of time she had worked for them as well as the different places where they had lived and to which she had had to move. In the document she kept repeating one phrase, namely 'been in service' (*in Stellung gewesen*). Apart from these details, she only mentioned her name, the place and date of her birth as well as the day of her confirmation. She used a pencil and separated each entry with lines. The pencil lines make the narration rhythmic and the verbal and visual staccato intensifies the changes and unrest in her life that are pinned down on paper, resulting in a powerful and impressive document. It emphasises the important role of work in people's lives. It also raises the question of whether there was nothing else but work that the author deemed worth mentioning, nothing else that she could remember or wanted to let others know or that she thought would be of interest to the doctors. The document she created gave the impression that she had always worked and been an industrious and diligent person; she might even have overworked herself. After years at the mental hospital, she must have known that doctors attached great importance to all aspects of work and patients' work attitude. From the doctors' perspective, work attitude was an indicator for the likelihood of recovery, and, as the medical records show, it influenced their medical (and personal?) assessment of patients on admission and during their time at the hospital.

On admission to an institution, a person's working life came to sudden halt. This was a source of unease especially for male patients, some of whom were worried about neglecting their business or duties and troubled by fears about the effect of the loss of earnings on their families. At the same time, work therapy imitated a kind of working life under the surveillance of attendants and doctors. Apart from the economic benefits and the therapeutic impact on inmates' condition and routine and on communal life in the institution, patients' reintegration into the labour market and the production process was hoped for, as the superintendent explained in a letter to the health authorities in 1930.[67] But because most of the patients at Langenhorn were considered chronically ill, this raises the question of whether the aim of rehabilitation could ever be widely reached, as had been the case during the First World War when patients were discharged from hospital earlier than initially expected.[68]

Potential rehabilitation was important not only for staff and the authorities, but also for patients. Some used the opportunities work therapy offered them to learn a trade such as shoe or cap making or to improve or maintain existing skills. Patients knew that they would be confronted with a difficult situation after their discharge from the mental hospital and wanted to be prepared. The high rates of unemployment during the Weimar period, which had adversely affected some patients even prior to institutionalisation, created much anxiety and insecurity, as is revealed in letters and case file entries. However, from the perspective of some patients the activities offered to them at Langenhorn – mainly agricultural, handicraft, and domestic work – were not always seen as helpful with regard to their employability following discharge. For example, when the doctor advised a bored and apparently idle inmate to employ himself in the cobbler's workshop or in tailoring, the patient pointed out that these activities may be beneficial for the institution but were of little use to him after his discharge from Langenhorn.[69] Instead he had taught himself shorthand writing and was hoping to find a job where he could make use of it. Given that the mental hospital was relatively close to the modern city of Hamburg, the patient's argument seems well justified. The work activities offered at Langenhorn and intended to enable patients' reintegration into the labour market, were outdated and not in line with changing occupational structures in conurbations such as Hamburg.

Patients who had worked as craftsmen prior to admission or who were unskilled had a different perspective on work therapy. In 1921, a young man, who had been a prisoner in Fuhlsbüttel, was sent to Langenhorn. He had worked as a shoemaker since the age of thirteen. Soon after his admission, he wrote a letter to the doctor asking if he could be moved to another ward in order to be able to work in the cobbler's workshop.[70] The young man noted that he was planning to become self-employed after his discharge and therefore needed to maintain his practical skills. He promised the doctor that he would be much calmer and more orderly once allowed to pursue his former trade.[71] The doctor consented and the patient was moved to the other forensic ward, where he worked as a shoemaker. A few months later the doctor confirmed that the patient did an excellent job and was 'willing, diligent and

The patient's view of work therapy

decent'.[72] The young man was released from Langenhorn in 1928. In this case self-interest and public interest overlapped and work therapy was successful in several ways. The doctor felt vindicated in his action, because the patient adjusted and worked well, the institution benefitted from a competent and engaged craftsperson, and the patient was able to hone his skills. As the doctor pointed out, the patient did an excellent job at making and repairing a large number of shoes for the institution. In 1925 alone 520 boots were made by patients in Langenhorn, and numerous shoes were repaired by them.[73]

In the case of the young man from Fuhlsbüttel, the patient was enabled to maintain not only his practical skills, but also his professional identity. He was not simply left to vegetate in a closed institution, but remained a shoemaker, whose skills were needed and appreciated. In this case, work therapy also seemed to foster a mutually appreciative relationship between the doctor and the hardworking and able patient. At the same time there were cases of inmates who were unable to work; who did not manage to retain their former occupational identity; who could not return to their former private and working lives; and who were increasingly – under the influence of the Great Depression, subsequent austerity measures and the ideology of National Socialism – seen as 'unworthy of life'.[74]

A safe place in uncertain times?

In January 1929, a young man aged twenty-one, who had worked at the port in Hamburg, was transferred from Friedrichsberg to Langenhorn.[75] He had previously enjoyed his work. At the mental hospital he worked mainly in the house and was described as diligent. After a few months he was told of his pending discharge, but in a letter to his father he explained that he did not want to leave Langenhorn for two reasons.[76] First, he feared that he would be unable to find a job, referring to the difficult times and working conditions, and arguing that everyone who had a job would try to keep it. His reasoning was not ungrounded, as between 1928 and 1932 the number of employed in Hamburg decreased by 60 per cent; being a port city, Hamburg was especially hard hit by the world economic crisis.[77] Second, he was worried that he would become a burden on his father.

Despite the letter, the father came to the mental hospital to pick up his son and take him home. After nine days, the son returned voluntarily to Langenhorn. He explained that conditions in Hamburg were too bad; he had been unsuccessful in finding work.[78] At his parents' place he did not even have a bed of his own and had nothing to wear. He therefore thought that it was better for him to return to the mental hospital. The director consented to his wish and so he stayed at the institution for one more year before being sent to Strecknitz near Luebeck, where he died of pneumonia in 1935, like many other patients who were transferred to this subsidiary of the institution at Langenhorn.[79]

Many notes and letters from patients with similar requests were kept in the Langenhorn records. During the Weimar period, marked by unemployment, poverty, inflation, and quasi civil-war conditions, an institution like Langenhorn was from the perspective of a number of patients and their families not just a place of control, expropriation, authoritarianism and confinement.[80] At this difficult period, mental hospitals were also perceived as places that offered patients security, a kind of stability and sense of belonging, which maybe tells us more about the wider socioeconomic situation than about conditions in institutions such as Langenhorn.[81]

There is also evidence that those patients who had been in the mental hospital for a long time especially feared that they would no longer be able to cope with life outside. For example, a patient, whose father had advised him to stay in the hospital, was longing for his release but was at the same time afraid of it. In a letter to the *Reichsstatthalter*, dated June 1934, he referred to the difficulties he envisaged being confronted with after his discharge because he had had no connection to the outside world for fourteen years ('*wo ich schon seit 14 Jahren nicht mehr mit der Außenwelt in Verbindung stehe*').[82] He asked who would give a job to a man aged thirty-four freshly released from a mental institution. Although he had worked in Langenhorn's bookbinder's workshop for ten and a half years, he doubted that he would be considered a professional by the outside world. Seven years earlier, in 1927, when his father had asked for his son's release from Langenhorn, the director had commented on the patient's lack of work aptitude and inability to compete with skilled workers on the labour market.[83]

Patients were motivated by the hope that working hard would lead to their release from the mental hospital. But when they realised that chances of getting employment were low in the world outside, their willingness to engage in work decreased, as is evidenced in some patients' letters.[84] Another patient, who was due for discharge, contended that he did not feel up to a life outside, that he still had to rest, and that he had no idea what life would be like if he had to leave Langenhorn.[85] He surmised that he would have to approach transition from the mental hospital to a life outside very slowly. The director accommodated his wish and allowed the patient to stay in Langenhorn, from where he began to look for work in Hamburg. After he had found appropriate work, he was discharged. He was one of the few whose search for work was successful. The procedure of letting inmates stay connected with the institution while they were looking for employment was encouraged at Langenhorn during the Weimar period. Those up for release were offered the possibility of leaving the asylum for a few days in order to look for work and then to return to get their discharge if they were successful. But not every patient was able to find work that way. One, who had already left the asylum, wrote a letter to the director requesting work as gardener or delivery boy at Langenhorn in order to prove that he was a good man, a man to marry, as he put it. The director refused his request, but expressed his sympathies with the difficulties that the former patient faced outside the hospital.[86]

High unemployment and fear of not finding a job after discharge was a constantly recurring topic discussed between doctors, family members and patients considered for discharge. One patient quoted his father's words that it was better for him to stay in the asylum where he would be cared for and given food and drink. The father had pointed to the high level of unemployment and the difficulties of finding a job.[87] The son felt that his father was cold-blooded and unsympathetic; he stayed on in the institution.

A still very common narrative in the history of psychiatry concerns the mentally ill person being held captive in an asylum against his or her will. With regard to the conditions during the Weimar Republic, it seems that this view of mental institution is not fully appropriate. Rather, as has been shown by Mark Finnane with regard to institutions in Ireland during periods of economic downturn and famine, patients and their families may have considered mental hospitals as places of refuge or 'asylums' in the true sense of the term.[88] However, things were to change soon. During the Nazi era wilful neglect and extermination of thousands of mentally ill patients became an even more sinister episode in the history of psychiatry.

Conclusion

Although patient work had been a crucial element in the treatment of the mentally ill since the beginning of the nineteenth century, its meanings changed during the Weimar Republic. This particular period was characterised by unemployment, poverty and social instability. At the same time, the ability and will to work became the essential criteria for the right to draw on government support measures. Patients at Langenhorn were on the whole well aware of the wider social conditions, and their perception of work inside the institution and their willingness to submit to work therapy were influenced by this awareness.

Work therapy at Langenhorn lacked some of the features that characterised work outside the walls of the institution. Patients did not usually receive a wage commensurate with their labours and the activities pursued at Langenhorn were not in line with changes in the labour market. Agricultural skills, for example, may have been vital for the internal economy of the institution, but not within the wider context of a modern port city. The scope for inmates' reintegration on their discharge from Langenhorn was therefore restricted, despite doctors' insistence on the rehabilitative role of work therapy. Nevertheless, work therapy can still be seen as a point of intersection between the state and the mental hospital. Due to the 'more active therapy', earlier boundaries between society and institutions became more porous – even from the perspective of the patients. The adoption of work as a central element within the organisation of the mental hospital initiated this process of dissolution, which was intensified by the conditions of the Weimar period.

Acknowledgement

This chapter draws on the research for a project funded by the German Research Foundation from 2012 to 2015, undertaken at the Department of History and Ethics of Medicine at the University Clinic Hamburg-Eppendorf (head of the project: Prof. Dr Heinz-Peter Schmiedebach; scientific researcher: Dr Monika Ankele, SCHM 1311/9-1). The project focuses on work therapy and family care during the Weimar period. The results of the project will be published in a monograph in 2016.

Notes

1 Alfred Birk, *Zur Frage der elektrischen Stadt- und Vorortsbahn in Hamburg* (Sonderdruck aus der 'Zeitschrift für das gesamte Lokal- und Strassenbahnwesen'; Wiesbaden: Verlag von J. F. Bergmann, 1904), p. 3.
2 Werner Jochmann and Hans-Dieter Loose (eds), *Vom Kaiserreich bis zur Gegenwart. Hamburg: Geschichte der Stadt und ihrer Bewohner* (Hamburg: Hoffmann und Campe, 1986), vol. 2, p. 23.
3 Printed matter from 23 February 1891, Organisationsplan von Oberarzt Dr. Reye, quoted by Arthur Kreßin, *Das Allgemeine Krankenhaus Langenhorn in Hamburg* (Hamburg: Wöll, 1950), p. 7.
4 See Staatsarchiv Hamburg (hereafter StAHH), 352-3, Sig. II L 15, Schreiben des Verwaltungsdirektors an die Gesundheitsbehörde (Writing from the administrative authority to the health authority) (18 November 1930); Schreiben des Betriebsrats an den Senator (Writing from the works council to the senator) (16 December 1930).
5 See, for example Salina Braun, *Heilung mit Defekt. Psychiatrische Praxis an den Anstalten Hofheim und Siegburg 1820–1878* (Göttingen: Vandenhoeck & Ruprecht, 2009); Heinz Schött and Rainer Tölle, *Geschichte der Psychiatrie. Krankheitslehren, Irrwege, Behandlungsformen* (München: C. H. Beck, 2006).
6 For different descriptions of asylums' directors and their remarks on architecture and location as meaningful elements of therapeutic acting see Johannes Bresler (ed.), *Deutsche Heil- und Pflegeanstalten für Psychischkranke in Wort und Bild* (Halle a. d. Saale: Marhold, 1910), vol. 1.
7 Christian Friedrich Wilhelm Roller, *Die Irrenanstalt nach allen ihren Beziehungen* (Karlsruhe: Müller, 1831), p. 190. See especially ch. 17 'Beschäftigung der Irren', pp. 178–92.

8 Ibid., p. 189.
9 Ibid., p. 190. '[D]aß die Bedürfnisse der Anstalt so viel möglich in ihr selbst, durch eigene Kräfte gewonnen werden.'
10 Gerhard Schäfer and Max Schubert, *Beschreibung der Staats-Krankenanstalt Langenhorn Hamburg* (Düsseldorf: Rhenania-Verlag Th. P. Braun, 1931), p. 3.
11 For the question of how to reach the city when the asylum was built in the outskirts as well as for the question what proximity and distance to a city could mean for an asylum at the beginning of the twentieth century, see Monika Ankele, 'Eine Chronik der Linie. Zur Annäherung zwischen Zentrum und Peripherie am Beispiel der Krankenanstalt Langenhorn bei Hamburg', in Thomas Müller (ed.), *Zentrum und Peripherie in der Geschichte der Psychiatrie. Interdisziplinäre Annäherungen* (publication forthcoming).
12 Theodor Neuberger, 'Langenhorn-Hamburg', in Bresler (ed.), *Deutsche Heil*, vol. 1, pp. 127–40.
13 StAHH, 352-8/7, Sig. 139, Staatskrankenanstalt Langenhorn. Kranken- und Diagnosestatistik für die Jahre 1893 bis 1925 (Health and diagnosis statistics from 1893 to 1925).
14 Emil Kraepelin, *Allgemeine Psychiatrie. Psychiatrie: Ein Lehrbuch für Studirende und Aerzte* (Leipzig: Johann Ambrosius Barth, 7th edn, 1903), vol. 1; Clemens Neisser, 'Die Bettbehandlung der Irren. Vortrag, gehalten in der neurologischen Abteilung des X. internationalen medicinischen Congresses', *Berliner Klinische Wochenschrift*, 38 (22 September 1890), 863–6.
15 For details about the application of prolonged bath treatment in the University Psychiatric Clinic Heidelberg under Emil Kraepelin around 1900, see Monika Ankele, *Alltag und Aneignung in Psychiatrien um 1900. Selbstzeugnisse von Frauen aus der Sammlung Prinzhorn* (Wien/Köln/Weimar: Böhlau, 2009), pp. 72–4. For a more detailed discussion of bed rest including the view of female patients on this method of treatment, see Monika Ankele, 'Begrenzter Raum. Das Bett in der Frauenpsychiatrie um 1900', *Zeitschrift für Kulturwissenschaften*, 2 (2008), 17–28.
16 Wilhelm Griesinger, 'Vorwort', *Archiv für Psychiatrie und Nervenkrankheiten*, 1 (1868/1869), 3–8. For the significance of Griesinger in reorienting psychiatry towards the natural sciences, see Eric J. Engstrom, *Clinical Psychiatry in Imperial Germany. A History of Psychiatric Practice* (Ithaca, NY: Cornell University Press, 2003), pp. 88–91.
17 Clemens Neisser, *Ueber die Bettbehandlung der akuten Psychosen und über die Veränderungen, welche ihre Einführung im Anstaltsorganismus mit sich bringt. Referat erstattet auf dem XII. Internationalen Medizinischen Kongress zu Paris am 6. August 1900* (München: Seitz & Schauer, 1900), p. 10.
18 Friedrich Utz (birth and death dates unknown), superintendent at the Bavarian asylum Gabersee, listed the patients' workdays per year; his statistics showed that numbers hit a low between 1905 and 1925 due to preference being given to bed rest and water therapy. Friedrich Utz, 'Die Arbeitstherapie', *Allgemeine Zeitschrift für Psychiatrie*, 92 (1930), 245–62.
19 For the psychiatric treatment of soldiers during the First World War, see Paul Lerner, *Hysterical Men. War, Psychiatry, and the Politics of Trauma in Germany*,

1890-1930 (Ithaca, NY: Cornell University Press, 2003); Maria Hermes, *Krankheit: Krieg. Psychiatrische Deutungen des Ersten Weltkriegs* (Essen: Klartext-Verlag, 2012); Philipp Rauh, 'Die militärpsychiatrischen Therapiemethoden im Ersten Weltkrieg und deren Nachkriegsrezeption', in Hans-Walter Schmuhl and Volker Roelcke (eds), *Heroische Therapien. Die deutsche Psychiatrie im internationalen Vergleich 1918-1945* (Göttingen: Wallstein Verlag, 2013), pp. 29-47. Hans-Georg Hofer, *War Trauma and Medicine in Germany and Central Europe 1914-1939* (Freiburg: Centaurus-Verlag, 2011).

20 Lerner, *Hysterical Men*; for an empirical study about the application of work therapy during the First World War see Hermes, *Krankheit: Krieg*.

21 Hans-Ludwig Siemen, *Menschen blieben auf der Strecke: Psychiatrie zwischen Reform und Nationalsozialismus* (Gütersloh: Van Hoddis, 1987); Lerner, *Hysterical Men*.

22 Hans Roemer, Gustav Kolb and Valentin Faltlhauser (eds), *Die offene Fürsorge in der Psychiatrie und ihren Grenzgebieten* (Berlin: Springer, 1927).

23 Hermann Simon, *Aktivere Krankenbehandlung in der Irrenanstalt*, Werkstattschriften zur Sozialpsychiatrie, vol. 41 (Bonn: Psychiatrie-Verlag, 1986 (reprint of the 1929 work)), pp. 6-7; Simon, 'Active Therapy in the Lunatic Facility (1929)', in Greg A. Eghigian (ed.), *From Madness to Mental Health: Psychiatric Disorder and Its Treatment in Western Civilisation* (New Brunswick, NJ: Rutgers University Press, 2010), pp. 271-5.

24 In these wards patients were under constant observation and expected to stay in bed even when they were not sleeping.

25 Simon, *Aktivere Krankenbehandlung*, p. 6.

26 *Ibid.*, p. 5.

27 Hermann Simon, 'Aktivere Krankenbehandlung in der Irrenanstalt', *Allgemeine Zeitschrift für Psychiatrie*, 87 (1927), 97-145.

28 For a detailed description of the five steps of work therapy formulated by Simon, see Simon, *Aktivere Krankenbehandlung*, pp. 25-7.

29 *Ibid.*, pp. 50-167, primarily pp. 60-2. 'Erst die Erziehung im weitesten Sinne des Wortes vermittelt ihm die Fähigkeit, sich in die geordnete Gemeinschaft einer größeren Anzahl von Menschen einzuordnen und damit auch selbst der Vorteile des Gemeinschaftslebens teilhaftig zu werden.' *Ibid.*, p. 61.

30 David F. Crew, *Germans on Welfare: From Weimar to Hitler* (Oxford: Oxford University Press, 1998), pp. 198-9; For the welfare system in Hamburg during the Weimar period, see Christiane Rothmaler and Evelyn Glensk (eds), *Kehrseiten der Wohlfahrt. Die Hamburger Fürsorge auf ihrem Weg von der Weimarer Republik in den Nationalsozialismus* (Hamburg: Ergebnisse Verlag, 1992).

31 Karl Heinz Roth, 'Ein Mustergau gegen die Armen, Leistungsschwachen und "Gemeinschaftsunfähigen"', in Angelika Ebbinghaus, Heidrun Kaupen-Haas and Karl Heinz Roth (eds), *Heilen und Vernichten im Mustergau Hamburg. Bevölkerungs- und Gesundheitspolitik im Dritten Reich* (Hamburg: Konkret-Literatur-Verlag, 1984), pp. 7-17; see also Uwe Lohalm, 'Hamburgs öffentliche Wohlfahrt in der Krise 1930-1933', in Rothmaler and Glensk (eds), *Kehrseiten der Wohlfahrt*, pp. 48-75.

32 Bernd Walter, 'Hermann Simon – Psychiatriereformer, Sozialdarwinist, Nationalsozialist?', *Der Nervenarzt*, 23:11 (2002), 1047–54. Especially when he put it into writing, in 1929 Simon added to the outline of his article, which had been published in the *Allgemeine Zeitschrift für Psychiatrie* in 1927, a chapter titled 'Experiences and thoughts of a practitioner about the psychotherapy of mental disease' (*Erfahrungen und Gedanken eines praktischen Psychiaters zur Psychotherapie der Geisteskrankheiten*) and published these two parts in a monograph.

33 Otto Brunner, Werner Conze and Reinhart Koselleck (eds), *Geschichtliche Grundbegriffe. Historisches Lexikon zur politisch-sozialen Sprache in Deutschland* (Stuttgart: Klett-Cotta, 1972), vol. 1, pp. 210–11.

34 For an English translation of the Weimar Constitution see http://en.wikisource.org/wiki/Weimar_constitution (accessed 9 February 2014).

35 In Germany the terms 'work therapy' (*Arbeitstherapie*) and 'occupational therapy' (*Beschäftigungstherapie*) were used synonymously.

36 StAHH 352-3, Sig. II L 15, Betriebsrat Langenhorn an den Senator (Writing from the employee organization Langenhorn to the senator), 16 December 1930.

37 StAHH 352-8/7, Sig. 16a, Jahresbericht über das Kalendarjahr 1926 (Annual Report for 1926), 1 February 1927.

38 StAHH 352-3, Sig. II L 15, Betriebsrat Langenhorn.

39 For the conditions of accommodation and working of the criminal inmates in the Langenhorn asylum, see Monika Ankele, '"Wie zusammen leben?" Die Patienten des "gesicherten Hauses" in der Staatskrankenanstalt Hamburg-Langenhorn', *Schriftenreihe der Deutschen Gesellschaft für Geschichte der Nervenheilkunde*, 20 (2014), 455–89.

40 StAHH 352-3 II, Sig. L 15, Schreiben an die Gesundheitsbehörde (Writing from the health authority), 28 August 1929.

41 StAHH, 352-8/7, Sig. 16a, Jahresbericht 1926: ' … daß nur solche Arbeiten ausgeführt werden, deren Ergebnis der Anstalt (es wird nicht für den Verkauf gearbeitet) Nutzen bringt; nicht lediglich aus ökonomischen Gründen, sondern auch, weil nur eine nutzbringende Arbeit, nicht eine spielerische Beschäftigung, auf die Dauer Befriedigung geben und eine heil-erzieherische Wirkung ausüben kann.'

42 For the influence of the authorities on the practice of work therapy, see Anna Urbach, 'Heilsam, förderlich, wirtschaftlich – Zur Rechtfertigung, Durchführung und Aneignung der Arbeitstherapie in der Landes-Heil- und Pflegeanstalt Uchtspringe 1894–1914', in Monika Ankele and Eva Brinkschulte (eds), *Arbeitsrhythmus und Anstaltsalltag. Arbeit in der Psychiatrie vom 19. Jahrhundert bis in die NS-Zeit* (Stuttgart: Franz Steiner Verlag, 2015), pp. 71–102.

43 In 1931 the welfare authorities paid for 90 per cent of the patients who were accommodated in an asylum where the charges were higher than that in welfare institutions. So for cost concerns, the welfare authorities proposed transforming Langenhorn into an alms-house under the authority of the welfare department. The director of Langenhorn as well as the health authorities reacted against this proposal. See StAHH 351–10, Sig. GF 32.15 (Bd. 1), verschiedene Schreiben (different writings), August to September 1931; for a detailed discussion concerning the

effects of the Great Depression on Hamburg's asylums and the controversy between the health and welfare authorities, see also Angelika Ebbinghaus, 'Aussonderung und Vernichtung in den Anstalten', in Angelika Ebbinghaus, Heidrun Kaupen-Haas and Karl Heinz Roth (eds), *Heilen und Vernichten*, pp. 136–46.

44 See, for example, StAHH 352-8/7, Sig. 126, writing from the shoemaker guild to the Great Senate (Hoher Senat), 12 December 1932; StAHH 353-II L 15, Schreiben der Gesundheitsbehörde an die Anstalt Langenhorn (writing from the health authority to the *Staatskrankenanstalt* Langenhorn), 19 December 1930, explaining the interests of the home for the blind relating to the manufacturing of brushes.

45 See anon., 'Die Behandlung der Arbeitstherapie im Reichstage', *Sanitätswarte*, 28:8 (20 April 1928), 134–6.

46 See, for example, StAHH 352-3, Sig. II L 15, Abschrift. Deutscher Verband für psychische Hygiene. Zur Frage der Arbeitstherapie in den Heil- und Pflegeanstalten. Stellungnahme zu der Denkschrift der Reichssektion Gesundheitswesen im Verbande der Gemeinde- und Staatsarbeiter (Transcript. German Association for Mental Hygiene. On the question of work therapy in mental hospitals. Advisory opinion on the memorandum from the *Reichssektion Gesundheitswesen* in the Association of Municipal and State Employees), Gießen, 29 July 1928. Signed: Sommer, Weygandt, Römer, Kolb, Simon.

47 StAHH 352-8/7, Sig. 16a, Jahresbericht 1926.

48 *Ibid.*

49 StAHH 352-6/7, Sig. 1609 (Abl. 1995/2).

50 See, for example StAHH 352-8/7, Sig. 15242, 17373 (both Abl. 1995/2).

51 StAHH 352-7/8, Sig. 166, Anfrageschreiben des technischen Büros (Request from the engineering office), 3 August 1931; Antwortschreiben (written reply), 5 August 1931.

52 StAHH 352-8/7, Sig. 112, Schreiben (writing), 6 July 1925; Faulstich explored the intentional starvation of patients in German psychiatric institutions during both wars, see Heinz Faulstich, *Hungersterben in der Psychiatrie 1914–1949. Mit einer Topographie der NS-Psychiatrie* (Freiburg im Breisgau: Lambertus Verlag, 1998); for the starvation of patients in Langenhorn during the First World War, see Kai Sammet, 'Burgfrieden und Totenstille – Die Irrenanstalt Hamburg-Langenhorn, die Verwaltung und der Hunger 1914–1918', *Zeitschrift des Vereins für Hamburgische Geschichte*, 89 (2003), 149–74. During the Second World War the *Kaiser Wilhelm Institut für Arbeitspsychologie* conducted nutrition experiments with forced workers to test the interrelationship between nutrition and work performance, see Irene Raehlmann, *Arbeitswissenschaft im Nationalsozialismus. Eine wissenschaftssoziologische Analyse* (Wiesbaden: VS Verlag für Sozialwissenschaften, 2005), pp. 185–90.

53 Maike Rotzoll, 'Rhythmus des Lebens. Arbeit in psychiatrischen Institutionen im Nationalsozialismus zwischen Normalisierung und Selektion', in Ankele and Brinkschulte (eds), *Arbeit in der Psychiatrie*, pp. 189–214; for a more detailed discussion about the 'T4 Euthanasia Programme', based on a quantitative and qualitative evaluation of patient records, see Maike Rotzoll, Gerrit Hohendorf, Petra Fuchs, Paul Richter, Christoph Mundt and Wolfgang U. Eckart (eds), *Die*

nationalsozialistische 'Euthanasie' –Aktion 'T4' und ihr Opfer. Geschichte und ethische Konsequenzen für die Gegenwart (Paderborn: Schöningh, 2010); Petra Fuchs, Maike Rotzoll, Ulrich Müller, Paul Richter and Gerrit Hohendorf (eds), 'Das Vergessen der Vernichtung ist Teil der Vernichtung selbst'. Lebensgeschichten von Opfern der nationalsozialistischen 'Euthanasie' (Göttingen: Wallstein, 2007).

54 StAHH 352-8/7, Sig. 13076 (Abl. 1995/2), letter from 29 May 1932.
55 See Ankele, 'Wie zusammen leben'.
56 See, for example StAHH 352-8/7, Sig. 15707 (Abl. 1995/2), Lebenslauf (curriculum vitae), undated (probably from 1927).
57 For a detailed discussion of communist politics in Hamburg during the Weimar Republic, see Ursula Büttner, Angelika Voß and Hermann Weber, Vom Hamburger Aufstand zur politischen Isolierung: kommunistische Politik 1923-1933 in Hamburg und im deutschen Reich (Hamburg: Lütcke & Wulff, 1983).
58 StAHH 352-3, Sig. II L15, Zeitungsausschnitt (newspaper clipping), anon., 'Schreckenstation Langenhorn' ('Langenhorn – ward of horror'), in KPD (Kommunistische Partei Deutschlands/German Communist Party) Wahlzeitung no. 3 (14 November 1929), n.p.; StAHH 352-3, Sig. II L 15, Zeitungsausschnitt, anon., 'Wir verblöden hier völlig' ('We are becoming completely stupid in here'), in Hamburger Volkszeitung no. 106 (30 June 1931); StAHH 352-3, Sig. II L 15, Zeitungsausschnitt, anon., 'Was man unter Arbeitstherapie versteht' ('On the meaning of work therapy'), in Hamburger Volkszeitung no. 258 (5 November 1931).
59 StAHH 352-3, Sig. II L 15, anon., Schreckenstation Langenhorn.
60 See StAHH 352-3, Sig. II L 15, and others, Schreiben des Direktors (letter from the superintendent), 24 November 1929; Schreiben der Gesundheitsbehörde (letter from the health authority), 3 December 1929.
61 StAHH 352-3, Sig. L II 15, Schreiben des Direktors, 24 November 1929, 'Natürlich nimmt man einen Kranken zur Beschäftigung ins Haus, um an ihm Hilfe zu haben, und nicht nur, um ihn damit therapeutisch günstig zu beeinflussen'.
62 See Monika Ankele, '"… daß diese Heilmethode auch von anderen als ärztlichen Gesichtspunkten aus bewertet und beurteilt werden muß." Zu den sozial- und gesellschaftspolitischen Debatten um die psychiatrische Arbeitstherapie in der Weimarer Zeit', in Ankele and Brinkschulte (eds), Arbeit in der Psychiatrie, pp. 157–185; Christian Ley, 'Beiträge der Reichssektion Gesundheitswesen im Verband der Gemeinde- und Staatsarbeiter zur Professionalisierung der Pflege zwischen 1918 und 1933' (Diplomarbeit, Fachhochschule Münster, 2006), http://christian-ley.de/Dokumente/Diplomarbeit.pdf (accessed 10 November 2013).
63 Ley, 'Beiträge der Reichssektion Gesundheitswesen', p. 49.
64 See Reichsversicherungsordnung (Social Insurance Code of the German Reich), 3. Buch Unfallversicherung von Stephan Moesle und Wilhelm Rabelling, 1. Abschitt § 544 (Umfang der Versicherung), quoted by StAHH 352-3, Sig. II L 15, Denkschrift zur Frage der 'Arbeitstherapie' in den Heil- und Pflegeanstalten unter besonderer Berücksichtigung der 'pflegerlosen Abteilungen' (hg. v. der Reichssektion Gesundheitswesen im Verband der Gemeinde- und Staatsarbeiter (memorandum on the question of work therapy in mental hospitals having a special regard to

non-attendant wards (published by the Empire Health Services Section of the Association of Municipal and State Workers)), Berlin 1927.
65 StAHH 352-8/7, Sig. 13302 (Abl. 1995/2), curriculum vitae, dated 8 February 1928.
66 For an outline of the history of Ricklingen, see 'Die Geschichte des Landesvereins im Überblick', http://landesverein.de/de/359/geschichte.html (accessed 9 February 2014). In 1929 an observer wrote that '[i]f slavery is still to be found anywhere in Germany, it is here [in Ricklingen]'. StAHH, SB I VG 24.23, Leitersitzungen (conference of the superintendents), 5 February 1923, quoted by Crew, *Germans on Welfare*, p. 199.
67 The Langenhorn asylum stated in a note from 1930 that they tried to bring patients back to the labour market after their release, see StAHH 352-8/7, Sig. 166, Schreiben der Anstalt an die Gesundheitsbehörde (letter from the *Staatskrankenanstalt* to the health authority), Hamburg, 13 March 1930.
68 Hans Roemer, 'Die sozialen Aufgaben des Irrenarztes in der Gegenwart', *Psychiatrisch-Neurologische Wochenschrift*, 45–6 (1920–21), 343–51, 344.
69 StAHH 352-8/7, Sig. 16052 (Abl. 1995/2), entry from 7 October 1929, 'Als ihm gesagt wurde, er solle sich doch mit nutzbringender Arbeit etwas beschäftigen wenn es ihm so zu langweilig sei, lehnt er diese ab und sagt: "Sehe ich denn so aus wie ein Arbeiter? Niemals werde ich aus ganz bestimmten Gründen in diesen Häusern eine Beschäftigung, sei es in der Schneiderei, Schusterei oder dergleichen anfassen. Das hat gar keinen Zweck, weil eine solche Arbeit gar keinen Nutzen für mein späteres Fortkommen hat. Ich will mich jetzt mit Stenographie beschäftigen und hoffe, darin so flott zu werden, dass ich sie später verwerten kann."'
70 StAHH 352-8/7, Sig. 13452 (Abl. 1995/2), letter to Dr Sierau (undated).
71 *Ibid.*
72 StAHH 352-8/7, Sig. 13452 (Abl. 1995/2), Abschrift eines Briefes von Dr. Sierau (copy of a letter from Dr Sierau), 6 September 1924.
73 StAHH 352/8-7, Sig. 125, transcript 6 January 1925.
74 For the increasing split of the working and the non-working patients in the 1930s, see Rotzoll, 'Rhythmus des Lebens'.
75 StAHH 352-8/7, Sig. 17815 (Abl. 1995/2).
76 *Ibid.*, transcript of a letter to the father, 2 October 1929.
77 See Ebbinghaus, 'Aussonderung und Vernichtung', p. 136.
78 StAHH 352-8/7, Sig. 17815 (Abl. 1995/2), entry from 28 October 1929.
79 For the history of the *Heilanstalt* Strecknitz, see Peter Delius, *Das Ende von Strecknitz. Die Lübecker Heilanstalt und ihre Auflösung 1941. Ein Beitrag zur Sozialgeschichte der Psychiatrie im Nationalsozialismus* (Veröffentlichungen des Beirats für Geschichte der Arbeiterbewegung und Demokratie in Schleswig-Holstein Bd. 2, zugl. med. Diss., Kiel: Neuer Malik-Verlag (Publications by the advisory council for the history of the labour movement and democracy in Schleswig-Holstein, vol. 2, at the same time medical dissertation, Kiel: Neuer Mailk Verlag), 1988.
80 See the increasing number of admissions to welfare institutions during the economic crisis in Germany.

81 See the report of attendants working in the *Heilanstalt Strecknitz* relating to the patients who were sent from the mental hospital at Langenhorn. The patients were described as completely neglected. Delius, *Das Ende von Strecknitz*.
82 StAHH 352–8/7, Sig. 14854 (Abl. 1995/2), letter to the *Reichstatthalter*, 21 June 1934.
83 *Ibid.*, letter from Dr Sierau, 26 January 1927.
84 See, for example, *ibid.*, letter from 29 May 1930.
85 StAHH 352–8/7, Sig. 13256 (Abl. 1995/2), entry from 13 May 1922.
86 StAHH 352–8/7, Sig. 13198 (Abl. 1995/2), letter from 12 May 1928.
87 StAHH 352–8/7, Sig. 14854 (Abl. 1995/2), letter to the *Reichstatthalter*, 21 June 1934.
88 Mark Finnane, *Insanity and the Insane in Post-Famine Ireland* (London, New York: Croom Helm and Barnes and Noble, 2003 [1981]).

12

They were 'improved', punished and cured: The construction of 'workshy', 'industrious' and (non-)compliant inmates in forced labour facilities in the First Republic of Austria between 1918 and 1933

Sonja Hinsch

Mathilde S., a twenty-one-year-old woman from Styria, was regarded as 'workshy'. She would roam the streets and beg. She also suffered from epilepsy. Her illness was considered to exacerbate her moral weakness. She was convicted for vagrancy and begging, had to serve one month in prison, then was detained and forced to work in a '*Zwangsarbeitsanstalt*' (forced labour facility). A stable lifestyle (*konsequente Lebensführung*) was thought to help her. It was even supposed to heal her epilepsy. This is what we can glean from the testimonies on Mathilde S., which were collected by the provincial government of Lower Austria about her detention in and release from the forced labour facility.[1]

The fate of Mathilde S. is that of one of the so-called '*Zwänglinge*' – those compelled to work in a forced labour facility – in the interwar period. There were five such facilities (two for men and three for women) in Austria until 1932. Subsequently, following legal reform, there were only three (two for men and one for women). Due to fragmentary sources, information on the number of detainees is only available for 1936. In the case of the two forced labour facilities for men, the combined average monthly number of inmates was between 258 and 303. In the case of the forced labour facility for women, it was twenty-nine.[2] People convicted as beggars, vagabonds, prostitutes and re-offenders were sent to prison, and some later taken to a forced labour facility until they were considered 'improved'[3] or, as defined in the '*Arbeitshausgesetz*' of 1932, until they had acquired a 'righteous' (*rechtschaffen*)[4] and hard-working or industrious (*arbeitsam*) attitude.[5] Prior to 1932, judges had to declare the admissibility of the internment. The actual decision about whether to detain a person was made by the Commission for Forced Labour Facilities and Borstals (CFLFB), which was part of the provincial government. After 1932 the judges themselves decided on detentions.[6] This implied a juridification of detention and also greater transparency in the decision-making process as the convicted person was present during the trial, which was not the case during the meetings of the CFLFB. Internment could last up to three years, in the case of re-offenders even five, without a fixed date of release. The workload was supposed to be so heavy that it could only be executed 'with the utmost effort'.[7] In the case of careless performance of work, inmates could be punished.[8] When internees tried to escape, they were often beaten, sometimes so hard that they needed medical treatment. They could also be shot, as was the case in some instances.[9]

Inmates' case files reveal the daily conflicts and negotiations between the judges, jurists, commissions, inmates, employees of the facilities and experts. We can glean how the law was interpreted and what different meanings were attributed to internment in forced labour facilities. Those sent to the forced labour facility were considered 'workshy' and the aim was to morally 'improve' them by means of steady, hard work in farming and other activities such as basket and doormat weaving. However, inmates were also characterised as 'dishonest', 'recalcitrant', 'violent' or 'badly behaved', and these derogatory labels were used to justify internment regardless of their perceived attitude towards work. A variety of sometimes contradictory aims and functions of internment coexisted, ranging from improvement to punishment and imprisonment. The secondary literature on forced labour facilities has highlighted the different – and fluctuating – aims and functions.[10] Ammerer, for instance, notes for Austria that the idea of moral improvement went along with other functions of forced labour facilities, such as the support of orphans and sick persons.[11] In the case of England and Ireland, admission to workhouses was voluntary; however, the disciplinary character of these is discussed in the secondary literature.[12] Ina Scherder points out that the workhouse also functioned as a hospital, an employment agency and a children's home.[13] Focusing on the different purposes of institutions in England, Ireland, Germany and Switzerland,[14] secondary literature on forced labour facilities and workhouses examines the relevant laws and regulations, staffing and the socio-demographic background of inmates and conditions in the institutions.[15] Research on Austria has tended to concentrate on the eighteenth to the mid-nineteenth centuries.[16] This chapter focuses on the hitherto neglected yet important period of the emergence of the welfare state (after the 1880s) and of a democratic Austria. It examines case files of internees, with particular attention being given to who was considered 'workshy', dangerous or to be improved. It will be argued that the varied aims of detention were not at odds with each other but part of the construction of moral deviancy, which was seen to require concerted action, i.e., discipline, punishment, imprisonment, locking up as well as attempts at 'improvement'. As the 'Instructions for Directors of the Styrian Forced Labour Facility Messendorf' put it:

The admitted persons shall be made to become aware of their immoral or thoughtless way of living. Their inclination towards bad habits and degeneracies shall be weakened and extinguished; they shall be brought to awareness of their duties towards God and human society, to fulfil these duties and get used to fulfilling them. This aim can only be achieved by precisely executing the house rules, by getting the inmate used to order, temperance, cleanliness, chastity, compatibility and continuous industriousness [*Arbeitsamkeit*].[17]

Here persons who qualified for detention were described as the opposite of those who engaged in steady work and led a moral life. In other words, steady work was part of a moral and socially compliant life.

Inmates of forced labour facilities were not usually diagnosed with a mental illness. However, the differentiation between different kinds of non-work within wider society and the construction of *Zwangsarbeitsanstalten* for those considered workshy rather than unemployed provides insight into the complex understandings of work and non-work during a period when patient work was considered an important part of mental hospital regimes. The description of internments in forced labour facilities therefore contributes to a better understanding of the wider context within which mental patients' work needs to be set.

Improvement

It is difficult to understand what 'improvement' meant in the context of detention. According to the 1885 law on forced labour facilities and borstals, a person could be interned until improvement was observed.[18] The law did not specify the meaning of improvement. The Vagrancy Act of 1885 was criticised at the time for not differentiating between begging due to necessity and begging on account of 'workshyness'. For example, Hugo Herz, a jurist and judge, held that the varied causes for begging were not taken account of.[19] According to the jurist and university professor Robert von Hippel, in contrast to the honest wayfarer, the vagrant would tramp because he or she did not want to work despite being able to.[20] People willing to work, who were in need and would beg occasionally, were to be distinguished from the workshy.[21] It was argued that 'workshyness' should be considered as a precondition for internment.[22] In the 1920 Act of Conditional Conviction (*Gesetz über die bedingte Verurteilung*)[23] for cases of re-sentenced criminals and in the '*Arbeitshausgesetz*' of 1932 for beggars, vagrants and prostitutes, the aim of internment was defined as getting internees 'used to a righteous and industrious life'.[24] By doing so, a distinction was implicitly made between people willing to work and those deemed 'workshy'.

However, in many cases, neither the internees themselves nor evaluations of their improvement were characterised in work-related terms. Other aspects were referred to. For example, improvement was assessed on the basis of behaviour, namely compliance with the institution's rules, as at Messendorf where good conduct was a criterion for an inmate's release.[25] Various descriptions of the internees' conduct referred not only to the time during their detention in the forced labour facility but also to their previous confinement in prison. In the case of Julius F., for example, the CFLB based their decision for his discharge on the following: 'Due to his faultless conduct and his remorseful self-examination during his time in prison, his willingness to improve is evident'.[26]

Ideas of improvement were also imbued with the ideal of bourgeois family life. An internee's intention to start a family was seen as evidence of improvement. Getting married and having children were considered as a change that would contribute to, if not guarantee, a person's improvement. Josefine Hi., for example, was not transferred to a forced labour facility, because not only was she 'not workshy' but also 'one could not give up hope that she would live in a righteous way having become a mother'.[27] Inmates and their relatives, too, claimed in their discharge requests that the internees were willing or obliged to care for their families. In such cases, gender-related differences can be identified. While men's duties were considered to involve providing an income for the family, the duties of women were seen to relate to household and childcare activities. Leopold Ha., for example, promised the provincial government to earn money for his family.[28] The mother of Ludwig K., another internee in Korneuburg, wrote to the provincial government: 'as soon as he has an income, he will dutifully support his family'.[29] By contrast, female internees' activities were described as contributory – but not financial – forms of caring. In his application for her release, the husband of Mathilde S. claimed: 'In my vocation I rely on her contribution because she has to mind my little household when I work. Apart from that, she helps me in the stone quarry.'[30] The mayor of Mathilde S.'s village supported the request because 'she had roved around in a workshy manner' but after having been married she would run the household, empathise with her ill husband and participate in his work.[31]

Industriousness

Even when we look at the contexts in which the terms 'workshy' and 'industrious' were used to label inmates, it is evident that something more than just the way of conducting work was at stake and formed an integral part of the meaning of work. Industriousness, for example, held further connotations, such as compliance and a socially acceptable aptitude. Not all forms of making a living were considered work, and not everyone earning a living was deemed industrious. Persons such as prostitutes and those working on and off may have been engaged in productive activities but were not considered as accustomed to an industrious life. 'Workshyness', so it was held, 'could be hidden behind any form of business'.[32] Likewise, 'fruitless business' could be a 'mask' for 'workshyness'[33] or be indicative of an 'emotional distance' from working.[34] Therefore, the mere description of the activities previously carried out by internees did not necessarily convey their propensity towards industriousness in the complex, over-determined way that it was understood. For example, male internees might formerly have made their living in agriculture, crafts, construction and mining, and as waiters, hairdressers, actors or dental technicians. Women likewise might have earned an income in agriculture, and also have worked as housemaids, in stone quarries, and as prostitutes. However, for the most part, prostitution was not regarded as a way to make a living but as a crime and immoral pursuit. It was construed as a dissolute livelihood that could not qualify as industrious work.

Other activities were designated as non-regular or random work. Leopold H., a former detainee in the forced labour facility of Korneuburg, was re-detained because he had acquired jobs by chance.[35] Inmates might have moved from job to job, become self-employed, or have had no socially acceptable work. They also might have been supported by their families or lived from begging and/or thieving. But, as Wadauer and Vana have pointed out, non-regular work and a variety of incomes were common in this period.[36] Skilled and unskilled work, casual work and forms of support were frequently combined to make a living.[37] Distinctions between workers, beggars and vagrants were therefore unclear.[38] This phenomenon was partly caused by the general problem of finding work. The official unemployment rate was very high, especially after the world economic crisis of 1929, when it reached 27.2 per cent in 1933.[39] However, non-work was evaluated in very different ways, at times leading to detention in a forced labour facility whereas in other cases it was not considered as a manifestation of 'workshyness'. In the case of Franz P. early parole was changed into a definite release from Korneuburg.[40] The provincial government argued that low wages had caused him to leave his former job. Thus Franz P. seemed to have valid motives. In one case, then, non-work was regarded as legitimate; in another, as illegitimate. The point was not whether the person was working or not working, but how he or she was doing in both cases – and what kind of work was being done. The activity also had to be of a virtuous kind, and the person performing diligently. In the case of Franz P. his mother promised that he would 'earn his bread in a righteous manner' and 'take the right path and earn his living through work and effort'.[41]

Regulations specified that the 'daily workload could only be achieved with the utmost effort'.[42] Diligence and willingness to engage in hard toil were important aspects of work in interwar Austria.[43] There were also others, such as the contemporary understanding of vocation as a combination of ability and enjoyment of an activity.[44] In the case of the unemployed, their aptitude and suitability for a job they had been trained for were preconditions for placement by the official labour allocation offices.[45] Juvenile inmates in borstals, who were interned under the same laws of 1885 as the adult inmates, had to be trained at the institution in an occupation commensurate with their abilities to increase their prospects of getting work on their release.[46]

Descriptions of (non-)industriousness were inherently linked to what was considered as (non-)compliance with social norms. Work was understood as demanding effort, abstinence and subordination, and constituted a criterion of social integration.[47] In contrast, specific forms of non-work were stigmatised. Josef Radauer, the director of a borstal, claimed that a slacker would not be able to differentiate between good and bad. He might become – when poor – a defrauder, thief or even a murderer.[48] Therefore, non-work could be linked to moral concepts such as dishonesty, neglect of one's duties and so forth. But this was not the case for every form of non-work. The aforementioned Franz P.'s temporary unemployment was socially and morally acceptable because he had given up his former work in the hope of gaining a better position with higher income.[49] This implies that there was a mutually constitutive process by which values of social and moral compliance were linked to legitimate non-work, and illegitimate forms of non-work to deviant behaviour.

Punishment and imprisonment

In a letter addressed to the ministry of justice, the administrators of the forced labour facility Suben wrote in 1933:

> We request the deletion of the first sentence of the house rules: 'The forced labour facilities are not prisons'. This sentence provokes anger among the inmates. They think that detention in a forced labour facility is much harder to endure than prison.[50]

According to institutional staff, the fact that internees did not know how long they would be detained was very difficult for most of them. Also, detainees often pointed out in petitions that they had already 'atoned' for their delinquencies. Reference to the fact that they had paid the penalty for a crime did not, of course, constitute an admission that a crime had been committed. It merely tells us that inmates believed that their argument for achieving release was strong and just.

Here one can see blurred distinctions between forced labour facilities and prisons. This problem also occurred with respect to the form of the procedure of internment. In procedural terms, a conviction by a judge was a precondition but not alone sufficient reason for the decision to detain someone in a forced labour facility by the CFLFB. The character of the convict also had to be examined. Detention could only be imposed if the person was not 'righteous' but might display a propensity to become so under constraint.[51] Yet, in practice, convictions were used as an argument in favour of detention. The process of detention, therefore, rarely differed from the process of imprisonment, as can be seen in the form of the CFLFB of Vienna: 'The Commission for Forced Labour Facilities and Borstals has ordered detention due to the decision of suitability of detention by the court'. The suitability of detention was thus justified by the convictions. In fact, the two authorities often delegated the actual decision to each other – the court delegated the decision to the CFLFB as the court only decided upon the admissibility, the CFLFB delegated the decision to the court as the CFLFB referred to the admissibility of detention in the justification of the detention. The only arguments left were the convictions, which – programmatically speaking – would not justify detention but only that the case was referred to the CFLFB.

Due to the moral construction of character – an integral part of the idea of improvement – there was no contradiction between a person's promise to lead an industrious (*arbeitsam*) life and atonement for a crime. At the same time, and in line with the precept that non-working, deviant persons should be improved, it was also demanded that 'incorrigible' persons be rendered 'innocuous' (*unschädlich*). As the criminal law expert, Robert von Hippel, notes in relation to forced labour facilities: 'Along with improvement, deterring someone or making them harmless play exactly the same role as in prisons.'[52]

Medicalisation

There was also disagreement among experts on whether a person was ill or deviant. Lutz Raphael uses the term 'scientification of the social', which denotes the increasing presence of medical scientists and their arguments in administration, industry, political parties, parliaments and social groups.[53] Physicians, in particular, had a vital role within forced labour facilities as they had to attest to inmates' suitability for detention. Their position was confirmed and regulated by the 1885 law on forced labour facilities and borstals, which stipulated that people should not be detained if they 'could not be used even for easy work', were mentally ill, had contagious diseases, or were pregnant.[54] Thereby, the role of physicians and psychiatrists was no mere formal prerequisite. The involvement of physicians and psychiatrists in forced labour facilities began in the late nineteenth century, followed by criminologists and psychologists in the twentieth century. According to Raphael they increasingly challenged legal experts' long-established authority.[55] Physicians and psychiatrists claimed for themselves a leading role in debates over the reform of forced labour facilities. The notion of vagabonds as individuals who are fully accountable for their actions competed with that of the vagabond as an ill person who was not a criminal (albeit still dangerous).[56] The competition between medical explanations and arguments in favour of forced improvement or punishment of persons considered criminally liable is illustrated in an article in a journal of forensic medicine, published in 1927:

> The contribution of the institution's physician is essential for the social recovery of the inmates. The aim of the prison regime is the transformation of an asocial or antisocial lawbreaker into a socially useful person. Nowadays, it is no longer believed that this aim can be achieved by getting the prisoners used to work ... It has been realised that it is a process of convalescence and recovery that is not only similar to the operations during the healing of physical and mental diseases, but in many respects merges with them.[57]

Physicians and psychiatrists repeatedly justified their authority claims in relation to their expertise, presuming that other protagonists in forced labour facilities would lack such knowledge. The 'common sense' of average staff was not considered sufficient.[58] These claims were widely accepted and popular in political debates. Psychiatrists conducted surveys on which the legislative authorities relied, and which will be discussed later. Thus, Julius Tandler, City Councillor for Welfare and Health, who was responsible for the authorisation of all detentions in forced labour facilities in politically left wing, 'Red Vienna', claimed that a physician should head the Ministry for People's Health (*Staatsamt für Volksgesundheit*). Eugenic ideas gained increasing influence. Eugenic measures such as sterilisation[59] were mooted by some for 'serious criminals, sexual offenders, idiots, serious epileptics, in short, inferior persons', based on the assumption that they would endanger the health of the nation by reproducing.[60] However, Tandler did not enforce negative eugenics programmes.[61] There is currently no evidence available that eugenic measures were implemented in forced labour facilities. However, there are phrases in the case files that refer to inmates as 'inferior', indicating that eugenic thinking was present in the institutions. While education was an integral part of the idea of youth, improvement was not always considered essential in the case of so-called 'asocial' persons. Controlling them was often seen as more important. Supporting them would be a eugenic error, according to Tandler.[62]

Yet other sources indicate that the influence of physicians and psychiatrists should not be understood as an indication of a unidirectional process whereby medical knowledge increasingly determined the practices of forced labour facilities. Rather, as Lengwiler and Germann point out, there was a mutually constitutive pattern of interaction between science and the welfare state,[63] a co-evolving process that raised awareness and established a shared understanding of normality.[64] This can be seen in the case of Paula E.[65] Staff at the forced labour facility at Wiener Neudorf described her as violent and hostile towards the guards as well as other inmates. They asked the provincial authorities to release Paula E. because her behaviour seemed to them to be due to mental illness. The institution's doctor, the public medical officer and a psychiatrist drafted expert testimonies; these did not pronounce her to be mentally ill. When Wiener Neudorf continued to complain about her, she was transferred to another forced labour facility at Lankowitz. It was argued that it was more likely that they could guarantee to maintain discipline at Lankowitz than at Wiener Neudorf because of the latter's outdated premises and equipment, which made it difficult to deal with defiant inmates.[66] During her stay at Lankowitz, Paula E. was eventually diagnosed as mentally ill by another psychiatrist and transferred to a mental hospital.

Paula E.'s file can be understood in various ways. According to Germann, the handling of her case can be seen as reflective of a rising awareness of the role of mental illness in cases of deviant behaviour.[67] The government's demand for medical certificates may also reflect a growing unease among bureaucrats about deciding upon internees' suitability for internment in the face of the increasingly acknowledged expertise in these matters of psychiatrists and physicians. Consultation with medical experts reassured officials in their decision making. Yet reliance on medical opinion was also used by administrators as a trump card to achieve their aims. The consultation by staff of the two institutions of medical experts in the case of Paula E., who had caused disciplinary problems at both Wiener Neudorf and Lakowitz, can also be understood as a way of getting rid of her.

In the process of the medicalisation of detainees, it is important to consider the role of inmates' behaviour. If they presented themselves in work-related terms (as working diligently, looking for and willing to work, but also as ill and unable to work), they were not likely to become subject to medicalisation. However, if the inmates tried to resist the institutional regime by escaping, going on hunger strike and threatening work routines and order with physical violence, they tended to be described in medical terms by the staff. There were also cases when inmates were classified in both medical and in work-related and moral terms. Medicine, morals and work were not considered as incommensurable. This was evident in relation to individual inmates and in scientific debate. For example, in 1914 the psychiatrists Ernst Bischoff and Erwin Lazar published a survey of the detainees of the institution at Korneuburg on behalf of the government of Lower Austria. Eleven types of detainees were distinguished. One group contained those who had been active in trade or commerce, but were later convicted on account of vagrancy and begging. They were said to be alcoholics, who had had an 'orderly family life'. Some suffered from *lues* (syphilis), tuberculosis or an organic disease. Due to their deficient ability to work, they were assumed to have a 'disinclination to work'. Another group was seen to consist of unskilled labourers, born to unmarried mothers and diseased parents. They were convicted of serious crimes and deemed to be mentally and physically healthy. Family circumstances, delinquency, alcohol consumption, physical and mental diseases, ability to work and ways of making a living were categories that referred to a range of social, medical, moral and other circumstances. They were combined in various constellations to delineate particular groups of inmates. For some, Bischoff and Lazar recommended work; for others, therapy. For yet others, detention in a forced labour facility was held to be a special form of amateur nursing and care.[68]

Bischoff and Lazar did not limit their diagnoses and recommendations to purely medical and psychiatric criteria. Similarly, in the case files inmates were variously described in medical, moral and work-related terms. Julius F., for example, who had dropped out of law school and been trained as an actor, would, according to his lawyer, become mentally ill if he had to perform unskilled work.[69] Mathilde S. was deemed 'workshy' due to the bad company she kept and, according to the mayor of the village she came from, 'suffering from epilepsy, she did not have enough moral strength to resist' such company.[70]

Conclusion

The construction of the meanings of 'workshy' and 'industrious' was multifaceted. Work did not just mean the performance of any kind of activity to earn one's living. Rather, it had to be a socially acceptable occupation and be pursued in a steady way. Being industrious also implied that a person fulfilled their duty towards the family, behaved honestly and remained sexually inconspicuous. Failing to commit to these values was punished by stigmatisation and criminalisation. If people failed to engage in acceptable work in an acceptable manner, they failed morally. Such failure was described both in work-related terms and in reference to intractable, dissolute and dangerous behaviour. Improvement was achieved through acceptable work, good behaviour and intentions, such as obeying the house rules and intending to marry and have children. Since workshyness was linked with attributes like dangerousness, detention in forced labour facilities aimed not only at improvement but also at punishment as well as incarceration to protect society. Even the distinctions between illness and immorality enforced by the increasingly prominent process of medicalisation were blurred in practice. Medical, work-related and moral terms coexisted alongside each other.

Acknowledgements

This chapter is based on research done for my dissertation. The research was conducted as part of the project 'Production of Work. Welfare, Labour-market and the Disputed Boundaries of Labour (1880–1938)' headed by Dr Sigrid Wadauer and financed by the European Research Council under the European Community's Seventh Framework Programme (FP7/2007–2013)/ ERC grant agreement no. 200918 and the Austrian Science Fund (FWF, Project Y367-G14) hosted by the university of Vienna.

I want to thank Sigrid Wadauer, Josef Ehmer, Alexander Mejstrik, Jessica Richter, Georg Schinko and Irina Vana for their comments. Last, but not least, I want to thank the editor, Waltraud Ernst, for her comments.

Notes

1 Provincial Archives of Lower Austria (hereafter NÖLA), Landesregistratur, XI, Karton 603 89 L.A. V1 L.A. VII4 1926, St.Zl. 384.
2 Ernst Seelig, *Das Arbeitshaus im Land Österreich: Zugleich ein Beitrag zur Neugestaltung des Strafrechts im Großdeutschen Reich (Sicherungsverwahrung und Arbeitshaus)* (Graz: Moser's Verlag, 1938), pp. 81–6. A comparison on a monthly or a daily basis is not possible due to the limitations of the sources.
3 Law on forced labour facilities and borstals: Gesetz vom 24. Mai 1885, betreffend die Zwangsarbeits- und Besserungsanstalten, Reichsgesetzblatt für die im Reichsrathe für die im Reichsrathe vertetenen Königreiche und Länder 1885/90, §9 (http://alex. onb.ac.at/cgi-content/alex?aid=rgb&datum=18850004&seite=00000210); Act of conditional conviction: Gesetz vom 23. Juli 1920 über bedingte Verurteilung, Staatsgesetzblatt für die Republik Österreich 1920/373 (http://alex.onb.ac.at/ cgi-content/alex?aid=sgb&datum=19200004&seite=00001555).
4 *Rechtschaffen* in German includes the meaning of being active or creating something.
5 Law on the placement of lawbreakers in an 'Arbeitshaus': Bundesgesetz vom 10. Juni 1932 über die Unterbringung von Rechtsbrechern in Arbeitshäusern, Bundesgesetzblatt für die Republik Österreich 1932/166, §1 (http://alex.onb.ac.at/ cgi-content/alex?aid=bgb&datum=19320004&seite=00000578).
6 Ibid.
7 Styrian Provincial Archives (hereafter StLA), LAA Rezens K 319 Gr III 3 1923, 'Hausordnung für die Zwänglinge in der steierm. Landes-Zwangsarbeitsanstalt zu Messendorf' (The house rules of the forced labour facility in Messendorf), § 22.
8 *Ibid.*, § 13.
9 StLA, LAA Rezens K 319 Gr III 3 1923, 'Instruktion über den Waffengebrauch der diensthabenden Aufseher' (Instructions for gun use by wardens), St.Zl. 2623.
10 See, for example, Gerhard Ammerer, 'Zucht- und Arbeitshäuser, Freiheitsstrafen und Gefängnisdiskurse in Österreich 1750–1850', in Gerhard Ammerer and Alfred Stefan Weiß (eds), *Strafe, Disziplin und Besserung. Österreichs Zucht- und*

Arbeitshäuser von 1750–1850 (Frankfurt a.M.: Peter Lang, 2006), pp. 7–61; Ina Scherder, 'Galway workhouses in the nineteenth and twentieth century: Function and strategy', in Andreas Gestrich, Steven King and Lutz Raphael (eds), *Being Poor in Modern Europe: Historical Perspectives 1800–1940* (Oxford: Peter Lang, 2006), pp. 181–97; Beate Althammer, 'Functions and developments of the Arbeitshaus in Germany', in Gestrich *et al.* (eds), *Being Poor*, pp. 273–97.

11 Ammerer, 'Zucht- und Arbeitshäuser', p. 29.
12 See, for example, Margaret Anne Crowther, *The Workhouse System 1834–1929: The History of an English Social Institution* (Cambridge: Cambridge University Press, 1981).
13 Scherder, 'Galway workhouses'.
14 See, for example, Virginia Crossman, 'The New Ross Workhouse Riot of 1887: Nationalism, class and the Irish poor laws', *Past & Present*, 179 (2003), 135–79; Inga Brandes, '"Odious, degrading and foreign" institutions? Analysing Irish workhouses in the nineteenth and twentieth centuries', in Gestrich *et al.* (eds), *Being Poor*, pp. 199–227; Scherder, 'Galway workhouses'; Wolfgang Ayaß, *Das Arbeitshaus Breitenau: Bettler, Landstreicher, Prostituierte, Zuhälter und Fürsorgeempfänger in der Korrektions- und Landarmenanstalt Breitenau (1874–1949)* (Kassel: Gesamthochschule, 1992), pp. 82–83, 119, 141–3, 151; Sabine Lippuner, *Bessern und Verwahren: Die Praxis der administrativen Versorgung von 'Liederlichen' und 'Arbeitsscheuen' in der thurgauischen Zwangsarbeitsanstalt Kachrain (19. und frühes 20. Jahrhundert)* (Frauenfeld: Verlag des Historischen Vereins des Kantons Thurgau, 2005).
15 Hannes Stekl, *Österreichs Zucht- und Arbeitshäuser 1671–1920: Institutionen zwischen Fürsorge und Strafvollzug* (Vienna: Verlag für Geschichte und Politik, 1978); Ayaß, 'Arbeitshaus Breitenau'; Christian Marzahn, 'Das Zucht- und Arbeitshaus: Die Kerninstitution frühbürgerlicher Sozialpolitik', in Christian Marzahn and Hans-Günther Ritz (eds), *Zähmen und Bewahren: Die Anfänge bürgerlicher Sozialpolitik* (Bielefeld: AJZ Druck & Verlag, 1984), pp. 7–68.
16 Ammerer, 'Zucht- und Arbeitshäuser'; Stekl, *Zucht- und Arbeitshäuser*; Helfried Valentinitsch, 'Das Grazer Zucht- und Arbeitshaus 1734–1783: Zur Geschichte des Strafvollzuges in der Steiermark', in Kurt Ebert (ed.), *Festschrift Hermann Baltl: Zum 60. Geburtstag dargebracht von Freunden und Kollegen* (Innsbruck: Universitätsverlag Wagner, 1978), pp. 495–514; Hannes Stekl, '"Labore et fame" – Sozialdisziplinierung in Zucht- und Arbeitshäusern des 17. und 18. Jahrhunderts', in F. Christoph Sachße and Florian Tennstedt, *Soziale Sicherheit und soziale Disziplinierung: Beiträge zu einer historischen Theorie der Sozialpolitik* (Frankfurt a.M.: Suhrkamp, 1986), pp. 119–47. Only Stekl's study on forced labour facilities in Austria analyses a longer period, up until 1920.
17 StLA, LAA Rezens K 319 Gr III 3 1923, 'Instruction für die Direction der steierm. Landes-Zwangsarbeitsanstalt in Messendorf' (Instruction for the directors of the forced labour facility), § 3.
18 Gesetz vom 24. Mai 1885/90, §9.
19 Hugo Herz, *Arbeitsscheu und Recht auf Arbeit: Kritische Beiträge zur österreichischen Straf- und Sozialgesetzgebung* (Leipzig/Vienna: Franz Deuticke, 1902), p. 35.

20 Robert von Hippel, 'Bettel, Landstreicherei, Arbeitsscheu und Arbeitshaus im Vorentwurf'. *Monatsschrift für Kriminalpsychologie und Strafrechtsreform*, 7 (1910–11), 449–70, 450.
21 Ibid., pp. 450–2.
22 Herz, *Arbeitsscheu*, p. 41; Hippel, 'Bettel', p. 451.
23 Gesetz vom 23. Juli 1920/373, § 21.
24 Bundesgesetz vom 10. Juni 1932/1667, § 1.
25 StLA, LAA Rezens K 319 Gr III 3 1923, 'Statut der steiermärkischen Landes-Zwangsarbeits- und Besserungsanstalt in Messendorf' (The statute of the forced labour facility).
26 Municipal and Provincial Archives of Vienna (hereafter WStLA), A1 M. Abt. 255 A 1928 Zl. 1–1226, Karton 11, St.Zl. a-762/28 1928, 'Wiener Magistrat im selbständigen Wirkungsbereich des Landes' (Provincial government of Vienna), Abt. 55, 17 December 1928.
27 NÖLA, Landesregistratur, XI, Karton 606 92 L.A. V1 L.A. VII4 1927 XI 1001-Schl, St.Zl. 1147, 'Niederösterreichische Landesregierung' (Provincial government of Lower Austria), 8 July 1925.
28 WStLA, A1 M. Abt. 255 A 1928 Zl. 1–1226, Karton 11, Geschäftszahl 732/1928, 'Leopold H. to the provincial government of Vienna', 13 June 1931.
29 NÖLA, Landesregistratur, XI, Karton 612 98 L.A. V1 L.A. VII4 1929 XI 951-Schl, St.Zl. 1078, 'Aloisia K. to the provincial government of Lower Austria', 20 December 1928.
30 NÖLA, Landesregistratur, XI, Karton 603 89 L.A. V1 L.A. VII4 1926, St.Zl. 384, 'Franz S. recorded by the Bezirkshauptmannschaft Mürzzuschlag', 1 March 1925.
31 NÖLA, Landesregistratur, XI, Karton 603 89 L.A. V1 L.A. VII4 1926, St.Zl. 384, 'Mayor', 23 February 1926.
32 Hugo Hoegel, *Die Straffälligkeit wegen Arbeitsscheu in Österreich* (Vienna: Alfred Hölder, 1899), p. 126.
33 W. J. Ruttmann, 'Arbeitsscheu', in Fritz Giese (ed.), *Handwörterbuch der Arbeitswissenschaften* (Halle a.S.: Carl Marhold Verlagsbuchhandlung, 1930), p. 372.
34 Ibid.
35 WStLA, A1 M. Abt. 255 A 1928 Zl. 1–1226, Karton 11, Geschäftszahl 732/1928, 'Wiener Magistrat im selbständigen Wirkungsbereich des Landes' (Provincial government of Vienna), 16 January 1930.
36 Sigrid Wadauer, 'Establishing distinctions: Unemployment versus vagrancy in Austria from the late nineteenth century to 1938', *International Review of Social History*, 56 (2011), 31–70, 42.
37 Irina Vana, 'Gebrauchsweisen öffentlicher Arbeitsvermittlung: Österreich 1889–1938' (PhD dissertation, University of Vienna, 2014), p. 390.
38 Wadauer, 'Establishing distinctions', p. 42.
39 Felix Butschek, *Der österreichische Arbeitsmarkt – von der Industrialisierung bis zur Gegenwart* (Stuttgart: Gustav-Fischer-Verlag, 1992), p. 83.
40 WStLA, M. Abt. 255 A1922 1 bis 600 A1 2, St.Zl. 246.

41 WStLA, M. Abt. 255 A1922 1 bis 600 A1 2, St.Zl. 246, 'Henriette P. to the provincial government', 17 August 1923.
42 Eduard Körner, 'Empfiehlt sich die Errichtung großer Landesanstalten oder kleinerer Bezirksanstalten? Verwendung der Zwänglinge außer der Anstalt', *Mittheilungen des Vereines der Beamten der österreichischen Landes- und Zwangsarbeits- und Besserungsanstalten*, 1:2 (1903), 5–13, 8.
43 StLA, LAA Rezens K 319 Gr III 3 1923, 'Hausordnung für die Zwänglinge in der steierm. Landes-Zwangsarbeitsanstalt zu Messendorf' ('House rules for the internees in the Styrian forced labour facility in Messendorf'), § 22.
44 Raimund Fürlinger, Beruf Berufswahl Berufsberatung Berufsfürsorge: Eine orientierte Schrift für Eltern, Erzieher, Lehrer und für die Jugend selbst (booklet, publisher unknown, undated); Fritz Karl Mann, 'Zur Soziologie des Berufs', *Jahrbücher für Nationalökonomie und Statistik*, 83:3 (1933), 481–500.
45 Gesetz vom 24. März 1920 über die Arbeitslosenversicherung, Staatsgesetzblatt für die Republik Österreich 1920/153, § 6.
46 Gesetz vom 24. Mai 1885/90, §13.
47 Walter Sperisen, 'Arbeitsscheu. Eine psychologisch-pädagogische Studie', *Beiheft zur Schweiserischen Zeitschrift für Psychologie und ihre Anwendungen*, 10 (1946), 31.
48 Josef Radauer, 'Einfluß der Arbeit auf die Erziehung', *Blätter für Zwangserziehung und Fürsorge*, 9 (1913), 109–27, 110.
49 WStLA, M. Abt. 255 A1922 1 bis 600 A1 2, St.Zl. 246.
50 Austrian State Archives (hereafter ÖStA), AVA, Justiz, Justizministerium (1849–1939), Arbeitshäuser Allgemein, Karton 4227, Zl. 270/33 (letter written by the administrators of the forced labour facility in Suben to the Ministry of Justice).
51 Seelig, *Arbeitshaus*, pp. 26–9.
52 Hippel, 'Bettel', p. 460.
53 Lutz Raphael, 'Die Verwissenschaftlichung des Sozialen als methodische und konzeptionelle Herausforderung für eine Sozialgeschichte des 20. Jahrhunderts', *Geschichte und Gesellschaft: Zeitschrift für Historische Sozialwissenschaft*, 22:2 (1996), 165–93, 166.
54 Gesetz vom 24. Mai 1885/90, § 6.
55 Raphael, 'Verwissenschaftlichung', p. 167.
56 Beate Althammer, 'Der Vagabund: Zur diskursiven Konstruktion eines Gefahrenpotentials im späten 19. und frühen 20. Jahrhundert', in Karl Härter, Gebhard Sälter and Eva Wiebel, *Repräsentationen von öffentlicher Sicherheit: Bilder, Vorstellungen und Diskurse vom 16.bis zum 20. Jahrhundert* (Frankfurt a.M.: Vittorio Klostermann, 2010), pp. 415–53, 433–52.
57 W. Gentz, 'Der Strafanstaltsarzt im Entwurf des Strafvollzugsgesetzes', *Deutsche Zeitschrift für die gesamte gerichtliche Medizin*, 10:1 (1927), 219–34, 228–9.
58 Ibid.
59 Doris Byer, *Rassenhygiene und Wohlfahrtspflege: Zur Entstehung eines sozialdemokratischen Machtdispositivs in Österreich bis 1934* (Frankfurt a.M.: Campus Verlag, 1988), p. 72.
60 Julius Tandler and Siegfried Kraus, *Die Sozialbilanz der Alkoholikerfamilien: Eine*

sozialmedisinische und sozialpsychologische Untersuchung (Wien: Verlag Gerold, 1936), p. 65.
61 Byer, *Rassenhygiene*, p. 54.
62 *Ibid.*, pp. 80–1.
63 Martin Lengwiler, 'Expertenwissen im Sozialstaat: zwischen Verwissenschaftlichung, Bürokratisierung und Politisierung', *Studien und Quellen: Zeitschrift des Schweizerischen Bundesarchivs*, 31 (2006), 167–90.
64 Urs Germann, 'Der Ruf nach der Psychiatrie: Überlegungen zur Wirkungsweise psychiatrischer Deutungsmacht im Kontext justizieller Entscheidungsprozesse', in Désirée Schauz and Sabine Freitag (eds), *Verbrecher im Visier der Experten: Kriminalpolitik zwischen Wissenschaft und Praxis im 19. und frühen 20. Jahrhundert* (Stuttgart: Franz Steiner Verlag, 2007), pp. 273–93.
65 NÖLA, Landesregistratur, XI, Karton 608 94 L.A. V1 L.A. VII4 1928 XI 351–900, St.Zl. 470.
66 *Ibid.*, 'niederösterreichische Landesregierung' (Provincial government of Lower Austria), 5 January 1927.
67 Germann, 'Psychiatrie', p. 282.
68 Ernst Bischoff and Erwin Lazar, 'Psychiatrische Untersuchungen in der n.-ö. Zwangsarbeitsanstalt Korneuburg', *Blätter für Zwangserziehung und Fürsorge: Organ des Vereines für Zwangserziehung und Fürsorge*, 10 (1914), 98–114.
69 WStLA, A1 M. Abt. 255 A 1928 Zl. 1–1226, Karton 11, St.Zl. a-762/28 1928, 'lawyer to the provincial government', 12 December 1928.
70 NÖLA, Landesregistratur, XI, Karton 603 89 L.A. V1 L.A. VII4 1926, St.Zl. 384, 'mayor', 23 February 1926.

13

Useful members of society or motiveless malingerers? Occupation and malingering in British asylum psychiatry, 1870–1914

Sarah Chaney

Occupation was a key feature of the nineteenth-century asylum system. On the one hand, providing residents with daily tasks was designed to counter the 'morbid introspection' thought to contribute to mental illness, while simultaneously aiding the running of the institution through free labour. The asylum itself functioned on the model of a work-based society: inmates were expected to contribute and earned privileges when they did so. This system was also designed to create 'useful members of society', preparing residents for life beyond the institution. Training in certain tasks, such as artisan labour, was expected to assist inmates on discharge. This emphasis on usefulness, however, was challenged on several fronts in the period 1870–1914, including the new economic view of 'malingering' in society and the development of a new psychological view of individual functioning, which saw external behaviour read as evidence of an internal mental state. This chapter asks: to what extent can we view the functioning of British asylums in these decades in relation to wider social and economic concerns about work?

Through the concept of malingering, an idea applied in both the psychiatric and industrial realm in this period, I explore how models of work within and outside asylums intersected and in what ways they differed. First, I outline the role of occupation in the late nineteenth-century asylum. The influence of 'moral treatment', a therapeutic regime based on environmental and social considerations, meant that alienists, or asylum psychiatrists, often made surprisingly little distinction between 'useful' and recreational occupation: both were thought to be curative. Indeed, these two types of activity were also thought to play a role in creating valuable citizens; a concern mirrored in early texts on the topic of malingering. In non-psychiatric texts of this period, there is evidence of a marked shift in the understanding of malingering from being a moral judgement about the avoidance of duty to a largely economic concern. This shift certainly had implications for understanding occupation within the asylum: not least because alienists contributed to debates around malingering with examples of self-inflicted injury throughout this period. Yet their suggestions that what they termed 'motiveless malingering' needed to be understood in relation to the psychological and emotional desires of the individual, rather than financial gain (a model which could not be applied in the context of unpaid asylum work), retained a moral emphasis. A study of attitudes toward occupation within psychiatry thus indicates that the 'useful citizen' of 1870–1914 was as much a moral as an economic concern, being framed by the political context of the Employer's Liability Act of 1880 and the Workmen's Compensation Act of 1906.

Occupation in the late nineteenth-century asylum

In his 1882 annual report to the hospital governors, Bethlem Royal Hospital superintendent George Henry Savage (1842–1921) lamented that '[a]nother year has passed, and we are no nearer solving the problem of occupation for the middle-class insane'.[1] What made this such a concern for the late Victorian British asylum doctor, and what was meant by it? Savage himself related employment to cure in a number of ways. His report continued:

> I look upon the airing-court passing of time as a necessity, but only half a good. The patients have so much fresh air, and some play rackets, lawn tennis, ball, &c., but the dull and moody ones loaf their time away, and grow more deluded or more demented. Very few cases of simple insanity, if treated early, are incurable; but to treat them properly requires constant personal attention, and an Asylum Medical Staff is rarely large enough to do much beyond supervise.[2]

Several contemporary concerns were reflected in Savage's remarks. What types of activities could be offered to patients? What impact did occupation have on mental symptoms? And what was the role of staff in providing or encouraging it? The types of work depicted here are primarily recreational pastimes. Indeed, in Bethlem's 'Return of Employment' two years previously, the vast majority of patients who were employed (just under half) were engaged in 'reading, writing, drawing etc.'[3] Given that the occupations most commonly represented among Bethlem patients were lower-middle-class professions, such as clerks and governesses, these activities might be seen as mirroring patients' lives outside the institutions and even empowering them to remain engaged in ordinary pursuits. Some patients actually set up journals while in the hospital; others (albeit a small minority) published books.[4]

Bethlem was very much a middle-class institution by the late nineteenth century, and Savage's words contrast in some ways with attitudes to work in pauper asylums of the same period.[5] Both the numbers employed and the types of occupation varied in these institutions. This is seen particularly clearly in instances when private and pauper asylums came under the same management. In Dumfries, Scotland, the private Crichton Royal Institution was overseen by the same medical superintendent as the charitable Southern Counties Asylum. In the superintendent's diary for 1880, James Adam (1834–1908) recorded that just 14 per cent of patients in the Crichton Royal were employed, while 60 per cent of their lower-class counterparts at Southern Counties were.[6] Manual labour was common in pauper asylums, and patients worked on the grounds, in the laundry, in workshops and on farms, enabling cash-strapped institutions to reduce running costs through the use of free labour.[7] At the Metropolitan District Asylum in Caterham, for example, a report for 1871–72 noted that the trenching and levelling of a piece of ground for a cricket pitch had 'been done solely by Patients' labour'.[8]

Patient work was thus a useful resource: even at Bethlem, inhabitants of both sexes were expected to assist attendants with housework on the wards. It is interesting to note that, while Savage considered male patients largely unable to work in the grounds, 'owing to the class of patients not being suited to heavy work', there was no similar expectation that they would be unable to perform household chores: social class perhaps had more of a bearing on occupation even than gender.[9] Indeed, Savage used occupational differences as a justification for segregating asylums by class. He noted:

> I have often had to insist on the importance of the class distinctions in Asylums, it is injurious to put domestic servants in the same ward with governesses and cultured ladies, the servants are not comfortable, and the ladies feel a loss of self-respect and often will not help themselves by doing ordinary ward work lest they too should be considered as servants. Asylum treatment is so eminently social that matters of this kind cannot be neglected.[10]

Savage's words here also point to the second issue related to occupation in asylums. Any form of work, however ordinary, was considered by many to be directly curative. The explanation for this notion is rooted in attitudes to selfhood in this period. The Victorian understanding of self emerged from the Enlightenment quest for self-knowledge, which itself followed on the rationalist discourse of seventeenth-century 'New Science'.[11] By the 1840s, however, belief in the intrinsic merits of self-knowledge and introspection had diminished. While the term self-conscious (as descriptive of an act of cognition and inward sense of reflection) dates from at least the seventeenth century, the earliest quotation given in the *Oxford English Dictionary* for the 'morbid' sense of the term is from 1834.[12] By the 1840s and 1850s, this gave rise to the psychiatric concept of 'morbid introspection' which, in later decades, developed into broader concerns about the potential dangers (to individuals and society) of 'self-consciousness' and the 'self-culture' of civilisation, as psychiatrists extended their remit beyond the asylum.[13] In the 1880s and 1890s, patients (as well as practitioners) were blaming introspection and self-consciousness for the onset of illness, suggesting that such associations had become widespread.[14] Young Arthur Browne, for example, was reported to have told the Bethlem medical officers that his delusions were 'probably due to self-consciousness & that he inherits that', while Nesta Luke was said to have attributed her illness directly to 'morbid introspection'.[15]

Occupation was one of the ways in which asylum superintendents aimed to counter this morbid introspection, which was considered responsible for exacerbating mental symptoms and, sometimes, the onset of illness itself. This explains why there was often not much distinction made between work-based and recreational pursuits. Annual reports frequently conflated the two, for both were considered valuable in drawing a patient 'out of himself and his narrowing feelings'.[16] The same understanding could also be found outside the professional realm. While George Boughton Hume was on leave of absence from Bethlem in October 1888, his wife Harriet wrote to doctors that she thought his condition had improved, offering as evidence: 'He has just started a little drawing which I imagine is an improvement.'[17] The social nature of asylum treatment, as described above by Savage, was an important element of this model. The aforementioned tables of employment at the Dumfries asylums also included a column listing those patients 'Dining in Association' (around two thirds of private patients and a third of pauper inmates). This was a particular innovation of James Adam's. In his first year at Dumfries, Adam established a *'Table d'hôte'* in every ward and, by year's end, claimed this had led to 'an increased tone of life and cheerfulness … among the ladies and gentlemen under their new social habits'.[18]

Both work and entertainment, it was claimed, could be substituted for other measures formerly used to prevent violence or self-injury, such as restraint. At the Crichton Royal Institution, James Adam described a patient, Mrs Blacklock, who had gouged out one of her eyes shortly after admission in 1875.[19] In October 1880, nine months after Adam became superintendent of the asylum, he reported that he had abolished the 'locked bed' from the institution, suggesting that Mrs Blacklock may have been under regular nightly restraint for five years. After visiting her during the following two nights, Adam declared that 'careful nursing and nourishing with a generous diet and a moderate amount of stimulant' had been substituted for restraint.[20] Mrs Blacklock's desire to injure herself was further countered by the activities in the asylum, so that she:

> Attends and enjoys the various amusements, and she enters with spirit and animation at times into the dances, she plays the piano, and altogether leads a life of as much composure and comfort as can be expected in a case of the kind, in which recovery cannot be hoped for.[21]

James Adam's conclusion on the case of Mrs Blacklock (written, as it was, as part of an article on 'self-mutilation') implied that entertainment and recreation had played a key role in preventing further episodes of self-inflicted injury. This reflects a wider emphasis on the importance of the social environment of the asylum in both care and cure.

Adam and Savage were not alone in viewing social interaction as a key element of asylum treatment. Descriptions of mental improvement in case records from 1880–1900 tended to be couched in terms relating to appearance, industriousness and interaction with others. Some forms of occupation (in particular, recreational pursuits) could thus be viewed as both preventing introspection and encouraging a person's interest in their fellows: a social ability which alienists considered was markedly diminished by insanity. As well-known author Daniel Hack Tuke put it in 1892: 'A departure from altruism and a leaning towards egoism, mark some of the early phases of mental affections.'[22] Cure, it was thought, could thus be measured by the level of interest and empathy individuals had for those around them.

Moral treatment and the creation of 'useful members of society'

Returning to the 'problem of the middle-class insane', there is one further aspect of Savage's report on occupation that deserves analysis: the proximity of his ideas to the ethos of moral treatment. A method of asylum treatment and governance often associated with the York Retreat around 1800, moral treatment continued to hold a strong resonance in the late nineteenth century.[23] The meaning of the term had, however, shifted during the intervening years, not least due to an increased emphasis on psychological models of mental health. In his 1892 essay, *Reform in the Treatment of the Insane*, Daniel Hack Tuke claimed that moral treatment was founded on the idea that the insane were not absolutely deprived of reason, and thus could be motivated by hope, feeling and honour. These same motivations he also highlighted in his description of psycho-therapeutics (explained as the influence of the mind upon the body for the treatment of illness).[24] While, by the 1870s, some physicians had come to view moral treatment as synonymous with the asylum environment, which encouraged rest and the removal from exciting influences, Tuke and his influential collaborator in the *Manual of Psychological Medicine*, John Charles Bucknill, claimed this was not the case. For Bucknill, rest was a physical therapy, similar to the mild air recommended for the treatment of consumption. Moral treatment instead came down to 'the influence of mind upon mind', and thus could be better described as 'intellectual and emotional treatment'.[25] Many of the methods by which this influence could be exerted, including education, diversion and attention, were also those Tuke saw as available to excite the imagination to effect cure through psycho-therapeutics.[26] This idea of 'influence', which, Bucknill claimed, could be exerted by attendants as well as doctors, could certainly incorporate coercive elements.

But in what ways did these physicians aim to influence their patients? Much of the language in texts from the 1880s and 1890s focused on the creation of 'useful members of society'. This was not necessarily a class-specific ideal, and similar phrases can be found in use at all the institutions so far referenced. The term 'useful' was multi-layered. One of its meanings was certainly to be economically productive. James Adam referred to efforts at Caterham to teach young residents a trade, through employment in the 'Tailors', Shoemakers' and Upholsterers' shops'.[27] Yet there remained a strong moral element to the educational efforts employed. Caterham was a so-called 'imbecile' asylum, and patients were largely those considered to be congenitally weak-minded. As Adam put it:

> Although, however, the bulk of the Patients now resident cannot be cured, they can be brought up to and maintained at a much higher mental and physical standard, and made useful members of society ... whereas by want of care and liberal treatment they would soon lapse into moral and physical degradation.[28]

Not only, then, was it important for patients to earn a living after discharge (as Adam claimed had been the case for some at Caterham). For a former patient to be 'useful', he or she must also not be deemed morally or physically degraded, an idea that chimed with contemporary understandings of racial degeneration.[29] These same attitudes continued to influence discussion post 1900, feeding into a perceived need to increase institutionalisation – and thus enforce moral obligations on the so-called 'weak-minded' – that led to the Mental Deficiency Act of 1913.[30]

The same moral and intellectual attitude to work was in place at Bethlem: an educated background was certainly not considered an excuse for remaining idle. When thirty-five-year-old Alexander Bruce was admitted in 1899, he was recorded as being of no occupation.[31] His friends complained that he constantly changed his residence and was unwilling to participate in family life. During his time at Bethlem, Bruce was reported to have told doctors 'that what he requires is a little discipline' and that he wanted 'to be "helped" to work'.[32] A letter subsequent to discharge was regarded as evidence of cure, for Bruce assured his former doctors that 'my intention in the future is to go with the stream & not against it. ... My experience here has quite enlightened me.'[33] Participating fully in society was thus seen as an important signifier of mental health. However, symptoms of mental ill-health were not thought necessarily to be a barrier to usefulness even outside the asylum. In a lecture in 1906, George Savage reflected on his early asylum experience, stating that he would then have thought anyone hearing voices required incarceration. However, since then, he had:

[S]everal examples of men suffering from these subjective nervous disorders who are earning their livings and are as free as you or I. ... it is interesting to have to note that there are some who, being hallucinated, still are capable citizens.[34]

While Savage likely had certain professional considerations in mind here – he was at that time in private practice, and keen to widen the field of those who might be treated by 'nerve specialists' outside the asylum – it is interesting that he urged greater freedom for certain asylum patients by using a model of work. Within an institution, patients might similarly be rewarded for assistance by greater freedom, such as leave in the grounds.[35] This idea of 'usefulness' as a measure of mental health was also widespread within the American mental hygiene movement, and promoted by those sympathetic to the needs of the mentally ill, including psychologist William James and former asylum patient Clifford Beers.[36]

Work and asylum life were so bound up together that patients sometimes requested career advice from their former doctors. In 1893, eight months after the young John Percy Ashton was discharged from hospital, cured, he wrote to Dr R. Percy Smith:

Do you know whether I could be anything else besides, or instead of, a farmer? Just before I was discharged you told my father you thought I liked the trade I am in now. I thought when you said it, you thought of something else as well.[37]

Ashton's question reminds us that occupation was a key part of late nineteenth-century identity and changing one's trade was not a decision to be undertaken lightly. Loss of occupation was a serious concern in terms of financial and social status, and often considered a reason why someone might enter an asylum in the first place. When Robert Beckford Govey, a middle-aged bank clerk, was admitted to Bethlem in 1882, the reason for his illness was listed as 'anxiety in business', and another mental breakdown the following year was attributed to 'Disappointment (loss of situation)'.[38] Opportunities to remain associated with a former occupation despite asylum internment could thus be regarded as empowering. In the 1850s, when society photographer Henry Hering took portraits of a number of Bethlem patients, George Johnston was pictured holding a sextant, emphasising his former position as ship's captain.[39] This was despite the fact that Johnston was incarcerated in the criminal department of the hospital, and his portrait was deemed to represent both his diagnosis and crime: subtitled as it was 'Mania. Homicide'. The style and format of the photograph, however, made both of these readings less significant than Johnston's occupation, presented as the key signifier of his identity.

Malingering:
The context of shifting attitudes towards the failure to work

Since occupation was seen as curative and economically useful, as well as a sign of improved mental state and quality of life, those who refused to participate in activities within asylums were viewed with suspicion. When thirty-eight-year-old clerk Walter James McMullen was admitted to Bethlem as a voluntary boarder in October 1889 (having previously been a certified patient), he was given a free place in the hospital for two months. Soon afterwards, however, the patient was described in disapproving tones: 'Lazy, quiet, does not work. Eats & smokes.' A week later, doctors were still more suspicious that McMullen was not a deserving case for treatment: 'He seems to be anxious to prove that he has numerous troubles & ill defined pains. ... Seems to be hypochondriacal & malingering.' A week later he was discharged uncured.[40] Yet if Walter McMullen was 'malingering' (that is, feigning illness), what had he not been cured of? Or was malingering considered to be an entirely separate category from his mental state?

By the early 1900s, some medical writers were claiming that malingering had 'reached a high level of perfection'.[41] Texts emphasised the role of the medical 'detective' to uncover those individuals deemed to constitute a social problem.[42] While this was certainly not a new idea for doctors, the last few decades of the nineteenth century saw a rapidly increasing interest in both the concept of malingering and use of the term itself. In three key medical journals (*Journal of Mental Science*, *British Medical Journal* and *The Lancet*), the number of articles containing the term soared from less than thirty in 1851 to nearly 300 in the first decade of the twentieth century. Similar levels of increase occurred in textbooks and newspapers.

But where did the concept of malingering come from? One medical correspondent to the *Oxford English Dictionary* – William Sykes MD – claimed to have 'traced this word down to almost the case of the Great French War'.[43] Like other writers in the 1880s and 1890s, Sykes was certain that malingering had entered the English language from the French verb *malingre* (to be sickly or weak), and that it gained an association with military conduct during the Napoleonic Wars.[44] This connection was made despite the fact that neither Sykes nor anyone else could find any French quotation using *malingre* in such a sense and, indeed, the term 'malingeror' in British texts pre-dated the Napoleonic Wars.[45] The idea thus rested on a prior assumption that military malingering had a French history, based on the fact that France was the first country to legally punish self-inflicted injury for the purposes of avoiding duty in a law of 1832.[46] This ruling subsequently became incorporated into military law in other nations.[47] Throughout the period 1870–1914 (and often beyond), commentators in French and English regularly referred to the origins of the concept of 'malingering' (however phrased) in the Napoleonic Wars.[48]

Yet military parlance alone does not explain the surge in interest in malingering in the last decades of the nineteenth century. Indeed, it was the increasing application of the concept to civilian populations that accounted for a large proportion of the increased use. A growing interest in civilian 'malingering' has been convincingly associated by historians with the rise of health insurance systems across Europe: the introduction of accident insurance in Germany in 1871 and the Employer's Liability Act of 1880 and subsequent Workmen's Compensation Acts in England.[49] Historical accounts of the emergence of these worker insurance schemes have portrayed them as representing a broad shift from a model of obligation (in which responsibility for accident and compensation lay with the employer, unless employee negligence could be proved) to one of collective responsibility. In the latter model, insurers would measure the statistical probability of an accident occurring against its severity to determine both the cost of insurance and any pay-out: a method that would seem to be free of judgement or blame. Yet the costs of such a system, and the means of assessing the worker's right to a claim, nonetheless made debates around malingering class-oriented from the outset. The malingerer was invariably the worker, not the employer, and he (and not his employer) would be the person accused of attempting to cheat the system. Thus physicians often became involved in such a system by policing it, whatever their personal political ideals.[50]

These concerns seemed to legitimise a distinction between deserving and undeserving recipients of relief, and can be (and have been) used to attack the concept of a welfare state as well as to support it.[51] Yet the background in military malingering also indicates another element in the late nineteenth-century context, suggesting that it was not as explicitly economic as many later writers have assumed, but also incorporated previous attention to 'duty'. We can see this particularly by comparing one of the earliest English medical texts on the topic with its counterparts nearly a century later. In 1835-36, the young Hector Gavin (1815–55) won a prize for his University of Edinburgh essay, 'On the feigned and factitious diseases of soldiers and seamen'.[52] Many later writers referenced Gavin's text, in particular the fact that, when the author revised his text in 1843, it now concerned 'chiefly' soldiers and seamen, and he also included a long list of other types of people who might be inclined to feign disease. These included prisoners, 'those of the lower classes of society who prefer idleness to industry', fanatics, sycophants, imitators, hysterics and 'persons not at all in poverty … who assume the semblance of disease from some inexplicable causes: these are chiefly females'.[53]

Many of Gavin's assumptions of the types of people inclined to malinger were repeated in later texts.[54] What changed, however, was the way in which these assumptions were framed. While Gavin's text had a strong moral emphasis on duty, the economic context was emphasised to a far greater extent in the early 1900s. This is not to say that Gavin did not consider that some malingerers might have a financial motive for their acts. However, his main concern was the moral impact on society of feigning disease. Thus, the role of the doctor for Gavin was twofold: to detect malingering, but also to find the quickest method to return the malingerer to his duty, through such measures as exciting shame or fear. Articles in psychological journals in subsequent decades draw similar conclusions. A piece in alienist Forbes Winslow's *Journal of Psychological Medicine and Mental Pathology* in 1856 placed military self-mutilation among a list of 'moral and criminal epidemics', through a section drawn from the author's *Anatomy of Suicide*.[55] Winslow's main concern in the later article was imitation, a factor he saw as responsible for historical and contemporary mental 'epidemics', from suicide and self-mutilation to spiritualist fanaticism. For Winslow, the moral aberration of one individual might be rapidly duplicated by his fellows, assisted by a sensationalist press, the laxity of spiritual teachers, the misuse of science and an ineffectual legislature.[56]

By the 1900s, however, malingering was largely couched in financial terms. One of the most outspoken writers on the topic was Sir John Collie (1860–1935). A lengthy background as medical examiner for various insurance companies in the late nineteenth century meant that Collie was appointed Home Office medical referee for the Workmen's Compensation Act. He published a number of guides for practitioners to help them determine whether or not compensation was justified, including the outspoken *Malingering and Feigned Sickness* (first published in 1913). The author claimed that he conducted around 2,000 medical examinations a year on behalf of two large public bodies and fifteen to twenty insurance companies. Of those he examined Collie considered that 25 per cent were fit to return to work.[57] Stemming from an insurance perspective, Collie's text was framed very differently from Gavin's. Whereas Gavin considered his historical examples as evidence that malingering was primarily associated with moral avoidance of duty, Collie's history of malingering was associated with legislative changes around compensation.

> The Common Law of England, which gave the right to obtain monetary compensation from negligent people, whether employers or otherwise, undoubtedly gave the first impetus to a more general adoption of the practice of making much out of little; the various Workmen's Compensation Acts have still further enlarged the field; and with the advent of the National Insurance Act, it is practically certain that it will become a matter for which all medical men must always keep their eyes open.[58]

Like Gavin, Collie began with assumptions about the psychology of human motivation, and fitted these into an explanation for malingering. What is striking to the historian is the way in which explanations altered. In the wake of the European unrest of 1830, Gavin and Forbes Winslow were most concerned with the way in which the acts of one individual might be duplicated by those around them, exemplified by the spread of malingering. However, in the capitalist-industrialist 1900s, an economic explanation of individual greed appeared the most likely one.

From an insurance perspective, malingerers in the period 1870–1914 were thus largely represented as working class. In 1889, George Thorpe, a general practitioner in Walthamstow, commented indignantly on the case of a seventeen-year-old servant he had treated. This 'healthy-looking country girl' visited Thorpe on several occasions with an inflamed hand.[59] The surgeon seems to have been suspicious from the outset, for '[h]er mistress informed me that the girl was not at all fond of work, and that she had a deal of trouble to get her to do it'.[60] When Thorpe examined the hand he discovered a needle, which he removed – a procedure that recurred several times over the next week. Eventually, Thorpe 'felt so disgusted with her that I advised her mistress to get rid of her at once, which was done, and the girl returned to the country'.[61] He concluded that '[i]t seems hardly credible that a person of her age could be so cunning, and would inflict so much pain upon herself to avoid work'.[62] This explanation nonetheless appeared to Thorpe to be the only possible one, given the girl's station in life.

Class-oriented definitions of malingering continued to appear in physicians' reports on working-class women who injured themselves in the early twentieth century.[63] Accusations of deception were not necessarily the only interpretations of working-class injury made by doctors. A liberal political bent might suggest a socio-environmental explanation. Scottish laryngologist, Sir James Dundas-Grant, for example, referred sympathetically (if patronisingly) to a 'poor lodging-house drudge' who had continued to return for hospital treatment following an operation, as scraps of bone were regularly found in the wound. Later, it was discovered that she was inserting the bone herself, an act Dundas-Grant judged a 'pitiful endeavour to obtain respite from the drudgery of her everyday existence [which] made her an object for commiseration rather than for blame'.[64]

Self-mutilation and 'motiveless malingering' in psychiatry

This interpretation of self-inflicted injury as malingering is an interesting one in light of the increasing attention paid to self-mutilation as a 'morbid impulse' in asylum psychiatry of the same period.[65] By the last two decades of the nineteenth century, the term 'self-mutilation' appeared in the indexes of psychiatric manuals, was the focus of journal articles, and had received a five-page definition in Daniel Hack Tuke's *Dictionary of Psychological Medicine*

(1892).⁶⁶ Alienists tended to incorporate a wide variety of acts under this headline term. In psychiatric and other medical literature one can find many descriptions of self-castration, eye enucleation, limb amputation, hair-plucking, knocking, burning and skin-picking, all of which were generally regarded to be distinct from suicidal acts. Many of these self-injurious acts were frequently characterised in asylum records and published papers as 'selfish'.⁶⁷ It might seem a sensible suggestion to associate this concern with contemporary writing on 'malingering': self-mutilation, after all, could render an individual economically unproductive. Yet there was an ongoing moral element to this discussion of self-inflicted injury, which was seen by many alienists as evidence of a morbid self-attention, and thus a wider failure to contribute to society than a simple refusal to work.

We can see this particularly in the psychological view of self-inflicted injury as an element of so-called 'motiveless malingering'. In 1870 (inspired not by economic legislation but by the high-profile death of the 'Welsh fasting girl', Sarah Jacob, the previous year)⁶⁸ the *British Medical Journal* (*BMJ*) published a series of articles on the topic of feigned disease and malingering.⁶⁹ An editorial remarked that investigation of this topic had hitherto been confined to the simulation of disease in order to escape military service. Although this was not strictly the case, these articles certainly pre-dated the financial incentives regarded as prominent by later writers. The majority of writers in the 1870s considered 'motiveless malingering' (as the *BMJ* termed it) to be an entirely new topic of medical enquiry. The very terminology used here indicates an important element of the debate. Motiveless malingerers were to be distinguished from those in whom the reason for self-inflicted injury was deemed obvious: evasion of duty or financial gain. By analogy to such contexts, however, the assumption was made that the asylum or 'nervous' patient *must* have an underlying motive for his or her injury. The term 'motiveless malingering' was thus adopted for distinction's sake, while:

> [B]y no means intending to imply that the will ever really acts without motive, but merely that in these cases the motive cannot be quoted beforehand as explaining the act, but has to be sought after the fact has been established by other means.⁷⁰

These motives were largely judged to be internal, and strongly associated with the mental state and emotional needs of the individual concerned.

An interesting example of this is the case of one young woman admitted to Bethlem in February 1893. Edith Mary Ellen Blyth was aged 30 and had been 'subject to hysterical symptoms for eleven years but never of unsound mind'.⁷¹ Now, however, Edith was diagnosed with melancholia, although many of her notes described her earlier hysterical symptoms. Of particular interest were the sores on the patient's limbs, which had appeared over the previous six years. After visits to 'over 20 doctors', these sores had eventually been ruled as self-inflicted.[72] On admission, a detailed description was given of Edith's physical state, and her methods of inflicting injury, primarily focusing on the case as one of deception.

> She has a number of scars on the left leg extending from the knee to the ankle, there are about 40 discrete ones, and others which have run together. ... She has similar old wounds on the left hip, the right thigh and on the extensor aspect of the right forearm. All these are self-inflicted and were done by scraping with a pair of scissors, and rubbing in ammonia afterwards. ... For the leg she has been seen by many medical men (by Broadbent, Christopher Heath, Jonathan Hutchinson, Treves etc.) and has undergone a course of the Weir-Mitchell treatment at Brighton. She was supposed to have some skin disease, this deception was continued till discovered by one of the surgeons (Treves) she was continually consulting.[73]

Yet the discovery that the injuries were self-inflicted did not appear to change the patient's behaviour, and Edith Blyth declared herself absolutely unable to control her impulses to injure herself. In hospital, she picked and bit at her hands, arms and fingers. On one occasion she was restrained with padded gloves, but when this failed to stop her biting herself the treatment seems to have been discontinued. Edith's doctors certainly noted the contradictions between their patient's acts, her declarations that she could not control herself and her good character, for '[s]he recognises that it is a disgraceful thing to have such injuries'.[74] Yet Edith's protests that 'she has done nothing wrong because she could not help it' do not appear to have been accepted.[75]

Cases like Edith's were described by practitioners as the type of malingerer who might 'assume their maladies without any ostensible object in sight, and often to the destruction, apparently, of their social happiness'.[76] The explanation for this was generally allied to insanity or associated nervous diagnoses such as hysteria. However, rather than dismissing self-mutilation as an insane (and therefore inexplicable) act, a number of alienists in the period 1870–1914 made concerted efforts to explain the actions of their patients – and, by comparison, to gain greater knowledge of human motivation in general. James Adam, for example, declared that he wished to throw:

> [A]dditional light ... upon the obscurity which surrounds the whole subject [through] an endeavour to trace some of the motives which have prompted to the commission of the acts at various periods of history, and under various religious conditions.[77]

Skin lesions, like those of Edith Blyth, were a particular focus in published papers. One physician in the 1930s reflected back on these cases as evidence that self-injury was directly expressive of the inner life of the individual: 'a reflection upon the skin of a disordered condition of the mind'.[78] Of the papers on 'motiveless malingerers' published in the *BMJ* in 1870, three dealt with 'feigned or hysterical diseases of the skin'. Similar examples appeared in dermatology textbooks and, at the end of the nineteenth century, this form of self-inflicted injury was the only one to receive a specific entry in Allbutt's *System of Medicine*.[79] Some physicians claimed that cases 'were nearly always of the nature of mechanical or chemical irritation of the skin', although others considered that lesions might appear spontaneously through a condition of mental distress: the effect of a peculiarly delicate state of both skin and imagination in neurotic individuals.[80]

Yet what were the most prominent explanations given by alienists for these forms of self-inflicted injury, and did these differ from those suggested for malingering in the same period? Self-mutilation was most commonly (although not exclusively) associated with diagnoses of melancholia, hypochondriasis, hysteria and moral insanity: all instances in which 'self-attention' was considered to be a particular concern. As evidence of the patient's mental state, self-injurious acts were frequently associated with a failure to work and socialise within the institution.[81] Thus, although considered to reveal the patient's mental state of introspection or self-consciousness, self-injury also continued to be considered evidence of moral and social lapses. In a paper on 'Insanity of conduct', published in the late 1890s, George Savage and Charles Mercier aimed to show 'that breaches of the conventional as well as the moral laws of society may be but symptoms of disorder or disease of the higher nervous system'.[82] Savage's examples in the paper concentrated on the 'malingering and mischief-making' he connected with hysteria and hypochondriasis.[83] Miss M., for example, a 'bright, pretty and accomplished' girl, had been sending threatening anonymous letters to relatives, 'saying many things which were not true. ... Beside all this, some time before, she had had a peculiar skin affection, which was proved to have been produced by herself by burning with hair-curlers'.[84]

Despite claiming Miss M.'s acts to be an instance of 'motiveless malingering', Savage nonetheless connected her self-injury with deception as well as her 'most supreme self-confidence': the inference being that her selfish instincts had won out.[85] This was more than just an issue concerning the individual. As in Forbes Winslow's article some forty years earlier, alienists in the 1890s and 1900s considered that the absence of altruism and social interaction (which both self-injury and refusal to work were considered evidence of) was a wider concern for society. Henry Maudsley, for example, associated the development from egoistic to altruistic sentiments with a shift in the individual's attitude from 'self-consciousness' to 'world-consciousness' (and *vice versa*).[86] Similarly, George Savage saw moral insanity as the form of mental disorder that was 'most dangerous socially' for such patients had 'no sense of truth or honesty, and no altruism'.[87] Malingering and self-injury, while interpreted economically by many physicians outside the asylum, continued to be viewed in the institution in relation to psychiatric understandings of the need for occupation in order to maintain physical, intellectual and moral health.

Conclusion

This chapter has argued that we cannot understand the meaning of work in the asylum in the period 1870–1914 without considering attitudes outside. Although many asylums were increasingly dealing with chronic cases in this period, the hope remained that work within an institution might produce useful members of society. Sometimes this might be by assisting with an outright cure and rehabilitation; in other instances, work could render inmates economically useful – and improve their wellbeing – without leading to discharge. Of course, this is not to say that the requirement to work was always welcomed by asylum patients. The model of occupation was heavily class-based, and the relevance and type of work depended on the status of the patient. The background of moral treatment ensured that recreation and employment were often considered equally useful forms of occupation, both in drawing inhabitants out of their 'morbid introspection' as well as fitting them intellectually and morally for social life beyond the institution. While occupation might be an obligation, it could also be empowering: narrowing the gap between asylum and society, despite laying expectations on the individual that they were required to fulfil should they wish to be discharged.

Attention to occupation in the late nineteenth century must also be seen in association with an economic and legal framework around work as a civic duty. This is particularly evident in contemporary attention to the perceived problem of malingering and the avoidance of work in civilian life. The increased interest within psychiatric circles in malingering, in particular through their attention to self-mutilation, encouraged a shift in understanding of the motivation it was assumed lay behind certain forms of malingering: from financial gain to a focus on the mental state of the individual concerned. This could be seen as challenging contemporary models of the social and political value of occupation. However, there was a strong moral context to this view of self-inflicted injury, even when there appeared to be no opportunities for any particular gain to be made by the individual through malingering. This makes most sense when we view self-mutilation within the context in which it emerged: the late nineteenth-century asylum emphasis on occupation as one of three key elements of recovery, with importance also laid on the physical appearance of the patient and his or her social interaction. Occupation was an important part of asylum life and therapy in the period 1870–1914. It was part of a much broader approach to asylum care and treatment that, it was claimed, was necessary in order to reintegrate patients into society. Sometimes (as happened at Caterham), even those deemed incurable could be rendered economically useful. The model of 'usefulness' could thus apply to the acute and 'curable' patients admitted to Bethlem as well as the incurable and chronic inmates that made up the population of many county asylums at this time.

Notes

1 George Savage, 'The Physician's Report for the Year 1882', in *General Report of the Royal Hospitals of Bridewell and Bethlem, 1882* (London: Batten & Davies, 1883), p. 41.
2 *Ibid.*, p. 41.
3 George Savage, 'The Physician's Report for the Year 1880', in *General Report of the Royal Hospitals of Bridewell and Bethlem, 1880* (London: Batten & Davies, 1881), p. 63.
4 Anon, 'Editorial', in *Under the Dome: The Quarterly Magazine of Bethlem Royal Hospital*, 1:1 (1892), 1–2; Bethlem Royal Hospital Archives (hereafter BRHA), CB/120, *Male Patient Casebook 1882*, entry 102 (Walter Abraham Haigh). Haigh also assisted both George Savage, and one of his successors Theophilus Hyslop, with their textbooks and is acknowledged in both.
5 Jonathan Andrews *et al.*, *The History of Bethlem* (London: Routledge, 1997), p. 119.
6 Wellcome Library, London (hereafter WLL), MSS.5517, diary by James Adam, 1880, entry for 2 January.
7 This was emphasised by Foucault in his classic work on moral treatment. Michel Foucault, *Madness and Civilisation: A History of Insanity in the Age of Reason*, trans. Richard Howard (London: Routledge, 1989). See more recent examples in Joseph Melling and Bill Forsythe, *Insanity, Institutions and Society, 1800–1914* (London and New York: Routledge, 1999); Andrew T. Scull, *The Most Solitary of Afflictions: Madness and Society in Britain, 1700–1900* (New Haven, CT: Yale University Press, 1993).
8 James Adam and William Cortis, *First Annual Report of the Committee of Management, Caterham Asylum* (London: Harrison & Sons, 1871), p. 16.
9 Savage, 'Physician's Report for 1882', p. 43. In 1880, just seven men were working in the grounds, but 27 out of 104 were contributing to household work (compared to twenty women out of the same total).
10 George Savage, 'The Physician's Report for the Year 1884', in *General Report of the Royal Hospitals of Bridewell and Bethlem, 1884* (London: Batten & Davies, 1885), p. 35.
11 Jerrold E. Seigel, *The Idea of the Self: Thought and Experience in Western Europe Since the Seventeenth Century* (Cambridge: Cambridge University Press, 2004); Rhodri Hayward, *Resisting History: Religious Transcendence and the Invention of the Unconscious* (Manchester: Manchester University Press, 2007); David Armstrong, *A New History of Identity: a Sociology of Medical Knowledge* (Basingstoke: Palgrave, 2002); Nikolas Rose, *Inventing our Selves: Psychology, Power and Personhood* (Cambridge: Cambridge University Press, 1996).

12 'self-conscious, adj.' *OED Online* (Oxford: Oxford University Press, 2013), www.oed.com.libproxy.ucl.ac.uk/view/Entry/175163?redirectedFrom=self-conscious (accessed 17 December 2013).
13 Michael J. Clark, '"Morbid introspection", unsoundness of mind, and British psychological medicine', in William F. Bynum, Roy Porter and Michael Shepherd (eds), *The Anatomy of Madness: Essays in the History of Psychiatry* (London: Routledge, 1988), vol. 3, pp. 71–101; George Savage, 'The influence of surroundings on the production of insanity', *Journal of Mental Science*, 37:159 (1891), 529–35; George Fielding Blandford, 'Prevention of insanity (prophylaxis)', in Daniel Hack Tuke (ed.), *A Dictionary of Psychological Medicine* (London: J. and A. Churchill, 1892), vol. 2, pp. 996–1002.
14 Edgar Sheppard, 'On some of the modern teachings of insanity', *Journal of Mental Science*, 17:80 (1872), 499–514, p. 502.
15 BRHA, CB/145, *Male Patient Case Book 1893*, entry 26; BRHA, CB/164, *Female Patient Case Book 1900*, entry 124. See also George Savage, 'Hypochondriasis and insanity', in Tuke (ed.), *Dictionary*, vol. 1, pp. 610–18; Henry Rayner, 'Melancholia and hypochondriasis', in Thomas Clifford Allbutt (ed.), *A System of Medicine* (London: Macmillan, 1899), pp. 361–81; Henry Maudsley, *Responsibility in Mental Disease* (London: Henry S. King, 1874), p. 298.
16 Savage, 'Hypochondriasis and insanity', in Tuke (ed.), *Dictionary*, vol. 1, p. 615.
17 BRHA, CB/128, Letter from Mrs Hume to Dr Smith, 28 November 1888, entry 27.
18 WLL, MSS.5517, 1880, entry for 3 December.
19 James Adam, 'Self-mutilation', in Tuke (ed.), *Dictionary*, vol. 2, pp. 1147–52, 1150.
20 WLL, MSS.5517, 1880, entry for October 2.
21 Adam, 'Self-mutilation', in Tuke (ed.), *Dictionary*, vol. 2, p. 1150.
22 Daniel Hack Tuke, 'Altruism', in Tuke (ed.), *Dictionary*, vol. 1, p. 83. For the same view, see Robert Jones, 'A lecture on mental unsoundness amounting to certifiable insanity and its diagnosis', *The Lancet*, 161:4162 (1903), 1572–6, 1575.
23 Anne Digby, *Madness, Morality, and Medicine: A Study of the York Retreat, 1796–1914* (Cambridge: Cambridge University Press, 1985).
24 Daniel Hack Tuke, *Reform in the Treatment of the Insane* (London: J. and A. Churchill, 1892), p. 36; Daniel Hack Tuke, *Illustrations of the Influence of the Mind upon the Body in Health and Disease: Designed to Elucidate the Action of the Imagination* (London: J. and A. Churchill, 1884), vol. 2, pp. 236–50.
25 John Charles Bucknill and Daniel Hack Tuke, *A Manual of Psychological Medicine* (London: John Churchill, 4th edn, 1879), p. 663.
26 Tuke, *Illustrations*, vol. 2, p. 282.
27 Adam and Cortis, *First Annual Report*, p. 17.
28 James Adam and William Cortis, *Third Annual Report of the Committee of Management, Caterham Asylum 1872–3* (London: Harrison & Sons, 1873), p. 16.
29 For more on degeneration theory and medicine, see Richard A. Soloway, *Demography and Degeneration: Eugenics and the Declining Birthrate in Twentieth-Century Britain* (Chapel Hill, NC: University of North Carolina Press, 1990); Daniel Pick, *Faces of Degeneration: A European Disorder, c. 1848 – c. 1918* (Cambridge: Cambridge University Press, 1989).

30 See the discussion following George Savage, 'On insanity and marriage', *Journal of Mental Science*, 57 (1911), 97–112. See also Anne Digby and David Wright (eds), *From Idiocy to Mental Deficiency: Historical Perspectives on People with Learning Disabilities* (London: Routledge, 1996).
31 BRHA, CB/160, *Male Patient Casebook 1899*, entry 16.
32 Ibid.
33 Ibid.
34 George Savage, 'An address on the borderland of insanity', *British Medical Journal*, 1:2357 (1906), 489–92, p. 491.
35 For example in the case of Walter Haigh, BRHA, CB/120, *Male Patient Casebook 1882*, entry 102, or Francis John Ambridge, CB/145, *Male Patient Casebook 1893*, entry 77.
36 See Clifford W. Beers, *A Mind that Found Itself: An Autobiography* (London: W. Heinemann, 1923); Emma Sutton, 'Re-writing "The Laws of Health": William James on the Philosophy and Politics of Disease in Nineteenth-Century America' (PhD Dissertation, University College London, 2012).
37 BRHA, CB/141, 'Letter from John Percy Ashton to Dr Smith, March 1893', *Male Patient Casebook 1892*, entry 96.
38 BRHA, CB/120, *Male Patient Casebook 1882*, entry 95; BRHA, CB/122, *Male Patient Casebook 1883*, entry 17.
39 BRHA, HPA-35, 'Portrait of G. J., a male criminal patient diagnosed with mania and charged with homicide', c. 1857–59.
40 BRHA, CB/131, *Voluntary Boarder Casebook, 1886–89*, entry 84.
41 Anon., 'Malingery', *The Lancet*, 165:4245 (1905), 45–6.
42 For the background on this, see Wolfgang Schaffner, 'Event, series, trauma: The probabilistic revolution of the mind in the late nineteenth and early twentieth centuries', in Mark S. Micale and Paul F. Lerner (eds), *Traumatic Pasts: History, Psychiatry, and Trauma in the Modern Age, 1870–1930* (Cambridge: Cambridge University Press, 2001), pp. 81–91; Greg A. Eghigian, 'German welfare state as a discourse of trauma', in Micale and Lerner, *Traumatic Pasts*, pp. 92–114; Joanna Bourke, *Dismembering the Male: Men's Bodies, Britain and the Great War* (London: Reaktion Books, 1996), ch. 2; Roger Cooter, 'Malingering in modernity: Psychological scripts and adversarial encounters during the First World War', in Roger Cooter, Mark Harrison and Steve Sturdy (eds), *War, Medicine and Modernity* (Stroud: Sutton, 1999), pp. 125–48.
43 Oxford University Press Archive (unnumbered), discarded slip for 'Malinger. Malingering' by William Sykes.
44 F. Chance, 'To Malinger', *Notes and Queries*, 5:122 (1888), 326–7; Herbert A. Strong, 'Malingering', *Notes and Queries*, 9:222 (1896), 252–3. See also Simon Wessely, 'Malingering: Historical perspectives', in Peter A. Halligan, Christopher Bass and David A. Oakley (eds), *Malingering and Illness Deception* (New York: Oxford University Press, 2003), pp. 33–41.
45 Francis Grose, *A Classical Dictionary of the Vulgar Tongue* (London: S. Hooper, 1788).
46 Roger Cooter also dates the bulk of material on malingering from this time,

although recognising earlier usage of the term. Cooter, 'Malingering in modernity', in Cooter *et al.* (eds), *War*, p. 128.
47 For background in France, see Julien Varet, 'Les automutilations de l'adolescence: Approche psychopathologique individuelle et lien social' (unpublished MD, Université Paris Val-de-Marne, 2007), p. 51; for Britain, see *Manual of Military Law* (London: Harrison & Sons, 1894), pp. 358–9.
48 For example, Charles Blondel's thesis was based in concerns stemming from the military crime of self-inflicted wounds. Charles Blondel, *Les auto-mutilateurs: ètude psycho-pathologique et mèdico-lègale* (Paris: J. Rousset, 1906).
49 Schaffner, 'Event, series, trauma', in Micale and Lerner, *Traumatic Pasts*; Greg A. Eghigian, *Making Security Social: Disability, Insurance, and the Birth of the Social Entitlement State in Germany* (Ann Arbor, MI: University of Michigan Press, 2000).
50 For example, Weber held socialist beliefs but nonetheless worked closely with insurance companies to assess claims. Frederick Parkes Weber, 'Remarks on the medical aspect of a system of compulsory instance of the working classes', *British Medical Journal*, 1 (1897), 388–9; See also WLL, Weber Collection, PP/FPW/B186 ('Life Assurance Claims, especially Early Claims') and PP/FPW/B360/1 ('Workmen's Insurance: Legislation and General Measures against Tuberculosis and all Preventable Diseases').
51 For a modern example of this, see Jack Kitaeff, *Malingering, Lies, and Junk Science in the Courtroom* (Youngstown: Cambria Press, 2007), p. 37.
52 Hector Gavin, *On Feigned and Factitious Diseases* (London: J. Churchill, 1843), p. 1.
53 *Ibid.*, p. 11.
54 For example John Collie, *Malingering and Feigned Sickness: With Notes on the Workmen's Compensation Act, 1906* (London: E. Arnold, 1917); Alexander McKendrick, *Malingering and its Detection under the Workmen's Compensation and Other Acts* (Edinburgh: E. & S. Livingstone, 1912); Arthur Bassett Jones and Llewellyn J. Llewellyn, *Malingering or the Simulation of Disease* (London: William Heinemann, 1917).
55 Forbes Winslow, 'On moral and criminal epidemics', *Journal of Psychological Medicine and Mental Pathology*, 9:2 (1856), 240–82, p. 268; Forbes Winslow, *The Anatomy of Suicide* (London: Henry Renshaw, 1840).
56 Winslow, 'On moral and criminal epidemics', pp. 281–2.
57 John Collie and Arthur Spicer, *Malingering and Feigned Sickness* (London: Edward Arnold, 1913), p. 7.
58 *Ibid.*, p. 1.
59 George Thorpe, 'A strange case of malingering', *The Lancet*, 134:3455 (1889), 1001.
60 *Ibid.*
61 *Ibid.*
62 *Ibid.*
63 For example Frederick Parkes Weber, 'Artificial skin eruption', *Proceedings of the Royal Society of Medicine*, 6 (1913), p. 115.
64 Anon., 'Discussion on functional and simulated affections of the auditory apparatus',

Proceedings of the Royal Society of Medicine (Otological Section), 6 (1913), 73–86, pp. 82–3.

65 William Carmichael McIntosh, 'On some of the varieties of morbid impulse and perverted instinct', *Journal of Mental Science*, 11:56 (1866), 512–33.

66 Adam, 'Self-mutilation', in Tuke (ed.), *Dictionary*, vol. 2, pp. 1147–52. For early examples of textbooks which utilised the term see G. Fielding Blandford, *Insanity and Its Treatment* (Edinburgh: Oliver and Boyd, 1884); James Shaw, *Epitome of Mental Diseases* (Bristol: John Wright, 1892). Articles include William J. Brown, 'Notes of a case of monomania with self-mutilation and a suicidal tendency', *Journal of Mental Science*, 23:102 (1877), 242–8; Eric Sinclair, 'Case of persistent self-mutilation', *Journal of Mental Science*, 32:137 (1886), 44–50.

67 Sarah Chaney, 'Self-control, selfishness and mutilation: How "medical" is self-injury anyway?', *Medical History*, 55:3 (2011), 375–83.

68 For more on the 'Welsh Fasting Girl', see Robert Fowler, *A Complete History of the Case of the Welsh Fasting-Girl, Sarah Jacob* (London: Henry Renshaw, 1871); Joan Jacobs Brumberg, *Fasting Girls: The Emergence of Anorexia Nervosa as a Modern Disease* (Cambridge, MA: Harvard University Press, 1988).

69 James Startin, 'Remarks on feigned or hysterical diseases of the skin', *British Medical Journal*, 1:471 (1870), 25–7; Charles Hilton Fagge, 'Notes on some feigned cutaneous affections', *British Medical Journal*, 1:476 (1870), 151–2; Thomas Flower, 'Feigned or hysterical disease of skin', *British Medical Journal*, 1:482 (1870), 307–8.

70 Anon. (editorial), 'Motiveless malingerers', *British Medical Journal*, 1:470 (1870), 15–16, p. 15.

71 BRHA, CB/146, *Female Patient Casebook 1893*, entry 26.

72 *Ibid.*

73 *Ibid.*

74 *Ibid.*

75 *Ibid.*

76 Anon., 'Motiveless malingers', p. 15.

77 Adam, 'Self-mutilation', in Tuke (ed.), *Dictionary*, vol. 2, p. 1147.

78 Henry MacCormac, 'Autophytic dermatitis', *British Medical Journal*, 2:4014 (1937), 1153–5, p. 1153.

79 Erasmus Wilson, *Lectures on Dermatology* (London: J. and A. Churchill, 1875); Henry Radcliffe Crocker, *Diseases of the Skin: Their Description, Pathology, Diagnosis and Treatment* (London: H. K. Lewis, 1893), p. 288; James Galloway, 'Feigned diseases of the skin', in Thomas Clifford Allbutt (ed.), *A System of Medicine* (London: Macmillan, 1899), pp. 937–9.

80 Galloway, 'Feigned diseases of the skin', p. 937; Wilson, *Lectures on Dermatology*.

81 For example in the case of Mary Stoate at Bethlem, outlined in Chaney, 'Self-control, selfishness and mutilation', pp. 377–8.

82 George Savage and Charles A. Mercier, 'Insanity of conduct', *Journal of Mental Science*, 42:176 (1896), 1–17, p. 2.

83 *Ibid.*, p. 2.

84 *Ibid.*, p. 3.

85 *Ibid.*, p. 3.
86 Henry Maudsley, 'The genesis of mind (II)', *Journal of Mental Science*, 8 (1862), 61–102, p. 67, p. 87. See also George Savage, 'Moral insanity', *Journal of Mental Science*, 27:118 (1881), 147–55, p. 147.
87 George Savage 'Mental diseases', in Allbutt (ed.), *System of Medicine*, p. 181.

14

Work and the Irish District Asylums during the late nineteenth century

Oonagh Walsh

Although integral to the life of the asylum, work – as occupational therapy (OT), as income generation, and as a means of evaluating a patient's recovery – has been little studied in its own right. Discussions of patient work parties, or the contributions made by particular cohorts towards the upkeep of the institution, tend to arise incidentally and as part of analyses of power relationships between staff and inmates. Yet in the period before the large-scale introduction of drug therapies and psychosurgery, work was the engine that ostensibly drove the Irish asylum, regulating patient movement, ordering the asylum day, and determining the extent of physical freedom allowed within and beyond the institution's walls. A willingness to work, and the capacity to obey instructions and complete tasks successfully, became a key means of indicating that a patient was ready to return to the sane world of productive labour.

This chapter will raise the principal issues surrounding work in the Irish District Asylums, and examine the manner in which employment, in a variety of guises, underpinned, and indeed at times forged, medical practice. The Connaught District Lunatic Asylum in Ballinasloe, County Galway (hereafter Ballinasloe Asylum), will be used as a case study to illustrate points that were relevant to the majority of the District Asylums at the end of the nineteenth century. This period is an important one in Irish psychiatric history. The early optimism of widespread cures through moral therapy had faded, and most institutions were badly overcrowded and under resourced. Pressing concerns over Home Rule, and a growing nationalist movement, saw social and medical concerns pushed far down the political agenda, and the asylums suffered as a consequence. Indeed, the dawning of the twentieth century, and the early years of the Free State, saw a period of stagnation for the old asylums, and little state intervention to improve the lot of the tens of thousands of inmates of the system throughout the country.

The original impetus behind the establishment of the Irish District Asylums was, officially, a desire to protect vulnerable, mentally ill individuals from abuse and exploitation in mainstream society.[1] However, in reality the Irish legislation prioritised public security over treatment, following an earlier English model of custody rather than cure. Under reforms in the 1830s, the English system had moved from the large-scale admission of lunatics to gaol, to direct admission to the asylum, thereby seeking to break the association between criminality and insanity. Ireland retained this destructive link throughout the nineteenth century, and indeed strengthened it through the passage of the Dangerous Lunatics Act of 1838.[2] Despite large-scale protests from the asylum inspectors as well as medical superintendents, the long-promised legislative reform actually reinforced the association, ensuring that Irish lunatics were regarded as not just 'mad' but 'bad'.[3] This factor, allied to the overcrowding that plagued almost every District Asylum in Ireland, ensured that the question of work and its benefits to patients and institution alike, received less attention than it deserved.

Work as physical therapy

The therapeutic value of work for the mentally disordered underpinned the patient–staff relationship, and was an important means of demonstrating mental recovery for both sides. Work was also quite literally built into the very fabric of the institution at Ballinasloe, as, from its opening, there was an expectation that patient labour would make a substantial contribution towards the asylum's running costs. Evidence from some of the well-established English institutions provided encouragement on this front, with several authoritative figures offering the prospect of significant financial as well as medical benefits from patient labour:

> Among the lower classes of the people, it will generally be found that useful occupation in the pursuits they have been most accustomed to is their best amusement, and such employment the most salutary mode of recreation that can be resorted to. One of the principal objects kept in view, in the direction of this Asylum, has been to obtain for the patients constant and regular employment, and for that purpose, not only farming and gardening, but all trades have been forced into the service: we have spinners, weavers, tailors, shoemakers, brewers, bakers, blacksmiths, joiners, painters, bricklayers, and stonemasons, all employed. All the clothing for the patients is manufactured and made by themselves; we bake our own bread, brew our own beer, and nearly one half of both male and female patients are constantly engaged in some kind of labour … it is a source of great saving to the institution; for notwithstanding that we have for many years received only seven shillings a week for each pauper, a fund has accumulated, which by the end of the year will exceed three thousand pounds.[4]

The vision conjured by William Ellis of happy, productive and profitable patients represented an ideal that proved difficult to achieve in Ireland. It was, of course, also reflective of core moral therapeutic principles that emphasised the importance of appropriate work roles for patients as the means of recovery. John Connolly, one of England's leading alienists, confirmed the importance of work for patients, stating: 'Bodily exercise in the open air cannot be estimated too highly; the same may be said of occupation, not too early resorted to.'[5] There was broad agreement, therefore, that work should form part of every recuperative patient's daily routine, but the practical issues inherent in equipping, supervising, training and controlling large numbers of inmates were not necessarily addressed.

The emphasis upon the importance of patients' contribution to their keep in the form of unpaid work was not merely an expression of the standard Victorian reluctance to encourage the 'indigent poor', but was born of necessity, and reflected the paucity of ratepayers in Ireland. The establishment of the District Asylums took place when Ireland was experiencing protracted economic stagnation.[6] The 1800 Act of Union had precipitated the decline of many once-profitable landed estates, and a steady increase in the pauper population ensured that wages fell steadily, reflecting an over-supply of labour for limited employment. In the 1830s, the average weekly wage paid to an Irish labourer was between two shillings and two shillings and sixpence, compared with eight to ten shillings for his counterpart in Britain.[7] Outside of the major cities of Dublin, Cork, Galway, Limerick and Belfast, there was little industrialisation and consequently, in contrast to the remainder of the United Kingdom, there was a relatively small pool of ratepayers. Thus the burden of support for Irish asylums fell disproportionately upon the aristocracy, who although they owned a startling 97 per cent of all land in Ireland, were frequently in possession of poorly managed and unproductive property.[8] The Irish District Asylums therefore operated in an environment where labour was cheap and readily available, making asylum patient labour relatively unprofitable, and the body of ratepayers (upon whom a tax was levied for the support of the asylums) was both small, and not especially wealthy. This created a rather different dynamic from that in mainland Britain, and was to have negative consequences upon the principle of full patient occupation.

Work as medical therapy

In the 1891 'Memorandum of Inspection' for the Ballinasloe Asylum, the question of work, and the beneficial nature of occupation for the patients, was discussed. The value of work as a means of distracting patients from their morbid thoughts, and providing a means of allowing maniacal patients to exhaust themselves, took explicit priority over the economic value of asylum labour. Noting that only seventeen acres were available 'for the employment of the inmates', the inspectors distinguished between exercise and work, by listing the airing courts separately from the farm, and bemoaned the fact that relatively few patients could avail themselves of manual labour. Work was seen specifically as therapy, with the asylum falling short of the standards prevailing in other institutions:

> It is needless to say that this small space can in no way afford occupation for the number of male patients resident in this Asylum. The importance of affording useful work for the insane is now considered of so vital importance in the treatment of insanity, that in nearly every European country, as well as in the United States, and in most of the British Colonies, farms are looked on as essential in connection with public Asylums.[9]

There was a recognition that not only did work offer therapeutic benefits to recuperative patients, but a lack of manual occupation led to high rates of relapse, especially among convalescent depressive patients. 'It is a vital necessity to keep melancholic patients occupied. Idleness and want of exercise has caused many to return to their state of stupor, following periods of recovery.'[10]

Work had other, less tangible, purposes in Irish asylums beyond the economic support of the institution, or the mere distraction of the patients from their mental conditions. It was used as a means of evaluating sanity, and was a key element in the assessment process. On admission, a careful note was taken of whether patients, especially men, had been gainfully employed prior to falling ill. Throughout their asylum stay, their willingness and ability to work productively in the institution was recorded, and all fell under the same necessity to labour productively for the greater good. Even idiots and imbeciles were required to contribute their labour in return for care and maintenance, fulfilling repetitive tasks on the farm and wards under the supervision of fellow patients as well as wardsmaids and keepers. It is ironic that the intellectually disabled, generally unable to secure gainful employment in the competitive marketplace outside the asylum walls, often found themselves making a genuinely useful contribution to the smooth running of the institution.[11] The patient case notes place a great deal of emphasis upon work, as much indeed as on mental states. A careful record was kept of how individuals approached their set tasks, and the terms 'willingly', 'cheerfully' and 'thoroughly' were used most often in cases that were close to discharge.[12] Equally, 'sullen', 'reluctant' and 'resentful' were attached to patients who were in fact completing their allocated work, but clearly under some duress.[13] Invariably this latter group was not deemed ready to be released.

There was a third category: those referred most often to as 'a drudge' or 'a mechanical drudge'. These patients were most often long-stay (many remaining all their lives in the asylum) and worked regularly, but with little enthusiasm or initiative. Thus, the manner in which work was performed, as well its successful completion, was equally important in assessing mental states.

Despite the relatively low value of patient labour, there is no doubt that the patients made a substantial economic contribution to the asylum. Indeed, their unpaid labour was an essential part of the institution's economy, without which it would have proved impossible to maintain buildings, operate the farm, clothe the inmates, or pay for goods and services locally. The development of the Irish District Asylums was predicated upon the somewhat optimistic belief that the institutions would be largely self-sufficient, growing their own crops, raising stock for milk and meat, weaving and spinning cloth for the manufacture of their own clothes, and maintaining buildings and equipment through the unpaid employment of skilled and semi-skilled inmates. The reality was rather different. In the rural asylums, the patient body was surprisingly homogeneous. The majority of admissions were agricultural labourers, both male and female, with a substantial number of domestic servants among the female intake. In 1892, for example, the overwhelming majority of admissions were drawn from the 'labouring class' and 'farming': the latter included farm owners as well as agricultural labourers. These two categories accounted for almost two-thirds of total admissions. However, if the 'no occupation or unascertained' category is removed from the total, then the percentage of labourers/agricultural labourers rises sharply to 82 per cent.[14] The range of skills and trades brought by other patients was narrow indeed: in 1892, only three tradesmen (shoemakers) and one 'artisan' (a woman, whose skill is not noted) were admitted. Although a small number of well-educated patients were included in that year's intake – two 'members of religious communities' and two 'students and teachers' – their talents could not formally be used in the service of the institution as the District Asylums did not provide any form of education for inmates.

The patient profile remained surprisingly static at the end of the nineteenth century. In addition to being a relatively unskilled, or at least non-specialised, body of men and women, they were also young and able-bodied, and therefore most in need of occupation. Between 1885 and 1890, for example, the largest admission group for males and females was twenty-five to thirty years of age, at 18 and 9 per cent of total admissions respectively. The overwhelming majority of patients were aged between twenty and fifty years of age, constituting 75 per cent of males and almost 70 per cent of females. The mean age of all admissions was thirty-nine for men and thirty-six for women. Thus, few of the patients were too young to work productively (there was a very small number of child admissions each year, averaging three individuals under the age of fifteen),[15] and although the asylum accumulated substantial numbers of the elderly and infirm, who were seldom taken out of the institution by their relatives, the Board of Governors were in the main responsible for large numbers of inmates who could reasonably be expected to work, but for whom there was little available employment.

Gender and work

Most asylums in Britain and Ireland included substantial acreages, and a priority was placed upon male occupation on the farm and surrounding parkland. At Ballinasloe, the institution had originally held only eleven acres of land, but by 1900 this had increased to over 100. This expansion was driven by the perceived need to provide work for the male patients, as well as increase home-produced food for the institution. Women were never considered for work on the farm, despite the fact that most had been agricultural labourers before admission. But in fact female patient work roles were rather more diverse, leading to a higher rate of occupation for women in asylums.[16] Their roles included helping the wardsmaids to clean and tidy the dormitories, as well as assist in changing bed linen. They worked in large numbers in the asylum's laundry: this was one of the asylum's busiest locations, owing to the continual changes of clothing and bed linen necessitated by the 'wet and dirty' patients. Women assisted in setting and clearing the refectories, and in helping fellow patients to eat. They wove cloth for a variety of garments, sewed and darned patients' outfits, and cleaned the institution from top to bottom, waxing, polishing and dusting the corridors, day rooms, offices and living quarters in every building. The scale of their industry was considerable and table 14.1, which lists the items produced almost exclusively by women patients in 1886,[17] gives an idea of their productivity.

Historians often (rightly) bemoan the limited economic and political opportunities available to women before the mid-twentieth century, and it is true that women were discriminated against extensively in almost every sphere. However, a highly gendered perspective on appropriate work roles for men and women operated, I argue, for the benefit of the latter as asylum patients. Their flexible adaptation to the work required within the asylum allowed them a much greater degree of occupation, which had a beneficial effect upon their mental states: the mental health inspectors were quite correct in identifying the negative impact upon male patients of absolute boredom and inactivity. Recuperative women patients had much greater freedom of movement throughout the institution as they worked, and a swifter return to the outside world. Women were much more likely to be released 'recovered' and 'cured' than were men, and their ability to work was an integral element in this factor.

Table 14.1 List of items produced by patients at Ballinasloe Asylum in a single year

Articles	Number
Shifts	733
Shirts	630
Sheets	407
Men's shoes	300 pairs
Dresses	290
Women's caps	281
Aprons	264
Flannel vests	189
Jackets	187
Bedticks	187
Vests	180
Pillow slips	131
Stockings	90
Bed bottoms	59
Overcoats	51
Caps	23
Petticoats	20
Tablecloths	20
Flannel drawers	15

Source: Compiled from table xxxi, 'Articles of clothing, bedding, &c., made by the patients during the year ended 31st December, 1886', *Annual Report* (Dublin: Alexander Thom, 1897), p. 30.

Economic value of work

In recent years, a good deal of discussion has taken in place in Ireland over the exploitative nature of many state and religious institutions. Bodies such as the Magdalen Laundries, which were quasi-penitential homes for unmarried mothers run by the Catholic Church, have been accused of effectively using their charges as slave labour by making work in their laundry a condition of residence.[18] In fact, a recent report has shown that the laundries made little profit, although the conditions for many of the women residents, some of whom spent their lives in one or another of the homes, were undoubtedly harsh and physically demanding.[19] Given the potential for economic exploitation that the asylums offered, with an often vulnerable patient population, an obvious question is that of the profitability or otherwise of patient labour.

An examination of the asylum's accounts immediately indicates that patient work offered a modest opportunity for profit. The Ballinasloe Asylum never came close to William Ellis' substantial profits from patient labour.

In 1886, the asylum's total income was £11,388. Of this, £5,345 was paid by the Grand Juries of the counties of Roscommon and Galway for the support of patients from those counties and a further £5,895 came from the Treasury in the form of four shillings per head Rate in Aid. The 'Farm and Garden Produce' came to a mere £68 16s 8d, the sale of pigs raised a further £63 13s 4d and the final £15 10s was ascribed to 'miscellaneous' income.[20] There was, of course, a substantial contribution to the work of the institution in unpaid patient labour, especially in maintenance, that cannot be estimated accurately, but in terms of income generation, patient work was not as profitable as many asylum superintendents liked to boast. The largest financial reward to be made from inmates came from the charges made on paying patients. However, the Ballinasloe Asylum was established for the care of pauper lunatics and there were few paying inmates. In 1886 only four such were admitted, contributing the princely sum of £75 in total.[21] Thus it can be stated that despite a large pool of free labourers, and the very small number of fee-paying patients, the asylum did not profit to any considerable degree.

Asylum patients were expected, as noted above, to take part in any occupation deemed suitable for them by the physician. But there were limits to what could reasonably be expected from any inmate, both in terms of their own capacity for work and the expectations of the asylum staff. Despite their rather lowly status, the asylums were in fact medical establishments, hospitals created with the intention of restoring admissions to full mental health. Thus, although they had much in common with the workhouse and prison worlds, they differed sharply in terms of the work that the residents could be coerced into doing. The attitude of the workhouse is embodied in its name: inmates were expected to labour in return for their keep, and only the very old and very young, or the physically incapable, were exempt from some manner of productive employment.[22]

Prisons similarly expected a high degree of work from their charges and this was a standard element of their sentences. 'Hard labour' was at the core of most prison stays and spanned a tremendous range of activity including stone breaking, work on docks (a dangerous occupation with high injury and mortality rates), road making and all manner of farm labour.[23] Strenuous and unpleasant work was part of the punishment, even if many of the prisoners were incapable of undertaking it.[24] Asylum inmates were not forced to work and were not be punished, at least officially, for a failure to obey an instruction to fulfil any given task. Equally, asylum patients were not sent out in work parties to provide cheap labour for local businesses or industries, as prisoners often were.[25] There would have been little demand for such services in any case. Wage rates were exceptionally low in the west of Ireland and, despite high levels of emigration from the province of Connaught well into the twentieth century, there was a surplus of labour that ensured wages remained at barely above subsistence levels.

The homogeneous profile of admissions noted above ensured that the Board of Governors could not depend upon the range of skilled labour that was available in other institutions in both urban Ireland and mainland Britain. The staff therefore included a large body of paid employees from outside the asylum walls, including a carpenter, tailor, painter and engineer, whose annual salaries ranged from £24 4s to £27 4s, with an additional £4 or so in kind in the form of accommodation and keep. While there had never been an expectation that the institution would function exclusively through free patient labour, it had been hoped and, indeed, expressly articulated by the Lord Lieutenant's Office that inmates would contribute towards their upkeep. Thus, there was an imperative to use patient labour where possible, even when it proved hardly worth the effort. In many cases, the necessity to keep patients under constant supervision as they worked meant that the task in hand was protracted and fraught with difficulties: the Board of Guardians heard many appeals from the institution's tradesmen that they were effectively taking on the keeper's supervisory role, and were unable to actually do the job they had been hired for:

> READ: the Manager's Report ... he [the asylum carpenter] asked that the patient assigned to him as his assistant be relieved of this task. In the past week, Michael M[__] has broken a jointer plane, and quarrelled with the Engine Man while at work in the sheds. His work is poor and he requires the most vigilant supervision, as he is constantly on the watch for the means to escape.[26]

The patient was relieved of his duties and no other inmate was assigned to the carpenter in his place. For the most part, patients chosen for asylum work tended to be pliant and reliable, especially those who were given any degree of responsibility. But the relationship between patients and permanent maintenance staff could be an uneasy one, which was often dependent upon the absolute submission of the former to the commands of the latter, with rapid complaints to the manager if conflict arose.

The use of patient labour also raised a degree of conflict in the local community, on two main levels. The first related to the tension between two diametrically opposed visions for the role of the asylum in Connaught. The institution itself was driven by a desire to be as self-sufficient as possible, and the large pool of unpaid labour at its disposal was a valuable resource towards this end. The therapeutic value of manual labour was an additional imperative towards patient occupation. However, local tradesmen and suppliers, as well as farm labourers, domestic servants and artisans, viewed the asylum as a valuable market for their goods and services and bitterly resented the institution's efforts to minimise costs through patient work and the development of the farm to supply crops and livestock for the asylum kitchens.

The Ballinasloe Asylum was situated in an economically deprived area of the midlands of Ireland, where throughout the nineteenth century the majority of the population teetered on the verge of starvation. The arrival of the asylum in 1833 proved an astonishing economic boon to the town, and to the surrounding area, pouring vast sums into the local economy in the form of wages, tenders and the rental of farm lands. The boost to the area proved life-saving at several periods, not least during the years of the Great Famine (1845–51), when the institution spent on average £3,000 per quarter in tenders and wages.[27] This ensured that the appalling effects of the famine were slightly ameliorated, and the expenditure of state funds via the institution replaced to a significant extent the normal transactions which had been eliminated through death and emigration. Indeed, even before the asylum opened, it was trumpeted as a potential boost to the region, as well as the most modern of medical institutions: 'The opening of the Connaught District Lunatic Asylum will transform this backward and remote district, bringing a humane refuge for the mentally distressed, as well as the not inconsiderable benefit of substantial economic investment.'[28] This argument was key in allaying local fears over the congregation of large numbers of lunatics in a relatively small town, and in countering assertions that the area would struggle to escape from the taint of the asylum. Despite some initial reservations, the extra-medical value of the asylum became rapidly clear and within a short period of time the local population regarded it with a proprietorial air.

Work and local politics

Throughout the nineteenth century, any attempt to source paid labour, materials or any supplies from beyond the immediate geographical area was met with fierce resistance. In order to maintain good relations with the community, the manager was instructed to source goods locally when possible, leading to a small number of suppliers prospering for many decades through the practice. The board of governors received regular petitions from vested interests regarding the supply of labour and goods to the asylum, petitions which often protested against the use of patient labour:

> We beg to bring to the board's notice the necessity of offering employment to those able and willing to take it. The use of inmates denies men the opportunity to fend for their families, and greatly speeds the departure of those who are forced to seek employment on foreign shores.[29]

As the nationalist movement gathered momentum from the 1880s onwards, the institution found itself under increasing pressure to both source locally made goods (as opposed to asylum produce), and employ local labour, as part of the Irish Revival's push to replace English imports with 'native' products.[30] The make-up of the asylum board was itself undergoing change in this period, with the Protestant Anglo-Irish elite, who had constituted the bulk of the membership, giving reluctant way to Catholic Nationalists. The latter were well connected to grass-roots activists who saw in the asylum a valuable means of consolidating political influence through the allocation of jobs and tenders. They were vociferously opposed to the use of patient labour and, once they secured a majority representation on the board, proceeded to expand the employment of paid labourers from the non-asylum workforce.

But it was not just the new political elite of Catholic Nationalists who used positions on the board to benefit themselves, and their supporters. The first board members were drawn from the landowning upper classes and merchant middle classes, who together monopolised economic authority in Ireland for most of the century. They exercised a system of political patronage on their own estates, and preferential employment practices in their businesses, drawn from centuries of favouring co-religionists and those with compatible political beliefs. This tendency carried seamlessly into asylum boardroom practice, with some breathtaking abuses of the privileges of board membership for private gain, and the enhancement of local political influence. One of the longest serving board members, Lord Clancarty, enjoyed considerable benefit from the operations of the asylum. He rented land to the asylum farm, sold timber from his estate for the expansion works in the institution, and supplied the limestone that was the institution's exclusive building material from his private quarry, as well as the sand used in the building's many construction projects. Although board members received no official remuneration for their service, Lord Clancarty at least extracted substantial profit from his privileged position on the board. He also played a rather contradictory role in terms of patient employment. On the one hand, he, along with the other board members, pursued a policy of using patient labour where possible. On the other, he recommended tenants from his estate for work in the institution in a variety of roles from keepers and nurses, to farm labourers and tradesmen. The tradition of landlord philanthropy that included placing one's tenants in employment remained strong in Ireland until the start of the twentieth century, and was especially important in maintaining Protestant and Unionist power bases. All applications for employment came before the board, and individuals including Clancarty provided character references for those personally known to them. It was rare for the board to reject an applicant recommended by a fellow member, giving tenants and parishioners (the Protestant Archbishop of Tuam was an ex-officio member, although he rarely attended the monthly meetings) a distinct advantage in employment, and further limiting the work available to residents in the asylum.

Non-working patients

Despite the emphasis placed upon work in the asylum, not all patients were viewed through the same functional prism. There were substantial numbers of inmates who were exempt from duties, despite in many cases being capable of undertaking a variety of responsibilities. They fell for the most part into three main categories.

The first is the most obvious one: the elderly, infirm or otherwise bedridden residents who were incapable of manual work. This encompassed a considerable range of individuals with a variety of diagnoses. Some were merely advanced in years, and were often suffering from senile dementia. A combination of age and an incapacity to follow instructions or complete tasks ensured that they were not considered suitable for work. Others were suffering from General Paralysis of the Insane, or had been injured in accidents, enfeebled through fever, or crippled with rheumatism and arthritis. In many cases, such patients simply lived the remainder of their lives in the asylum and were eventually buried in the institution's graveyard; permanent residents in every sense. Others, especially those who were in generally fair physical condition, were moved if at all possible to the workhouse. One might interpret this constant movement as a means of shedding unproductive workers who were unlikely to leave the asylum or make any significant financial contribution to it, but in fact they were transferred in order to free up desperately needed beds. This cohort proved restless indeed: constantly shuttled between the workhouse and the asylum, with no prospect of returning to the world outside either set of walls.

The second group of patients who were rarely expected to labour in the asylum comprised most of the puerperal maniacs. These women were often admitted to the asylum in great distress. Most were indeed maniacal and had threatened or attempted suicide as well as having harmed a child. In the early stages of their treatment, they were never required to work at any of the usual female occupations. More interestingly though, they were rarely asked to work even when they were in recovery. Given that they were all relatively young women (of childbearing age) this was unusual. Yet a close examination of their records shows that the asylum authorities had a surprisingly enlightened attitude towards their particular diagnosis. Recognising that, in fact, many of these patients were malnourished and exhausted from a continual cycle of pregnancy, birth and nursing, they were allowed to rest following admission and discharged only when they had recovered physically. Thus they were (exceptionally among able-bodied patients) allowed to rest in bed, and were prescribed the 'hospital diet' in order to build up their strength. This was sumptuous in comparison with the normal diet of Irish female labourers, and included meat, vegetables, wine and spirits, a far cry from the buttermilk and potatoes that still made up most of the diet in the impoverished west of Ireland. Even when these patients became calm and biddable in the asylum, they were not expected to work in the physically demanding environment of the laundry or on the farm: rather, they were assigned to the sewing room, or given light cleaning duties in the main asylum buildings, and not on the wards. Thus work, although vital to the asylum's survival, was not expected from all inmates. Indeed, the institution was capable of making distinctions between those who under normal circumstances would have been expected to labour as part of their recovery (the able-bodied young female), and those whose bodies required support and rest before embarking once again on the debilitating path of motherhood.

The third group that was largely exempt from the prevailing work ethic was the epileptics. These are a fascinating, and sadly neglected, asylum cohort in Britain as well as Ireland. Constituting, on average, one in ten of the patients throughout the nineteenth century, these individuals were not mentally ill in the sense of suffering under the common diagnoses of mania, melancholia or dementia, or congenital afflictions including imbecility or idiocy.[31] Owing to the unpredictable nature of their seizures, they were rarely allocated work, and as they were often injured in falls were frequently confined indoors where supervision was easier. They led often unhappy and stressful lives: not insane, yet incurable, and frequently admitted following the loss of employment as a result of their illness. Despite a willingness to work, they were rarely permitted to follow any specialised occupation, and their plight was difficult indeed.

Work as privilege

The term 'work' often implies duties reluctantly undertaken in exchange for pay, or in the case of many asylum patients for bed and board, given the limited therapies available. But work in the asylum was regarded by many patients as a reward for good behaviour and as confirmation that they were valued members of the institutional community. Work became a means of validating one's recovery and, in some cases, one's identity. The circumstances under which many patients had been admitted were often highly traumatic: one patient was brought 'bound, gagged and struggling, for he refused to accompany the constables quietly'.[32] The ease of committal offered by the Dangerous Lunatics Act ensured that violence, or at least the threat of violence, was an integral element in most warrants. Whether a violent act had been executed, or the patient had merely threatened it, was irrelevant: the patient was arrested and brought to the asylum under armed constabulary escort. This was often a humiliating and distressing experience, and many began their stay with a sense of dislocation from their workaday selves, a fact bemoaned loudly and repeatedly on admission. 'He tells me he is a man of some standing in his community, with a twenty acre farm and four servants: he should not be treated as a common lunatic or criminal.'[33] This is particularly the case with male patients, many of whom had been the sole breadwinner as well as patriarchal head of household, and they found their demotion to irrational lunatic a troubling transition. In these cases, work at a higher level of responsibility within the asylum was a means of recovering their real selves and demonstrating to the medical staff that the disturbed individual brought before them was in fact a man, on a level with themselves. Jobs of especial responsibility and importance were therefore contested, and patients fought to ensure that they secured and retained them. Positions of responsibility as assistants to the clerks, or as managers of staff quarters, were especially prized. The importance of these posts is also seen in their withdrawal for poor behaviour: patients could be 'demoted' from the relatively privileged world of indoor work to the lowest level of outdoor work party for infractions. In one case, a patient who had held the position of valet to the manager was returned to the farm following a violent argument with another patient. He 'wept and begged' to be allowed to resume his duties, as he 'cannot bear to be treated as a common labourer, when he had organised the Manager's apartments so well'.[34] The removal of such responsibilities was traumatic indeed, and indicates how important certain types of work were within the institution. Just as in the outside world, men ranked each other according to responsibility and status and clung fiercely to the distinctions between the vast mass of unskilled workers and the few given access to the asylum's inner sanctums.

Conclusion

Work in the Irish District Asylums served many, often conflicting, purposes. Although primarily used as a means of supplementing the often meagre financial support offered by the State, its uses went far beyond this simple purpose. Work took the form of occupational therapy, was used as a test of sanity, and as proof of insanity. Its distribution among the patients, and its removal as both punishment and reward, indicates the importance it held in the institution. As in the outside world, work helped to establish status, and also reflected the changing political, economic and social context within which the asylum operated. It was, indeed, central to the success of the institution, but its changing use over the course of the century gives us a good deal of insight into the complex nature of institutional care in Ireland.

Notes

1. Sir Robert Peel, in particular, was concerned with the exploitation suffered by 'lunatics at large', and saw the asylums as a means of protecting them. See also Brendan Kelly, 'Mental health law in Ireland, 1821 to 1902: Building the asylums', *Medico-Legal Journal*, 76 (2008), 22.
2. Criminal Lunatics (Ireland) Act 1838 (1 & 2 Vict. c. 27).
3. The Act was amended in 1867.
4. Letter from William Ellis to Andrew Halliday, 30 November 1827, in Andrew Halliday, *A General View of the Present State of Lunatics and Lunatic Asylums in Great Britain and Ireland and in Some Other Kingdoms* (London: Thomas and George Underwood, 1828), p. 93.
5. John Connolly, *The Treatment of the Insane Without Mechanical Restraints* (London: Smith, Elder, 1856), p. 68.
6. Joel Mokyr and Cormac Ó Gráda, 'Poor and getting poorer? Living standards in Ireland before the famine', *The Economic History Review*, 41:2 (1988), 210–15.
7. *Third Report of the Commissioners for Enquiring into the Condition of the Poorer Classes in Ireland* HC 1836 [43] 30 1, p. 4.
8. William E. Vaughan, *Landlords and Tenants in Mid-Victorian Ireland* (Oxford: Clarendon Press, 1994), ch. 1.
9. 'Ballinasloe District Asylum: Memorandum of Inspection on the 3 March, 1891', in *Annual Report of the Ballinasloe District Lunatic Asylum* (hereafter *Annual Report*) *for the Year 1891* (Dublin: Alexander Thom, 1892), p. 8.
10. National Archives of Ireland (hereafter NAI), 'Board of Governors' Minutes, Ballinasloe Asylum', 8 May 1889.
11. See Oonagh Walsh, 'A person of the second order: The plight of the intellectually disabled in nineteenth-century Ireland', in Laurence M. Geary and Oonagh Walsh (eds), *Philanthropy in Nineteenth-Century Ireland* (Dublin: Four Courts Press, 2014), pp. 161–80.
12. NAI, Case notes nos 3412, 3518 and 3434.
13. Almost without exception, these terms carried a broader judgement on a patient's willingness to positively engage with the life of the asylum by agreeing to work. In these cases, the physician's focus was upon work as a test of ability to be discharged as much as it was upon a necessary task to be completed.
14. *Annual Report for 1892* (Dublin: Alexander Thom, 1893), p. 19.
15. The Irish District Asylums were established for the care of 'able-bodied adults' only. The physically ill or incapacitated were to be housed in the workhouses. Children were not regarded as 'fit subjects' for the asylums and, indeed, fears were often expressed regarding the physical safety of children in these institutions.
16. This was a consistent pattern. In 1863, for example, only 12 out of 178 male patients could find work on the asylum farm, largely owing to the small acreage. But sixty-one of the female patients were at work all day at 'needlework and knitting, in the laundry and cleaning the asylum'.
17. The shoes were produced by male cobblers, and some of the heavier garments were made by male tailors.

18 See www.magdalenelaundries.com/what.htm for details of one of the advocacy group's concerns (last accessed 30 January 2015).
19 Martin McAleese, *Report of the Inter-Departmental Committee to Establish the Facts of State Involvement with the Magdalen Laundries* (Dublin: Department of Justice and Equality, 2013), ch. 20.
20 *Annual Report for 1886*, 'Abstract of accounts' (Dublin: Alexander Thom, 1887).
21 One of these had failed to maintain payments, and was £12 10s behind the annual charge of £20 by the end of 1886.
22 Thomas Edward Jordan, *Ireland's Children: Quality of Life, Stress, and Child Development in the Famine Era* (Westport, CT: Greenwood Press, 1998), p. 65.
23 Russell P. Dobash, 'Labour and discipline in Scottish and English prisons: Moral correction, punishment and useful toil', *Sociology*, 17:1 (1983), 2.
24 Seán McConville, 'The Victorian prison: England, 1865–1965', in Norval Morris and David J. Rothman (eds), *The Oxford History of the Prison: The Practice of Punishment in Western Society* (New York: Oxford University Press, 1995), p. 122.
25 It became more common in the later twentieth century for asylum patients to work on local farms, or as casual labourers, both individually and in work parties. The wages they received were held for their use by the hospital and were either paid upon discharge or piecemeal to pay for cigarettes and small necessities.
26 NAI, 'Draft Minutes of the Board of Governors', 29 September 1880.
27 NAI, 'Account Books', 1845–50.
28 *The Western Star and Ballinasloe Advertiser*, 29 October 1830.
29 NAI, 'Rough Board of Governors Minute Book', 12 April 1879.
30 Timothy G. McMahon, *Grand Opportunity: The Gaelic Revival and Irish Society, 1893–1910* (New York: Syracuse University Press, 2008), p. 140.
31 *Annual Report for 1878* (Dublin: Alexander Thom, 1879), p. 15.
32 NAI, Committal Warrant no. 8720, 1 December 1892.
33 NAI, Case notes, no. 1973, 29 October 1898.
34 NAI, Case notes, no. 1921, 4 May 1893.

15

From work and occupation to occupational therapy: The policies of professionalisation in English mental hospitals from 1919 to 1959

John Hall

From the early nineteenth century, some form of regular and meaningful occupation for patients in English mental hospitals had been seen as central to their management, for at least three reasons: first, as a continuing legacy of the humanitarian ideals of moral treatment; second, since a pattern of regular daily activity was seen as conducive to less disturbed behaviour (not necessarily as therapeutic); and, third, as the use of patient work in utility departments kept hospital costs down. This chapter examines new ideas, identifiable from the end of the First World War, about the role of mental hospitals and the place of the range of occupations and activities provided for patients in them. It does not address how patients and their families experienced these various administrative and clinical changes: patients in public hospitals had little effective voice in how they were treated, although patients in private hospitals had some choice in where and how they were looked after.

The new range of activities required new sets of skills that were not possessed by the existing hospital staff, so new staff groups were recruited and later formally trained. These developments, and the accompanying shifts in terminology and rhetoric used to justify occupations as therapies, led to new professional groups, one of which, occupational therapists, strove throughout the period to establish hegemony over other groups who were also supervising patient activities. These changes, both to a wider range of occupations and to new staff groups, took place in an administrative and clinical context overseen between 1913 and 1959 by a statutory regulatory body, the Board of Control for England and Wales.[1]

The institutional and administrative framework

Until the late seventeenth century the mediaeval Bethlem Hospital in London was the only separate institution for mentally ill people in England. Other 'lunatics' remained in their community of origin, or were confined in prisons or workhouses. Privately owned madhouses, often managed by lay people, then grew in number from the late seventeenth century.[2] Following the early example of the Bethel Hospital, a charitable hospital established in Norwich in 1713, a number of voluntary asylums were founded later in the eighteenth century, managed as charities by Boards of Governors in the same way as the general hospitals and infirmaries founded in the same period.

In 1808, for the first time, local magistrates were permitted (but not required) to establish public asylums, funded by local taxation, and in 1845, under the Lunatic Asylums Act, each borough and county was required to provide accommodation for pauper lunatics. Thus, from 1845 a two-standard pattern was set which was to last until after the Second World War. The publicly funded mental hospitals, essentially for the poor, were linked to the broader provisions of the New Poor Law, which continued to provide workhouses for older and other disabled people. The attitudes underpinning the poor law influenced public and administrative attitudes towards the insane poor, and extended to attitudes regarding appropriate activity within the asylums. As Bartlett put it: 'the asylum tried to instil the ethics of work and morality into its charges'.[3] Independent charitable mental hospitals (known formally as registered hospitals) and small private nursing homes were for the financially better off, but while the great majority of the English hospitals were publicly funded, the smaller number of charitable hospitals played a disproportionally large role in the developments included in this chapter.

The separate Lunatics Act of 1845 established a national monitoring body, the Board of Lunacy, which set national standards of practice. Through successive legislation the powers of the commissioners of the Board, some of whom were legally qualified, some medically qualified, and some lay people, were increased, attempting to ensure that those standards were met. These Acts of Parliament also specified the responsibilities of the medical superintendents of the hospitals, who were not only the senior clinicians but also effectively the overall managers of the hospitals.

In 1841 the Association of Medical Officers of Asylums and Hospitals for the Insane was founded as a national body for medical staff working in these hospitals. It later became the Medico-Psychological Association and, in 1926, the Royal Medico-Psychological Association (RMPA). Nearly all of the presidents of the RMPA were medical superintendents and the medical commissioners of the Board were appointed from senior medical superintendents. The career of Sir Hubert Bond (1870–1945) illustrates this trend: after working in four different mental hospitals, he was from 1903 medical superintendent of two hospitals, before becoming in 1912 a commissioner in lunacy, thereafter remaining a commissioner with the Board until his retirement in 1945, being president of the RMPA from 1921 to 1922. He also became the first president of the English Association of Occupational Therapy.

So, from the mid-nineteenth century policies for these hospitals were formulated by collaboration between a statutory body and a medical professional body, which together controlled most aspects of mental hospital practice, although the local boards of visitors of the county and borough councils controlled the finances of the public hospitals, typically trying to keep costs down.

The position in 1913

In 1913 the Mental Deficiency Act was passed, which for the first time in England required separate hospitals to be provided for people considered to be mentally defective, as opposed to mentally ill. In the same act, the previous Board of Lunacy for England and Wales was replaced by a new statutory body, the ominously named Board of Control, which survived as a separate regulatory body, even after the introduction of the comprehensive state-funded National Health Service (NHS) in 1948, until finally disbanded in 1960.

The Board of Control created a vast amount of paperwork, including annual reports with detailed statistical appendices and other publications – such as their 1933 *Memorandum on Occupation Therapy* – which illustrate the wide-ranging interest of the Board in the development of services.[4] The medical superintendents of both public and registered hospitals produced annual reports for their own management committees and boards of governors, respectively, which in turn were sent to the Board of Control, usually including comments on developments within their hospital in the preceding year. They and their medical colleagues also publicised these as articles in the *Journal of Mental Science*, the official journal of the RMPA.

These three sources together, supplemented after 1936 by the publications of the English Association of Occupational Therapists, provide an overview of the range of work and activities in the mental hospitals, together with the staff groups who worked there, and, crucially, illuminate the tensions between them, the increasing range of professional organisations representing them, the contested nature of some of those developments and the hidden social class and financial factors influencing those developments.

During the latter half of the nineteenth century the public asylum system had grown steadily, both by the building of more asylums and by extensions to existing buildings, so that by 1914 there were ninety-seven publicly funded county and borough asylums in England and Wales, with 101,538 inmates, most of whom were paupers. There were fourteen registered (or charitable) hospitals, including the Bethlem, with 2,625 patients in total.[5] These figures demonstrate an important difference between the two categories of hospital: the registered hospitals were on average only about one-sixth of the size of the public hospitals. Significantly, a unique research-oriented mental hospital for acute cases only, the Maudsley Hospital in London, managed by London County Council, was opened to psychiatric patients after the First World War in 1922.[6] There were also sixty licensed houses under medical control, and a number of very small nursing homes, mostly with less than ten beds.

Most of the chapters in this book describe or imply common practices within European and North American countries, regarded as a central element of asylum regimes, which typically included working in service departments, such as hospital kitchens, or providing labour in hospital gardens and farms. Many of these tasks were monotonous and boring, and some were physically demanding: laundry work for women and farming work for men often involved heavy lifting and long exposure to damp and cold conditions. But the varying social and financial contexts of the different categories of English institutions, and hence the differences in the activities and work that could be provided, mean that it is misleading to talk about anything like *the* work or occupational therapy (OT) provided in England and Wales. The Board of Control 1933 memorandum explicitly recognised that departments of the hospitals served as 'treatment centres as well as providing material service'.[7]

Change in English mental hospitals from 1919 to 1959

The outbreak of war in 1914 had meant that the new administrative procedures of the Board of Control were not fully implemented until the cessation of hostilities in 1918.[8] From 1919 the Board became an active policy-making body, issuing detailed policy and good practice guidance alongside the annual reports: thus it was not solely an inspectorial and regulatory body. The Board operated through its commissioners, who were required to visit each institution regularly, so the commissioners and other senior officers of the Board – such as the senior architect – became a well-informed group on the state of mental hospitals and psychiatric provision in the country.

The network of publicly funded county and borough mental hospitals, charitable registered hospitals, and private licensed houses and nursing homes continued essentially unchanged during the inter-war period. The principal medical treatments (apart from 'tonics' and essentially palliative procedures) offered in the earlier part of the post-war period were sedative medicines. The leading British psychiatric textbook of the period referred to the use of three categories of drug (bromides, chloral and paraldehyde) as sedatives for the management of the patients' current behaviour, without the expectation that they were treating the underlying condition.[9] Indeed, Henderson and Gillespie stated in 1944 that there were no specific treatments for schizophrenia.[10]

The essentially palliative procedures included a range of hydrotherapies (such as Turkish, Russian and prolonged immersion baths). Other treatments were directed at the physical illnesses of the patients, which in public hospitals often included major chronic conditions such as tuberculosis and recurrent epidemics. Bed rest was stressed for both melancholia and schizophrenia. For the former 'the first essential [was] to promote complete rest in bed'.[11] The main components of the treatment of melancholia were given as OT, care for the physical state of the patient, hydrotherapy, drugs and 'talking over the problem'.[12]

From 1935 four new physical treatments were introduced in quick succession, which at the time were seen as revolutionary. Insulin coma therapy (a form of drug-induced coma) was introduced by Sakel in 1935, leucotomy (a neurosurgical operation) was introduced by Moniz in 1936, and convulsions (physical shaking) induced by the drug Cardiazol were introduced by Meduna in 1937, followed by electrical induction of convulsions in 1938 by Cerletti and Bini. In a comprehensive overview of British psychiatry published in 1944, only two additional interventions were mentioned in the chapter on schizophrenia, involving the use of nitrogen inhalations and intravenous sodium amytal, both of which were 'disappointing'.[13] Fresh hopes were raised after the war by the new generation of psychotropic drugs synthesised by French pharmacologists, with the first, chlorpromazine, distributed for clinical trials in 1951.[14] Thus, before 1935, while it was acknowledged by psychiatrists that there were no known specific effective treatments for psychiatric conditions, the language and rhetoric of treatment and therapy was maintained and extended to non-specific activities.

New ideas in mental health

The end of the First World War led to a number of changes to the organisation of healthcare in Britain. In 1919 a Ministry of Health was established for the first time for England and Wales, and ministerial responsibility for the Board of Control was transferred from the Lord Chancellor (the chief *legal* officer of the government) to the new Minister of Health. A new General Nursing Council formed in the same year created a standard pattern of training and put the registration of nurses on a statutory basis, signalling wider opportunities for state-recognised professional advancement for women.

A number of ventures reflected new ideas and growing public interest in mental illness. The New Psychology of Sigmund Freud and his colleagues, especially Carl Gustav Jung, grew in influence, and was widely accepted both within medical and religious circles, although in England psychoanalytic methods never reached the dominance within professional psychiatry that they achieved in the United States.[15] The Tavistock Clinic was established in London in 1920, a charitable and increasingly influential out-patient clinic promoting psychodynamic psychotherapy.[16] The mental hygiene movement, founded in America in 1909 by Clifford Beers, grew in Britain, promoting better public understanding of mental health issues. The First International Conference on Mental Hygiene, held at Washington, DC, in 1930, was widely reported in Britain, including a lengthy series of articles in the *Journal of Mental Science*.[17]

A Royal Commission on Lunacy and Mental Disorder sat from 1924 to 1926, in part because of a highly critical account of conditions at one Manchester mental hospital, written by a psychiatrist who had worked there.[18] Their report made a number of recommendations to liberalise mental health practice, and the resulting 1930 Mental Treatment Act opened the way for more progressive treatment regimes, including the opening of psychiatric out-patient clinics.[19] The first Child Guidance Clinics in Britain were set up in London in 1927 and 1928, demonstrating new concerns about vulnerable children and their families. The Commonwealth Fund of New York directly funded both the formation of a national Child Guidance Council and training for child guidance staff, which led directly to the creation of a new mental health profession, psychiatric social work, with a distinctive training starting in 1929, and a professional association formed in 1930.[20]

Taken together, these developments illustrate shifts towards more effective co-ordination of both healthcare policy and the training of healthcare professions, more critical and creative approaches towards standards of institutional care, an openness towards American practices, and the beginnings of early intervention outside closed institutions.

New ideas in occupation

Against this background, the introduction of craft activities at Gartnavel Royal Hospital in Glasgow in 1919, by the leading Scottish psychiatrist Dr David Henderson, has been seen as the first 'whole-hearted' adoption of a modern concept of OT in Britain, although there is ample evidence of craft activities before this date.[21] Henderson had been influenced by his visit to the American psychiatrist Adolf Meyer in 1908,[22] and he promoted widely his ideas on the introduction of OT to Britain through the British medical press.[23] In a 1924 *Lancet* article he said the work of an occupational teacher was best suited to a 'well-educated intelligent, refined type of girl'![24]

During the 1920s and early 1930s there was widespread action in England to increase the range of occupation. In January 1922 the Board of Control convened a conference on lunacy administration, attended by the medical superintendents and chairmen of visiting committees, which considered a wide range of concerns, including occupation of patients, and recognised the policy of the strictest economy in the asylums.[25] The annual report of the Board for 1931 noted the high standard of the best American hospitals, making use of occupation therapists, but noted that that standard required lavish staffing.[26]

The interest of psychiatrists in occupation is best illustrated by the several visits organised by a committee of the RMPA between 1929 and 1934 to mental hospitals in Germany and Holland, specifically to see how occupations were organised. Dr Hermann Simon's system at Gütersloh in Germany was seen to involve a transformation of the hospital regime so the entire institution became a 'vast occupation centre'.[27] By contrast Professor Van der Scheer, working at Santpoort in Holland, emphasised the role of the medical officers in detailed planning of the activity programme for individual patients.[28] Considerable prominence in the discussion of these visits was given to the overall goal of totally overcoming the problem of the refractory patient.

The annual conference of the RMPA in 1934 included several sessions on OT: in the vote of thanks for the presidential address it was noted that 'a good matron was, ipso facto, an occupational therapist', and in one discussion session the chairman of the Board of Control (Laurence G. Brock) distinguished between 'curative' therapy for recoverable cases, and 'non-curative' therapy for non-recoverable cases.[29] Advertisements for private establishments in the *Journal of Mental Science* included details of the activities they offered; an annual report for St Andrew's Hospital Northampton took thirteen pages to list 650 recreational events during the year.[30]

All of these developments contributed to the thinking behind the 1933 *Memorandum on Occupation Therapy* issued by the Board, a significant early policy document in the history of occupation.[31] One core message of the memorandum was that OT was to be seen as an institution-wide approach, not simply as an agglomeration of individual procedures. The memorandum mentioned both of the two training courses then in existence (at Dorset House, in Bristol, and the Maudsley, in London) and also considered the need for the training of existing nurses and for the employment of technicians. The Board actively sponsored interest in other treatments, later including the physical treatments of insulin coma therapy, leucotomy and convulsive therapy.

The impact of the Second World War

As in the First World War, many medical, nursing and other staff joined the armed forces for the duration of hostilities, and the government again commandeered some 30,000 mental hospital beds to provide emergency beds. The Second World War also stimulated demand for rehabilitation facilities for wounded military personnel, but as a then recently trained occupational therapist recalled, during the war 'in the psychological field, occupational therapists, without the materials required for the usual craft work, turned the patient's interests to other and what might be termed more mundane but realistic occupations' – including semi-skilled war work.[32]

Among the rehabilitative initiatives for service personnel were new approaches to organising psychiatric in-patient settings, known as 'therapeutic communities', which emphasised the flattening of authority hierarchies within the wards, and so implicitly gave more therapeutic authority to non-medical staff.[33] Additionally, the importance of activity directly related to 'resettlement' to independent living and employment was realised, leading both to the need for patients to relearn (or learn) domestic self-help skills and to the wider introduction of industrial therapy (IT), using commercial working practices in sheltered centres, and leading to industrial therapists forming their own professional organisation, the British Institute of Industrial Therapy. IT attempted to replicate both the tasks and structures of outside work, but in practice most of the tasks provided were of an unskilled or semi-skilled nature, with only limited provision of secretarial work. Recent historical research by Vicky Long suggests that the design and delivery of IT, too, was limited by financial constraints, as had been found at the Maudsley before the war.[34] One pioneering unit at Belmont Hospital used both therapeutic community and rehabilitation methods, with workshops and permanent disablement resettlement officers: the staff there believed that 'occupational therapy, as it is now usually practised, cannot claim the rehabilitative effect of productive group work'.[35]

Another development was the perception of creative artistic activities – engagement in graphic and plastic art, listening to and participating in music, reading and performing plays – as therapies distinct from OT, and with the potential for interpretation of the creative process or product from a psychotherapeutic viewpoint – initially informed by psychoanalytic theory. Although these activities were not themselves new, they were increasingly practised as distinctive creative therapies – art, music and drama therapies – with their own professional organisations and each with their own training. Art therapy in Britain, for example, dated from 1942 through the work of Adrian Hill, whose ideas were introduced into long-stay mental hospitals by Edward Adamson after his discharge from military service at the end of the Second World War.[36]

One consequence of these changes was that, for the first time, the total numbers of psychiatric in-patients in England and Wales began to reduce from the peak level of 155,000 in 1955. These initiatives contributed to a progressive shift in the objectives of occupation away from hospital-based work and activity regimes, such as promoting a calm hospital environment, towards simulating conditions outside the hospital, preparing patients for real-life living and employment.[37]

All of these forms of patient activity – OT, IT and creative therapies – then came to be subsumed under the umbrella concept of multi-disciplinary rehabilitation, especially for longer-term patients.[38] The new rhetoric of active rehabilitation was exemplified by the widely read 1959 publication *Institutional Neurosis* by the charismatic psychiatrist Russell Barton, with his seven-step plan to encourage activity.[39] Ideas of rehabilitation included the possibility of therapies taking more account of patients' own wishes and concerns.

On the one hand, the war disrupted existing patterns of in-patient care but, on the other hand, it created new clinical priorities. These new perspectives on the organisation of in-patient regimes were adopted by psychiatrists returning from military service, who had clinical experience outside pre-war conventional institution-based psychiatry. They were now working in the changed social circumstances of the British welfare state after 1948, the National Health Service Act 1946 also having the effect of absorbing ten of the fourteen registered hospitals into the NHS (implemented in 1948), the four remaining hospitals (including St Andrew's Hospital Northampton, together with the OT training school there) continuing as purely private institutions.

Medical influence and control

Individual medical superintendents carried both managerial and legal responsibility for virtually every aspect of the life of their hospital until 1960, including patterns of occupation, and without their consent no new treatments could be introduced into a hospital. The 1933 Board of Control memorandum had stressed that all occupations were to be 'under medical direction'.[40] The first British textbook on OT, directed principally at mental nurses, was written by the medical superintendent of the North Riding Mental Hospital at Clifton Hospital in York, Dr Iveson Russell, in 1938.[41]

Junior doctors learned largely by informal apprenticeship under a superintendent, but would also read the *Journal of Mental Science*, and books such as Henderson and Gillespie's textbook.[42] This included a chapter on OT that was virtually unchanged through the ten editions from 1927 to 1960, but did not clearly advocate the employment of occupational therapists. Henderson and Gillespie's book was supplanted as the leading British psychiatric textbook in 1954 by Wilhelm Mayer-Gross, Eliot Slater and Martin Roth's *Clinical Psychiatry*, which emphasised the benefits of group activities, but characterised OT in Britain as 'being more of *pastimes and hobbies* [emphasis in the original] than of rough manual work, as on the European continent'.[43]

However, the advent of the NHS reduced the prestige of medical superintendents' posts and after the war 'it was increasingly evident that recruits of the requisite standard were not coming forward to become medical superintendents'.[44] Similarly, the greatest problem of the mental hospitals under the early NHS was the shortage of nursing staff, with stagnation in recruitment and dilution of the quality of staff.[45] As David Clark, who was Medical Superintendent at Fulbourn Hospital near Cambridge, has shown, the reality was that all staff, doctors, nurses and therapists, had to work together to bring about change, and those psychiatrists in the forefront of therapeutic innovation worked hard to identify staff who could work *with* them.[46]

There was accordingly a tension in the mental hospitals between the formal authority of doctors and their dependence on having sufficient numbers of staff with the appropriate knowledge and skills to implement their plans. While doctors sought to expand the range of activities undertaken by patients, this could only happen if skilled staff were available to supervise the patients undertaking them. Staff working in the hospital utility departments were skilled only in the work of their department and they could not be diverted from their essential tasks in the kitchens, laundries and farms.[47]

Training in occupational therapy

It was a widely held view among medical superintendents that the standard of education of most attendants was poor – this is confirmed by historical accounts of British psychiatric nursing – and they were not necessarily capable of supervising a wider range of activities.[48] From the 1920s utility department staff and mental nurses were supplemented by 'occupation officers', craft and trade teachers, and instructors, whose job was to widen the range of activities, although they had not received any specific training.[49] The next major initiative was to introduce formal training in the skills thought desirable.

The first trained occupational therapist to practise in Britain was Margaret Fulton, who was appointed in 1925 to the Aberdeen Royal Asylum (a Scottish Royal Hospital); she had trained in America.[50] The first training course in England for practice in OT was set up by Dr Elizabeth Casson at Dorset House in Bristol (table 15.1).

Casson had been one of the RMPA visitors to Santpoort in 1929. She had previously worked at a registered hospital, Royal Holloway Sanatorium, and had also visited American craft centres, before buying Dorset House, a large house in a fashionable area of Bristol, with money loaned by her family. In 1929 it was opened as a private mental nursing home for twenty-five women only, with an active programme of craft activities central to the milieu of the institution. A year later, in 1930, Casson then started there the first school of OT in Britain, with another American-trained occupational therapist, Constance Tebbitt, as the first principal.[51]

The students had no prior experience in the mental health field. Casson

Table 15.1 Dates of foundation of the first six occupational therapy training courses in Britain

Date	Name	Type of institution
1930	Dorset House, Bristol	Private psychiatric nursing home
1932	The Maudsley Hospital, London	Acute psychiatric teaching hospital
1935	The London School	Private business
1937	Astley Ainsley, Edinburgh	Scottish physical rehabilitation centre
1941	St Andrew's Hospital, Northampton	Registered mental hospital
1942	The Retreat, York	Registered mental hospital

Source: The data are compiled from Wilcock, Occupation for Health, pp. 519–23.

came from an artistic family, and ideas and activities derived from the arts and crafts movement were prominent in the course, thus setting a precedent for the strong craft-based content of the other early training courses. The accounts of the community life at Dorset House, with an emphasis on each member of the community feeling 'an integrated part of the whole' and with no 'social or professional distinctions between members of staff', are strongly reminiscent of the later post-war therapeutic communities, such as Belmont Hospital in Surrey, led by Maxwell Jones.[52]

The second English training school to open was at the Maudsley Hospital in 1932, which had been planned as a teaching and research unit and did not accept long-term patients.[53] The report of the Maudsley's medical superintendent for 1935 makes it clear that the main organiser of the course was Dr Thomas Tennent, then deputy medical superintendent of the Maudsley Hospital, who had also worked with Adolf Meyer in America.[54] Recruitment of the students was aimed at those who were already mental nurses. From 1935 the nearby, but organisationally completely separate, Camberwell School of Arts and Crafts provided teaching in craft work for the course. The report also directly expressed concerns about the costs of the new service; in some instances patients paid for their own materials. The other chief difficulty was the absence of any suitable quarters. This report is significant because of the detail it gives of the practical challenges which had to be overcome in establishing both the activities and the training, and also because of the absence of concern that patient occupation should pay for itself.

The educational committee of the RMPA were aware of the two earlier courses and, led by Dr Russell, they decided in 1934 to introduce a Certificate in Occupational Therapy for Mental Nurses. This certificate was intended to 'enable the holders to organise the work in a large division of a mental hospital'.[55] It is interesting to note that the implication of this objective is that the certificate would be designed for work in the larger public hospitals, but nothing further is recorded of this plan.

The third English school based in a psychiatric setting (and the fifth British school) was opened in 1941 at St Andrew's Hospital, Northampton (then and now the largest of the registered hospitals), in part to compensate for the wartime staffing shortage.[56] By this point Thomas Tennent had moved from the Maudsley Hospital to become medical superintendent at St Andrew's, and on taking up post there in 1938 had immediately appointed not only staff to supervise OT but also 'ladies' companions' and 'gentlemen's companions' (untrained people of a social class similar to the patients) who worked in the OT sessions. The training course began by Tennent approaching the local College of Art for help in instruction in arts and crafts and half of the first intake in 1941 were former students from the college.

The fourth English school based in a psychiatric setting started in 1942 at The Retreat at York, also a registered hospital, and the original base for the development of 'moral treatment'. The conventional image of the hospital, based on the earliest years of its work, does not apply to this later period.[57] Uniquely, the course extended over four years, and combined both a mental nursing qualification with an OT course, although there appears to have been less emphasis on craft work. The course only lasted until 1949, closing because it could not attract enough students to meet the requirements of the Occupational Therapy Association's training regulations.[58]

None of the actual training courses were based in a publicly funded institution, and, apart from the Maudsley, they catered for fee-paying patients from a higher social class than the patients typically admitted to the public hospitals. One aspect of the activities provided in these settings was that they had to be attractive to potential patients and their families, apart from their therapeutic benefit, and this may explain in part the emphasis at Dorset House, and at the Maudsley and St Andrew's Hospitals, on arts and crafts activities.

The creation of formal training courses stimulated the formation of professional associations. The Association of Occupational Therapists (covering England and Wales) was formed after informal suggestions from Dorset House students in 1935, leading to informal discussions between staff from different hospitals, with formal inauguration of the Association in 1936.[59] Paradoxically, the Scottish Association of Occupational Therapy was formed in 1932, before the first training course in Scotland opened in 1937 at the Astley Ainslie Institution in Edinburgh.[60] This contrasts with the direct linkage between the start of the first training course in England for psychiatric social workers in 1929, and the formation of the Association of Psychiatric Social Workers in 1930.[61]

The Association of Occupational Therapists was thus founded when there were only three training schools in the whole of Britain: the courses at Dorset House, the Maudsley and at the privately owned London School based in premises on Tottenham Court Road.[62] The development of mental health services in Wales lagged behind England, although legislatively the position in Wales was the same as in England, with the Board of Control responsible for the mental hospitals. The first mental hospital to be built in Wales was the North Wales Hospital at Denbigh opened in 1842.[63] The massive population growth in South Wales from the middle of the nineteenth century resulted in mental hospitals being built there from later in that century, but there were never any registered hospitals in Wales, and the first OT training course in Wales was only started in 1964 at Cardiff.

One of the first acts of the Association was to agree a definition of an occupational therapist:

> Any person who is appointed as responsible for the treatment of patients by occupation, and who is qualified by training and experience to administer the prescription of a Physician or Surgeon in the treatment of any patient by occupation.[64]

By 1938 the Association had prepared an examination syllabus and the first examinations had been taken. Initially students could train to work in either the psychiatric or physical medicine side, or both, but from the late 1940s all students were required to be qualified in both. In 1939 it was estimated that there were only sixty-four occupational therapists working in English mental hospitals – in other words, only just over half of all such hospitals had a qualified therapist – but it is not clear in what ways the presence of an occupational therapist by itself changed the pattern of activities in hospitals as a whole.

This inevitably meant that the additional demands for the provision of therapeutic and rehabilitative activities during the Second World War could not be met by qualified staff, so improvised short courses were introduced for both service and civilian staff.[65] At the end of the war the association then faced the difficult task of assimilating these staff into the accepted training systems, so a new range of people, particularly men, entered OT as a profession without their first experience of training being at one of the conventional training courses. A range of training options, and special exemptions on the basis of other experience, continued until well after the end of the Second World War.

Mental nurses continued to play an ongoing part in the provision of occupation, and were also seen as recruits for training, supplemented after the war by growing numbers of industrial training officers recruited from skilled tradesmen with industrial experience, and small numbers of separate art therapists. But even by 1968 staff involved in providing occupation for patients were still 65 per cent nursing staff, 18 per cent OT staff and 17 per cent industrial staff. Within any one hospital patient activities were supervised by a number of groups of staff, with a range of work experience before entering hospital employment and with widely differing experience of training.

Issues in the development of occupation in English mental hospitals

Several influences came together after the First World War to change attitudes towards mental illness and mental institutions. These resulted in a number of initiatives to improve the conditions in both public and private psychiatric hospitals and homes. During this period British psychiatrists were actively learning from practice in other countries – it is striking how many of the key innovators cited here – Henderson, Casson and Tennent – were influenced directly by the American social psychiatrist Adolf Meyer.[66] The RMPA actively visited centres of good practice in Germany and the Netherlands and reported their findings widely. The Board of Control encouraged good practice through their memoranda and guidelines, alongside their statutory monitoring and policy-making roles, working closely with the RMPA.

Increasing attention was paid by English psychiatrists to both the overall empirical and clinical objectives of occupation in mental hospitals, and to the specific activities required to achieve them. At least five broad objectives can be discerned – the first four emerged in a rough time sequence, with the fifth being emphasised at a number of points in time, not least when formal training began from 1930:

1 Occupation as an element of institutional management, to reduce levels of disturbed behaviour in hospital residents.
2 Occupation as an element of an ordered and varied waking day.
3 Occupation to increase the range of skills of patients.
4 Occupation to prepare for community living and work.
5 Occupation as individualised creative activity.

The early identification of the tension between institutional regimes and meeting the needs of individual patients is noteworthy. Associated with this range of objectives was the semantic confusion created by the multiple meanings and boundaries of the rhetoric of occupational *therapy*, which in one sense was intended to be inclusive and in another referred to only one element of activity within a mental hospital. The term could refer to essentially managerial and palliative block institutional routines and also, in another sense, to individualised therapeutic programmes. Laws has drawn attention to the contested nature of beliefs about 'therapeutic' work, and the non-linear ways in which paradigms have shifted.[67] She suggests that 'conceptions of therapeutic work have been faced with a host of recurrent tensions: between economically viable employment and specifically "therapeutic" occupations; between the competing requirements of protectionism and reality'.[68] Elizabeth Casson, in giving her account of the beginnings of Dorset House, made no mention of the contribution of OT to the finances of institutions.[69]

The RMPA strove to control most training activities in the psychiatric field as, apart from the nurse training system that they had provided from 1891, they also considered offering a certificate in OT for nurses, in addition to the individual training schools mentioned.[70] Medical superintendents and other psychiatrists were the main initiators of new developments and, through their writing of textbooks and professional articles and working through both their professional body and the national statutory machinery, they encouraged new practices and new forms of training, most obviously in a small number of privileged private and research institutions in England and Scotland. While Elizabeth Casson is rightly seen as the initiator of formal training in OT, the significant role of Thomas Tennent (himself a President of the RMPA) in setting up training both at the Maudsley and at St Andrew's Hospital at Northampton has been overlooked.

It has not previously been pointed out that four of the first six training initiatives in OT in Britain originated in English voluntary or private psychiatric settings: in two registered hospitals (the York Retreat, and St Andrew's Hospital Northampton), in one private psychiatric nursing home in Bristol (Dorset House – for women only), and in the unique Maudsley Hospital in London. Most of the early Scottish developments (at the Royal Edinburgh Hospital, the Glasgow Royal Mental Hospital and the Aberdeen Royal Cornhill Hospital) were in the Scottish Royal Hospitals, comparable to the English registered hospitals. The registered hospitals and nursing homes were also in competition with each other for business, and prided themselves on having higher standards of accommodation and staffing: the quality of their provision for occupation would have been part of their implicit advertising.

None of the first training courses were in public mental hospitals, although they provided the overwhelming majority – over 95 per cent – of psychiatric beds in England. The costs of providing accommodation, staff, equipment and materials for the enhanced range of activities, and for training, were significant. Evidently the medical superintendents and managers of public mental hospitals, with their income derived from public taxation, did not feel able to justify this expense.

So, a presumably unintended consequence of the early English training courses being rooted in private or charitable institutions was the attention paid to activities only possible in better-resourced institutions, catering for patients from a wealthier social class. This was in contrast to the limited range of occupations that were possible in the larger publicly funded hospitals. This raises the question of how well prepared the graduates of those courses were when starting work in the less well-equipped and funded public hospitals. Together with the limited capacity of the training courses, inadequate to meet even minimal staffing targets by 1939, this probably contributed to the evident reservations of some leading psychiatrists, such as the 1954 caustic remark by Mayer-Gross and his colleagues already cited, about the relevance of the 'new OT' to their own therapeutic goals.

A number of different staffing and training assumptions underpinned the new training courses, which were of different duration, intended for different groups (nurses and/or non-nurses), and initially for different client groups, with different training routes in either psychiatric or general medical work. While the first training course began in 1930, not until eight years later, with the agreement of a common national training syllabus in 1938, was it clear that a distinct professional group would be established. It is perhaps surprising that formal training in OT in Britain was not started until 1930, given that the RMPA mental nurse training had started in 1891, with further national developments in nurse training from 1919, and with the, then, Chartered Society of Trained Masseuses (now physiotherapists) having initiated training from 1895.[71] But, together with the entry of both social workers and psychologists into the mental health field through the child guidance clinics,[72] the training courses contributed to the widening range of jobs available to educated women, and illustrate the social-class and gender factors influencing both the provision of activities and who supervised them.

The professionalisation of OT, begun by the formation of the English Association in 1936, was followed by professionalisation of both creative therapists, with their own training courses, and industrial therapists. As nurses controlled wards, and hospital 'artisans' and tradespeople controlled the utility departments, so industrial, occupational and creative therapists controlled the spaces they occupied within the hospital, the latter often on the fringes of the hospital campuses, marginal to the control of psychiatrists and nurses. Inevitably there were ongoing contests between the different groups, and the professional organisations representing them, in striving to achieve hegemony in the field. The concept of 'boundary rhetoric', defined by Shapin as 'a way of defining a practice, of protecting it from unwanted interference and excluding unwanted participants, of telling practitioners how to behave', is useful in analysing the 'politics of demarcation and alliance' so apparent in this field.[73]

In 1960 and 1961 three events took place that changed the professional, legal and physical environments in which these activities continued. With the passing of the Professions Supplementary to Medicine Act in 1960, OT became regulated by government, so therapists at last had an assured position within the NHS. With the implementation in 1960 of the 1959 Mental Health Act, the Board of Control, which from 1948 had operated within the new nationally co-ordinated management framework for all hospitals rather than liaising with individual county and borough councils and governing bodies, was disbanded. By that act the powers of medical superintendents were abolished, with individual consultant psychiatrists then becoming responsible for their own patients. And the then Minister of Health, Enoch Powell, announced in 1961 that the large mental hospitals in which these activities took place would eventually close.[74] It took fifty years for them finally to do so.

Conclusion

This chapter has mapped the developments of work and OT in the mental illness field in England between 1919 and 1959. The perspective offered here is to place the changes in practice in the occupation of psychiatric patients in the context of wide-ranging public, governmental and professional medical concerns to improve mental health services, informed by the impact of new ideas in mental health. Although a rhetoric of OT underpinned the training courses initiated from 1930, the Second World War created new priorities and objectives, and led to other professional groups, and a new encompassing rhetoric of rehabilitation. Wider changes in the pattern of mental health services since 1959 have prompted a shift of scholarly historical attention away from the dominant focus on institutional practice, towards more dispersed models of provision associated with the fragmentation of long-accepted concepts of mental disorder as illness, and hence away from medical dominance.[75]

Notes

1 The chapter examines developments in England only. Scotland had separate legislation for the regulation of mental hospital practice and a separate classification of mental hospitals, crucially distinguishing the better-funded 'Royal' Hospitals from hospitals administered by civic authorities. Although the legislation discussed applied to both England and Wales, the Welsh situation will not be discussed.
2 William Parry-Jones, *The Trade in Lunacy* (London: Routledge & Kegan Paul, 1970).
3 Peter Bartlett, *The Poor Law of Lunacy* (London: Leicester University Press, 1999), p. 246.
4 Board of Control, *Memorandum on Occupation Therapy for Mental Patients* (London: His Majesty's Stationery Office (hereafter HMSO), 1933).
5 Board of Control, *The First Annual Report of the Board of Control for the Year 1914* (London: HMSO, 1916).
6 Edgar Jones, Shahina Rahman and Robin Woolven, 'The Maudsley Hospital: Design and strategic direction, 1923–1939', *Medical History*, 51 (2007), 357–78.
7 Board of Control, *Memorandum on Occupation Therapy*, p. 8.
8 Board of Control, *The First Annual Report*.
9 David Henderson and Robert D. Gillespie, *A Textbook of Psychiatry* (Oxford: Oxford University Press, 1st edn, 1927), p. 121.

10 Henderson and Gillespie, *Textbook of Psychiatry* (6th edn, 1944), pp. 328–30. Ten editions were published.
11 *Ibid.*, p. 285.
12 *Ibid.*, p. 286.
13 See the chapter on schizophrenia by Wilhelm Mayer-Gross and Norman P. Moore, in Gerald W. T. H. Fleming (ed.), 'Special number: Recent progress in psychiatry', *Journal of Mental Science*, 90:378 (1944), 231–55, 252.
14 John W. Dundee, 'A review of chlorpromazine hydrochloride', *British Journal of Anaesthesia*, 26 (1954), 357–79.
15 Graham Richards, 'Britain on the couch: The popularisation of psychoanalysis in Britain 1918–1940', *Science in Context*, 13:2 (2000), 183–230.
16 Henry V. Dicks, *Fifty Years of the Tavistock Clinic* (London: Routledge & Kegan Paul, 1970).
17 Jonathan Toms, *Mental Hygiene and Psychiatry in Modern Britain* (Basingstoke: Palgrave Macmillan, 2013).
18 Montagu Lomax, *Experiences of an Asylum Doctor* (London: George Allen & Unwin, 1922).
19 Hugh Pattison Macmillan (chairman), *Report of the Royal Commission on Lunacy and Mental Disorder* (London: HMSO, 1926). Also known as the Macmillan Report.
20 Noel Timms, *Psychiatric Social Work in Great Britain (1939–1962)* (London: Routledge & Kegan Paul, 1964).
21 Ann A. Wilcock, *Occupation for Health: A Journey from Prescription to Self Health* (London: British Association and College of Occupational Therapists, 2002), vol. 2, p. 96.
22 David K. Henderson, 'Life and work', *Scottish Journal of Occupational Therapy*, 30 (1957), 7–10.
23 For example, David K. Henderson, 'Occupational therapy: A series of papers read at a meeting of the Scottish Division held at the Glasgow Royal Mental Hospital on Friday, May 2, 1924', *Journal of Mental Science*, 71 (1925), 59–80.
24 From our own correspondents. 'Scotland: Occupational therapy in early mental disorder', *Lancet*, 206 (1924), 621.
25 Anon. (editorial), 'Lunacy administration: Conference of Medical Superintendents and Chairmen of Visiting Committees', *British Medical Journal*, 1:3187 (1922), 149–51.
26 Board of Control, *The Eighteenth Annual Report of the Board of Control for the Year 1931* (London: HMSO, 1932).
27 A. E. Evans, 'A tour of some mental hospitals of western Germany', *Journal of Mental Science*, 79 (1933), 150–66.
28 A. E. Evans, 'Report on the RMPA study tour of Holland', *Journal of Mental Science*, 75 (1929), 192–8.
29 Anon. (editorial), 'Notes and news from the Annual RMPA Conference', *Journal of Mental Science*, 80 (1934), 775, 777.
30 Anon., *Annual Report for St Andrew's Hospital Northampton* (Northampton: St Andrews Hospital, 1934).

31 Board of Control, *Memorandum on Occupation Therapy*.
32 Evelyn M. MacDonald, 'History of the Association: Chapter IV 1942–1945', *Occupational Therapy*, 20 (1957), 30–33, 32.
33 Nick Manning, *The Therapeutic Community Movement: Charisma and Routinisation* (London: Routledge & Kegan Paul, 1989).
34 Vicky Long, 'Rethinking post-war mental health care: Industrial therapy and the chronic mental patient in Britain', *Social History of Medicine*, 26:4 (2013), 738–58.
35 Maxwell Jones, 'Industrial therapy of patients still in hospital', *Lancet*, 2 (1956), 985.
36 Diane Waller, *Becoming a Profession: History of Art Therapy in Britain, 1940–82* (London: Tavistock, 1991).
37 Nancy Wansbrough and Agnes Miles, *Industrial Therapy in Psychiatric Hospitals* (London: King Edward VII's Hospital Fund for London, 1968).
38 Douglas H. Bennett, 'The historical development of rehabilitation services', in Fraser N. Watts and Douglas H. Bennett (eds), *Theory and Practice of Psychiatric Rehabilitation* (Chichester: Wiley, 1991).
39 Russell Barton, *Institutional Neurosis* (Bristol: John Wright, 1959).
40 Board of Control, *Memorandum on Occupation Therapy*.
41 John Iveson Russell, *The Occupational Treatment of Mental Illness* (London: Baillière, Tindall & Cox, 1938).
42 Henderson and Gillespie, *Text Book of Psychiatry*. This included a nine-page chapter on occupational therapy, which was identical, word-for-word, between 1927 (1st edn, pp. 475–83) and 1955 (8th edn, pp. 669–77).
43 Willy Mayer-Gross, Eliot Slater and Martin Roth, *Clinical Psychiatry* (London: Baillière, Tindall & Cassell, 1st edn, 1954), p. 282.
44 Charles Webster, *The Health Services Since the War* (London: HMSO, 1988), vol. 1, p. 332.
45 *Ibid.*, vol. 1, p. 334.
46 See David H. Clark, *Administrative Therapy* (London: Tavistock, 1964).
47 *Ibid.*
48 Peter Nolan, *A History of Mental Health Nursing* (London: Chapman & Hall, 1993).
49 Wilcock, *Occupation for Health*, vol. 2, pp. 105–9.
50 *Ibid.*, vol. 2, pp. 110–15.
51 Elizabeth Casson, 'Dr Casson tells how the Dorset House School of Occupational Therapy came into being', *Occupational Therapy*, 18:3 (1955), 92–4.
52 Constance Owens, 'Recollections 1925–1933', *Occupational Therapy*, 18:3 (1955), 95–7; Maxwell Jones, *The Therapeutic Community: A New Treatment Method in Psychiatry* (New York: Basic Books, 1953).
53 Jones et al., 'The Maudsley Hospital'.
54 London County Council (hereafter LCC), *The Maudsley Hospital Denmark Hill SE5 (University of London). Medical Superintendent's Report from 1st January 1932 to 31st December 1935* (London: LCC, 1936), pp. 39–40.
55 Anon. (editorial), 'Report of the Educational Committee', *Journal of Mental Science*, 80 (1934), 766.
56 Jane Evans, *From Priory Cottage to Park Campus: The Story of Occupational Therapy Education in Northampton* (Northampton: University of Northampton, 2007), p. 4.

57 Anne Digby, 'The changing profile of a nineteenth-century asylum: The York Retreat', *Psychological Medicine*, 14:4 (1984), 739–48.
58 Wilcock, *Occupation for Health*, vol. 2, pp. 522–3.
59 *Ibid.*, vol. 2, pp. 157–9.
60 *Ibid.*, vol. 2, pp. 156–7.
61 Malcolm Payne, *The Origins of Social Work* (Basingstoke: Palgrave, 2005), p. 43.
62 Wilcock, *Occupation for Health*, vol. 2, pp. 519–20.
63 Pamela Michael, *Care and Treatment of the Mentally Ill in North Wales, 1800–2000* (Cardiff: University of Wales Press, 2003). This is itself the first academic study of a Welsh mental hospital.
64 Wilcock, *Occupation for Health*, vol. 2, p. 162.
65 *Ibid.*, vol. 2, pp. 191–2.
66 *Ibid.*, vol. 2, p. 96. See Eunice E. Winters (ed.), *The Collected Papers of Adolf Meyer: Psychiatry* (Baltimore, MD: Johns Hopkins University Press, 1951), vol. 2.
67 Jennifer Laws, 'Crackpots and basket-cases: A history of therapeutic work and occupation', *History of the Human Sciences*, 24:2 (2011), 65–81.
68 *Ibid.*, p. 78.
69 Casson, 'Dr Casson tells how', 92–4.
70 Anon. (editorial), 'Report of the Education Committee', *Journal of Mental Science*, 80 (1934), 766.
71 Jean Barclay, *In Good Hands: The History of the Chartered Society of Physiotherapy, 1894–1994* (Oxford: Butterworth-Heinemann, 1994).
72 John Stewart, *Child Guidance in Britain 1918–1955* (London: Pickering & Chatto, 2013).
73 Steven Shapin, 'Discipline and bounding: The history and sociology of science as seen through the externalism–internalism debate', *History of Science*, 30 (1992), 333–69, 335.
74 Enoch Powell, 'Address to the National Association of Mental Health Annual Conference', in *Annual Report of the National Association for Mental Health* (London: NAMH, 1961).
75 See Volker Hess and Benôit Majerus, 'Writing the history of psychiatry after 1945', *History of Psychiatry*, 22 (2011), 139–45; John Turner *et al.*, 'Mental health services in England, 1959–2007: Practitioner memories and historian's narratives', *Medical History* (in press).

16

Work is therapy?
The function of employment in British psychiatric care after 1959

Vicky Long

As the contributions to this volume demonstrate, work and occupation have long formed part of mental healthcare. Yet in the post-war era, the adoption of the policy of psychiatric deinstitutionalisation transformed the nature and intended functions of employment for people with mental health problems within British psychiatric hospitals, and beyond. This chapter focuses on industrial therapy (IT), which hospitals increasingly embraced as part of rehabilitation programmes designed to prepare long-stay patients for discharge. Seemingly distinct from the more established occupational therapy (OT), IT involved patients undertaking industrial sub-contract work in spaces designed to resemble a factory environment.

This chapter will commence by outlining the drive towards psychiatric deinstitutionalisation in post-war Britain, and the development of psychiatric rehabilitation as a means of re-equipping long-stay patients with the skills necessary for independent living, in which occupation was seen as crucial. The chapter then turns to consider two earlier developments which informed the design and ethos of IT; namely, the system of rehabilitation designed to meet the needs of disabled soldiers during the Second World War, and occupation and employment schemes developed for people with learning disabilities. Over the course of the 1950s and 1960s, most British psychiatric hospitals established an industrial therapy unit, and this chapter will explore the operation of these units and the creation of complementary extramural facilities. The chapter then evaluates the tensions between individual therapeutic needs and labour-market requirements which came to the fore in IT, before examining how the industrial therapy model came under pressure due to changing social and economic circumstances in the late twentieth century.

Psychiatric deinstitutionalisation and psychiatric rehabilitation in Britain

Psychiatric deinstitutionalisation in Britain is best seen as a slow and uneven process, rather than a rapid transformation. While the 1957 Report of the Royal Commission on the Law Relating to Mental Illness and Mental Deficiency urged relocating mental healthcare from hospitals to community settings, it was not until 1986 that the first psychiatric hospital in Britain closed.[1]

The recommendations of the 1957 Committee were given a legislative foothold by the 1959 Mental Health Act and the 1960 Mental Health (Scotland) Act, which enabled local authorities to provide a range of community-based services. However, in 1961 the Minister of Health, Enoch Powell, announced a far more decisive shift in policy: existing mental hospitals should be eliminated, in-patient care should be cut back, and psychiatric beds should in future be situated in small clusters within general hospitals. Projecting that the need for psychiatric beds would drop from more than 150,000 to around 80,000 over a sixteen-year period, regional hospital boards were asked to review their provisions and to curtail any further investment in the infrastructure of the mental hospitals.[2]

The shift from intramural to extramural care was predicated on the grounds that developments in treatment methods and the expansion of out-patient provisions would lead to a sustained decline in the number of people requiring lengthy in-patient treatment. Yet many healthcare practitioners were sceptical that these developments would have much of an impact on long-stay patients, and Ministry of Health officials did not advance any concrete proposals as to how this patient cohort should be managed.[3] As 70 to 80 per cent of the patients in mental hospitals in England and Wales in 1964 had been resident for more than two years, this posed a substantial stumbling block to Powell's proposals.[4] Nor could it be assumed that this problem would rapidly be resolved through patient mortality, as a 1961 study of the in-patient population of Menston Hospital revealed that many long-stay patients were relatively young and unmarried, with few contacts in the community. Moreover, the low staffing levels and limited occupational and therapeutic opportunities available within the hospital further compounded the challenges of discharging such patients.[5] The psychiatrist David Clark, who worked at Fulbourn Mental Hospital between 1953 and 1983, recalled that by the 1960s:

> [W]e were just beginning to realise that the process of regaining social competence was far harder for long-term patients from mental hospitals than we had at first thought ... Many long-stay patients were too crippled (either by their long incarceration or by their original psychotic disorder) to manage the transition on their own.[6]

The transition from institutional to community-based care is often attributed to the development of biomedical therapies, most notably new drug treatment. Yet these therapies targeted clinical symptoms, and could do little to re-equip long-stay patients with the social skills needed for independent living. Mental healthcare workers therefore turned to the newly emerging field of psychiatric rehabilitation to resolve this dilemma. As Clark observed in his memoir, rehabilitation had traditionally been associated with the practices of restoring function in disabled war veterans, but was subsequently applied to chronic physical illnesses in the 1950s and psychiatric conditions in the 1960s.[7] While rehabilitation was a medicalised process, it evolved to cater for the needs of disabled people and focused predominantly on social and economic as opposed to medical matters. As Fraser Watts and Douglas Bennett explained, psychiatric rehabilitation examined the interaction between the person and his or her social environment, and sought to enhance patients' ability to function by building on their capacities, so as to facilitate their social adjustment. 'The basic sciences to which rehabilitation needs to look are largely the social and behavioural sciences rather than biological sciences,' they argued.[8]

For long-stay patients below the age of retirement, employability was identified as a crucial social competency that could play a significant role in enabling an individual to live independently in the community. However, a number of psychiatrists queried whether the existing means of occupying patients in hospitals could sufficiently equip patients for jobs in the labour market. Patients either tended to be occupied in tasks that contributed to the running of the hospital, such as cleaning, laundry, farm work and food preparation, or in occupational therapy. OT was often viewed as a source of diversionary activities, rather than a means of producing marketable items for the open market, although it could still yield tangible benefits for institutions.[9] Denis Martin, a psychiatrist at Claybury Hospital in Essex, argued in an influential 1955 article, which outlined the process and problems of institutionalisation in psychiatric hospitals, that hospitals' occupational regimes contributed towards institutionalisation. Those patients who undertook work to maintain the hospital helped keep running costs down, which Martin argued fuelled a conflict of interest, for 'the transfer of a patient from one type of work to another for therapeutic reasons may be strongly resisted because he is, in the language of the clinical notes, such a "good worker"'. OT departments ran the risk of 'becoming production houses for the hospital', evaluated by the number of useful items produced for the hospital, rather than their therapeutic value to patients. Even when this was not the case, Martin complained, OT departments sought to distract patients from their problems, and in so doing fostered patients' dependency upon the hospital by encouraging patients to ignore, rather than solve, their problems.[10]

The origins of industrial therapy

The developing practice of IT owed much to the system of rehabilitation devised for physically disabled veterans of the Second World War, but also took inspiration from methods of occupying and employing people with learning disabilities. The wartime system of rehabilitation had evolved to maximise efficiency by returning injured soldiers either to military service or the civilian workforce. As a consequence, vocational rehabilitation formed an integral part of soldiers' rehabilitation.[11] Similar initiatives during the course of the First World War had not led to any long-term provisions for disabled people. However, in 1941 the Ministry of Labour appointed an inter-departmental committee, which in 1943 published its recommendations on the rehabilitation, training and employment of all disabled people.[12] The post-war shortage of labour power made action on this issue seem particularly desirable, and the government rapidly enacted the Committee's recommendations in the 1944 Disabled Persons (Employment) Act. Under the terms of this act, employers were obliged to hire a proportion of registered disabled staff, while new disablement resettlement officers were tasked with assisting registered disabled people into employment. The newly created body Remploy was to provide sheltered work, while industrial rehabilitation units were established to restore the working capacity of disabled people, and to allow individuals to retrain for new occupations where a return to their former occupation was deemed impossible. The template for these units was the Egham Rehabilitation Centre, based in a country house, which opened as a residential unit in 1943.[13]

Between 1948 and 1951, a further thirteen industrial rehabilitation units were opened within existing government training centres, which were based in industrialised areas. This choice of location meant that the units exchanged the country feel of Egham for a conventional factory environment. Attendees either received a recommendation from a doctor, or were unemployed persons whom disablement resettlement officers believed would benefit from a course of industrial rehabilitation. Upon admittance, a medical officer evaluated attendees to identify the extent of the disability, its impact upon working capacity, the level of remedial exercises required, and whether the individual was capable of returning to his or her former occupation. Units were managed by a rehabilitation officer, and courses typically ran for six to eight weeks, extending up to a maximum of twelve weeks. They were equipped with a gymnasium, supervised by a remedial gymnast, and with workshops and outdoor grounds, in which attendees' aptitude for different types of occupation could be evaluated by occupational supervisors and a vocational officer. A social worker provided assistance with domestic, financial and social matters which threatened to undermine attendees' resettlement, while a disablement resettlement officer focused on securing employment for attendees at the end of their course.[14]

These provisions did not formally exclude psychiatric disorders, but they were framed very much with physical disability in mind. Nevertheless, psychiatrists began to explore whether their patients could benefit from these provisions, and, indeed, whether these provisions could be implemented in an adapted way within psychiatric hospitals to further the goal of psychiatric rehabilitation. One pioneer in this field was Maxwell Jones, who had developed a transitional community to help rehabilitate former prisoners of war. Jones later wrote that these men's rehabilitation was 'enormously helped by the ready response of over sixty employers who were willing to engage our patients in various kinds of work'.[15] In Jones' view, OT in mental hospitals could provide an outlet for emotions, and thus served some therapeutic purpose. Yet, he claimed, OT 'cannot claim the rehabilitative effect of productive group work, which is capable of leading to better contact with reality, to behaviour more in accordance with social standards, and to the foundations of self-esteem'.[16] Impressed by Jones' work with former prisoners of war, the Ministry of Labour established an industrial neurosis unit at Belmont Hospital under Jones' directorship in 1946, which targeted those whom Jones described as 'unemployed "drifters"'.[17] Patients were classified on leaving the unit as suitable for open employment, suitable for sheltered employment, or unemployable.[18] The unit initially sought to train attendees in particular trades, such as bricklaying, plastering, carpentry, hairdressing, tailoring and gardening, but found that patients were more responsive when given the opportunity to improve the environment of the hospital, for example by repairing furniture or redecorating buildings.[19]

Although Jones came into conflict with the Ministry of Labour over the selection of patients for his unit in the early 1950s,[20] he nevertheless publicly endorsed the industrial rehabilitation services offered by the ministry for disabled people, and urged other psychiatrists to exploit these provisions for their patients. In 1955, 1 per cent of the individuals admitted to a Ministry of Labour industrial rehabilitation unit had a diagnosis of mental deficiency, 3 per cent of psychoses, and 12 per cent of psychoneuroses. In a 1956 article, Jones described an ongoing experiment through which patients at mental hospitals, psychiatric clinics and colonies for mental defectives were accepted onto courses within industrial rehabilitation units. Of a cohort of 208, 130 were placed into employment or further training. At a six-month follow up, 65 per cent of the patients who had completed the course and who could be traced were either employed or in training.[21]

The adoption of IT in mental hospitals also appears to have stemmed from earlier experiments on means of occupying people with learning disabilities, undertaken by Aubrey Lewis' Occupational Psychiatry Research Unit at the

Maudsley, a body which later evolved into the Social Psychiatry Research Unit. This body was established in 1947 with funding from the Medical Research Council, and one of its three initial focal points was the working capacity of people diagnosed as mentally ill or defective.[22] Lewis observed that notwithstanding the desire to prevent the exploitation of these people as 'slave labour', it was customary to train and employ people diagnosed as mentally defective in crafts, while mental hospitals occupied some of their patients in tasks relating to the upkeep of the hospital. In his view, it was time to investigate the working conditions under which such patients would perform best. 'There is no evidence that the activities usually available in occupational therapy departments ... are more beneficial than normal occupations of the remunerative kind would be,' Lewis argued, suggesting that, 'the supposed economic and political objections to such work have been given undue weight.' He proposed evaluating the outcome of such an experiment by measuring individuals' outputs, alongside their mental health and social adjustment.[23]

Lewis' unit undertook its investigation at Darenth Park, a large institution for people with learning disabilities which was located in Kent. By 1949, the unit had conducted cognitive, personality and aptitude tests on 100 patients at this institution. Lewis concluded that 'in this institution there are many patients of an intelligence level equal to much of the unskilled work carried out in ordinary factories'.[24] In a progress report produced by the Unit for the Medical Research Council, Lewis explained how individuals in institutions for mental defectives were 'seldom occupied or trained in such a way as to fit them for self-supporting work in industry'.[25] He described the establishment of workshops at Darenth Park, in which patients, supervised by nurses, either undertook the hand-trimming of plastics, or the assembly of cardboard packaging, and were paid on a piece-work basis. The initial findings of this research, Lewis claimed, suggested that individuals diagnosed as mentally defective 'work better when given a routine job (in contrast to a common view among experts in mental deficiency that unstable mental defectives need variety and constant change in occupation)'.[26] Lewis reiterated this view two years later, observing that 'vocational guidance and selection are of minor importance'. 'Our experience,' he noted, 'indicates that in addition to the jobs usually prescribed for defectives repetitive work in factories is suitable for many patients.'[27]

Lewis described how patients had been trained to do factory work in a workshop in the institution, before being sent on licence to work for private companies. Many female patients, he believed, would also do better in factory work than in domestic service. With this in mind, Lewis argued that the training in skilled and semi-skilled work provided by mental deficiency institutions and local authority craft centres did not do enough to equip individuals diagnosed as mentally defective for the unskilled work available to them in community settings. He believed that workshops should prepare patients for the conditions they would find in the industrial workplace. Sheltered workshops, claimed Lewis, were 'valuable training centres for defectives who have faulty work habits or attitudes or who are very slow, but capable of being speeded up ... defectives respond readily to incentives, including financial incentives'.[28] Financial incentives, indeed, appeared to be a driving factor in the experiment overall: one memorandum observed that the mental defectives who secured employment as a consequence of the unit's work netted the Treasury £16,500, and that the potential gains were large, given that there were some 45,000 individuals diagnosed as mentally defective who were estimated to be capable of securing employment.[29] The unit's findings were publicised to the medical community via a series of articles in the early to mid-1950s.[30]

The development of industrial therapy for psychiatric patients

Psychiatric hospitals began to re-examine how patients were occupied within hospitals as part and parcel of broader programmes of hospital reform and psychiatric rehabilitation. In 1954, for example, David Clark introduced a programme of 'occupation and liberalisation' in the male wards of Fulbourn Hospital. The programme sought to occupy as many patients as possible by graduating levels of activity for different patient cohorts: habit-training groups were instituted for incontinent and demented patients, for example. Efforts were made to select jobs which would suit individual patients, assist their recovery and contribute towards the life of the hospital, and a graduated system of pay and reward was introduced. A deputy chief male nurse, appointed as occupation officer, interviewed patients, studied working arrangements, transferred patients between different types of occupation and set pay rates. Although the programme led to an increase in the discharge rate of patients who had been resident in the hospital for less than a year, Clark observed that there had been no significant change in the discharge rate of patients who had been resident for more than a year.[31] Clark drew his inspiration from a 1953 World Health Organization Report, which emphasised the need to engage patients in 'planned and purposeful activity', advocating a series of graded activities catering for different groups of patients. Observing how vocational guidance and sheltered workshops had facilitated physical rehabilitation by providing patients with new work skills, the report suggested that similar provisions would benefit the rehabilitation and social resettlement of psychiatric patients.[32]

Between 1955 and 1956, a study undertaken at Banstead Hospital sought to investigate whether long-stay patients could benefit from participating in an industrial workshop. These experiments were undertaken by members of the Medical Research Council's Social Psychiatry Research Unit, the organisation which had just a few years earlier investigated the capacity of people with learning disabilities to undertake industrial work. Reporting on the study in a 1956 article, the authors argued that the therapeutic value of work in preventing deterioration in psychiatric patients had been recognised since the nineteenth century, yet the absence of objective studies of the therapeutic benefits of work therapy stymied the development of the field. The Banstead study established an industrial workshop for a group of twelve male patients aged between twenty-six and forty-six. All the patients had a diagnosis of schizophrenia, and had been resident for between four and twenty-two years. Unlike Clark's earlier experiments, the workshop was overseen by a supervisor who had never hitherto set foot inside a psychiatric hospital, but possessed a 'firm but good-natured disciplinary leadership'.[33] Within the workshop, patients were engaged in the folding of cardboard boxes, supplied by a firm which had for several years been contracting out work to a sheltered workshop in a mental deficiency hospital. Although this work was repetitive, unskilled and poorly remunerated, the authors found it advantageous as no specialist equipment was required, and it enabled investigators to measure the daily output of each patient. To incentivise the patients participating in the study, earnings were distributed according to output. Few patients, however, exceeded earnings of £1 a week, the threshold at which patients forfeited sickness benefit and became liable to pay taxes. The authors reported that the persistence of schizophrenic symptoms sometimes led to disruptive episodes in the workroom, but stressed that such incidences were fairly isolated and of short duration. After twelve months, three of the patients had been discharged, one had absconded, seven had been transferred from closed wards to open wards, and one remained on a closed ward. The workshop programme was subsequently expanded to involve a further twenty male patients and thirty female patients. Summarising their experiment, the authors concluded that 'many long-stay patients are capable of reaching normal levels of rate of work at comparatively unskilled tasks', although the low cap on earnings before tax was exceeded and the resultant withholding of benefits served as a disincentive.[34] The authors also believed that attendance at the workshop improved patients' social behaviour; although they cautioned that the custodial and authoritarian attitudes of older male nurses towards patients could slow progress.

The Banstead study, which in many respects duplicated the earlier investigations into the occupation of mental defectives, established the template for the industrial workshops which spread rapidly throughout British psychiatric hospitals. The number of hospitals reported to have an industrial unit rose from twenty-one in 1957,[35] to fifty-eight by 1959[36] and one hundred by 1967, leaving only twenty-two psychiatric hospitals without such a unit.[37] Rather than attempting to identify and meet patients' individual vocational skills and attributes, these units tended to deliver repetitive unskilled work, measuring success in terms of output and enhanced discipline. Indeed, some writers contended that the very monotony of the work and the disciplinary character of the workshop was a virtue, on the grounds that chronic psychiatric patients lacked the inner energies and emotions needed for more complex work. This logic inverted the conventional wisdom of industrial psychology, which viewed repetitive, monotonous work and characterless working environments as causes of neurosis among hitherto healthy workers.[38] It also suggests that attitudes towards learning disability, embodied within the experiments of the Occupational Psychiatric Research Unit, subsequently coloured approaches to the vocational aptitudes of people suffering from mental illness.

These new IT units were established as a supplement to, or in place of, OT, and incorporated industrial features, such as factory lighting and seating, continuous belt processes, time sheets and time clocks. John Denham, a consultant psychiatrist at Long Grove Hospital in Epsom, noted that an IT unit was cheaper to furnish than an OT unit. 'Just a bare room with a minimum of furniture is required,' he wrote. 'The more factory-like the surroundings, the higher the patient's output.'[39] The comparatively low costs involved in setting up an IT unit doubtless appealed to psychiatrists given the low budgets assigned to psychiatric hospitals in this era.[40] Indeed, while 30 per cent of units were located within purpose-built spaces, 47.5 per cent were situated in parts of the hospital converted for the purpose and a further 22.5 per cent were based in the wards.[41] A survey undertaken in the early 1960s found that 60 per cent of units were managed by a nurse rather than an industrial supervisor.[42] While some units functioned 'on a full commercial footing', others 'appeared to be basically occupational therapy departments finding outlets for their work'.[43] Working hours rarely exceeded thirty hours a week and patient workers tended to receive low hourly or weekly rates of pay rather than normal piece rates.[44]

A draft hospital building note for a rehabilitation centre for psychiatric patients produced by Rudolf Freudenberg, head of the mental health section at the Ministry of Health, illustrates the composite nature of these new spaces.[45] In a traditional industrial workspace the nature of the work processes undertaken determined layout; Freudenberg, however, stressed the need for a flexible space which could be adapted for IT, OT and training in home making. The psychiatric context also shaped security and decor. Patients 'should not be kept in one confined area unless this is absolutely essential', Freudenberg urged. Envisaging a unit which could serve the needs of disparate patient groups, he suggested some rooms 'require finishes suitable to industrial workshops', while others (presumably intended for patients who were older, or more severely ill) 'require finishes and decoration comparable to those found in ward day rooms'.[46] In other respects, the industrial dimensions of the space predominated. Thus, Freudenberg stressed the importance of good lighting and ventilation, suggesting that advice be sought from the Factory Inspectorate regarding safety precautions. Mirroring the development of welfare spaces within model factories, Freudenberg advocated a canteen and rest room.[47]

As psychiatric deinstitutionalisation gathered pace and the locus of care gradually shifted from the hospital to the community, the focus began to shift from inter- to extramural provisions. However, the Ministry of Labour capped the intake of people with a mental disorder into its rehabilitation centres at 20 to 25 per cent, on the grounds that people suffering from a mental illness needed a longer course of rehabilitation, were at a high risk of relapse and were difficult to resettle into employment.[48] A similar pattern existed in the provision of long-term sheltered work for severely disabled people believed to be unable to enter open employment, organised by the government body Remploy. In 1976, 20 per cent of Remploy's workers suffered from a mental disorder, of which 9.4 per cent were listed as suffering from a mental illness, and 10.4 per cent were described as having a learning disability.[49] This sharp demarcation between physical disability and mental disorder puzzled some researchers, as many individuals with physical disabilities who attended the Ministry's rehabilitation units were found to also suffer from psychological disorders.[50] In 1949, one of the Ministry's own medical advisors examined a cohort of fifty industrial rehabilitation unit attendees. Forty-six of these attendees were registered as having a physical disability, and four as having a psychological disability, yet the advisor found that seventeen of the fifty had a psychological disability, and a further twenty-six were disabled due to a combination of physical and psychological factors. Reviewing his findings, the advisor observed that mental disability tended to 'assume an organic title'.[51]

Faced with Ministry of Labour obstruction, a number of psychiatrists established extramural services, often in collaboration with external partners. Dr Donal Early was an early adopter of IT, introducing industrial work at Bristol's Glenside Hospital in 1957. However, he feared that 'if industrial work in hospitals … becomes an end in itself', there was a risk that patients would adapt to the repetitive work, settle down and become further institutionalised. IT, he insisted, 'must be therapeutic, and its aim must be the return to the community of a useful and acceptable citizen'.[52] Hoping to enable more patients to secure employment in open industry following their discharge, Early collaborated with local industries to establish the Industrial Therapy Organisation in 1960, which provided sheltered employment in premises fitted out as factories.[53] During the first five years of the organisation's activities, 25 per cent of cases gained employment in open industry and a further 19 per cent secured a post in sheltered employment.[54] Seeking to increase the number of former patients employed in open industry, Early pioneered the sheltered working group, in which a group of former patients who might otherwise be employed in a sheltered workshop instead worked together within an otherwise open industry. The Department of Employment subsequently dubbed these working groups 'enclaves', a term which Early objected to on the grounds that it connoted 'a territory surrounded by foreign domination'.[55] Other IT organisations were established in Epsom, Thames, Wirral and Ulster, although by 1978 only the Epsom group was still operating.[56] Birmingham, meanwhile, founded an Industrial Therapy Association in 1963, which established a factory outside the grounds of Birmingham's All Saints Hospital in 1965 to recreate 'an authentic working environment involving the realities of working life such as daily travel, arriving on time, meeting production targets and meaningful activity'.[57]

Industrial therapy after 1975

Rising levels of unemployment and the process of hospital rundown and closure had an impact upon the nature and scope of IT. The process of deinstitutionalisation gradually amended the purpose of IT within psychiatric hospitals, as the less-sick patients were discharged, leaving behind people with more intractable problems. While industrial therapy units had originally been established to 'preserve or re-establish outside interests and standards by providing work of an industrial nature', one 1975 article in the *British Journal of Psychiatry* observed that they often 'merely offer the patient activity and occupation'.[58] IT, in other words, had become a means of occupying chronic long-stay patients within institutions, rather than a means of rehabilitating and discharging patients. Indeed, some psychiatrists argued that it was unrealistic to expect all psychiatric patients to secure employment in the open market, and suggested that there was a need to provide more permanent sheltered work for patients who suffered from more severe and enduring forms of mental disturbance.[59] Sheltered work had long been seen as an appropriate resource for people with learning disabilities, and this suggestion illustrates how the concepts of chronic mental illness and mental disability converged in the 1960s and 1970s. John Wing, for example, believed that social disabilities posed more of a barrier to the discharge of long-stay patients than any residual clinical symptoms. On these grounds, he used the term 'long-term mental disablement' to encompass 'those who are disabled by reason of mental retardation, dementia … and chronic mental illness'.[60] Wing explained that, 'To refer to those disabled by chronic schizophrenia as "mentally ill" induces an expectation that medical treatment is the chief factor determining the type of residential or day care needed, whereas it is generally agreed that social needs are often more important'.[61]

In the long term, deinstitutionalisation led to a decline in the number of long-stay in-patients, and transformed the demographic of this patient cohort. There was no practical need to re-equip the elderly patients who increasingly made up the numbers of long-stay patients with workplace skills. Meanwhile, newly admitted patients spent much shorter spells in hospital: they were consequently unlikely to become institutionalised, and often did not spend long enough in hospital to make use of its IT unit. Units sited within hospitals closed down as the process of hospital rundown took hold, while the community-based day centres which developed in their wake often focused on recreational as opposed to work-orientated activities.[62]

Changing economic circumstances also fuelled the decline of industrial therapy. With the decline of the industrial sector and the rise of the service sector, there was an increasing disparity between the work undertaken within IT units, and the types of work available in the labour market, which now required different skills from those imparted within IT units. This challenge was compounded by rising levels of unemployment. IT had been pioneered in an era of full employment, and had sought to re-equip psychiatric patients for an inflexible labour market; little heed had been paid to patients' own aspirations or interests, although in part this reflected the challenges facing psychiatrists who struggled to create diverse and interesting work opportunities for their patients.[63] However, as unemployment began to rise from the late 1970s onwards, many began to question the viability of securing employment for former psychiatric patients, and indeed whether there was any point in persisting with occupational rehabilitation if few former psychiatric patients could realistically be expected to secure work in open industry.[64] If it had been difficult for people suffering from mental disorders to secure a job in an era of full employment, it become far more of a challenge by 1986, when unemployment levels in Britain reached 11.2 per cent.[65] By 1977, the percentage of attendees at the Department of Employment's Employment Centres[66] who ultimately secured employment was 25 per cent; back in 1946, 70 per cent of attendees had been placed in employment.[67] One response was to suggest that psychiatry should no longer be concerned with patients' employment. This attitude was often reinforced by the argument that the cost of operating sheltered workshops outweighed the cost of unemployment benefits.[68] Although rising levels of unemployment stymied efforts to secure employment for people who suffered from mental disorders and consigned many to an impoverished existence on benefits, it did offer one consolation: unemployment had now become a commonplace experience, and was no longer a marker of mental disturbance. As one service user explained in the early 1990s, it was now easier to conceal his history of schizophrenic breakdowns because people he met automatically attributed his unemployment to the state of the labour market.[69]

The plummeting chances of a person with a serious mental health condition securing a job led some to challenge the long-held assumption that former patients should adapt to the labour market. Highlighting the discrimination facing former psychiatric patients in the labour market in 1990, for example, Gerald Midgley argued that efforts to re-equip individuals who failed to tackle the discrimination innate in the labour market were doomed to failure, and suggested that more efforts should be made to effect social and political change.[70] The principle of social inclusion which currently dominates mental health policy, meanwhile, militates against the provision of separate facilities and services to aid the employment of people with mental health issues, on the grounds that solutions should focus on integrating service users into the labour market, rather than providing segregated sheltered facilities. In line with this logic, government subsidies were withdrawn from Remploy. Of the fifty-four Remploy factories operating in 2011–12, forty-eight had closed by December 2013, and the remaining six had been sold.[71]

Conclusion

The transfer of psychiatric care from institutional settings to the community prompted psychiatrists to develop new ways of occupying their patients which would facilitate this process. The very title of the new practice developed to accomplish this – industrial therapy – promised to unite work and therapy in a modern reworking of work therapy. IT aspired to meet the needs of the contemporary labour market and a rapidly changing mental health sector. In practice, however, IT focused on work, at the expense of therapy. It frequently boiled down to the provision of repetitive, unskilled work, which was intended primarily to re-equip long-stay patients with the skills necessary to function in the workplace; patients' own interests and aptitudes were a lesser consideration. In this respect, IT diverged from the practice of OT, duplicating instead the mechanistic approach to rehabilitation for people with physical disabilities which was implemented after the Second World War. The unemployment of psychiatric patients in an era of full employment was seen as a 'medico-social rather than an industrial problem'.[72] Yet this did not mean that IT focused on enhancing patients' psychological wellbeing; rather, it meant that patients should adapt to the conventions of the workplace. While IT sought to facilitate patients' discharge from hospital by fostering their capacity to function independently, it perpetuated some of the aims and objectives which had characterised its earlier incarnation as a practice designed for people with learning disabilities, and consequently contributed to a growing conflation of disability and chronic mental disorder.

As levels of unemployment rose, and psychiatric hospitals closed, the system of IT collapsed. The industrial sector declined, employment opportunities for people with mental health issues fell and the costs of employing people in sheltered workshops came under fire. The unemployment of people with mental health issues was now viewed as an industrial problem – a regrettable yet natural consequence of the labour market – rather than a medico-social problem which required intervention from mental healthcare workers.

Notes

1 Report of the Royal Commission on the Law Relating to Mental Illness and Mental Deficiency (1957), Cmnd 169.
2 Kathleen Jones, *Asylums and After. A Revised History of the Mental Health Services: From the Early 18th Century to the 1990s* (London: Athlone, 1993), pp. 159–61.
3 For more information on the Ministry of Health's attitude see Vicky Long, *Destigmatising Mental Illness? Professional Politics and Public Education in Britain, 1870–1970* (Manchester: Manchester University Press, 2014), pp. 115–17.
4 John K. Wing, Douglas H. Bennett and John Denham, 'The industrial rehabilitation of long-stay schizophrenic patients: A study of 45 patients at an industrial rehabilitation unit', *MRC Memorandum No. 42* (London: Her Majesty's Stationery Office, 1964), p. 1.
5 Charles P. Gore and Kathleen Jones, 'Survey of a long-stay mental hospital population', *The Lancet*, 2:7201 (1961), 544–6.
6 David H. Clark, *The Story of a Mental Hospital: Fulbourn 1858–1983* (London: Process Press, 1996), p. 218.
7 Ibid.
8 Fraser Watts and Douglas Bennett, 'Introduction: The concept of rehabilitation', in Fraser N. Watts and Douglas H. Bennett (eds), *Theory and Practice of Psychiatric Rehabilitation* (Chichester: Wiley, 1987 [1983]), pp. 3–14, 13.
9 Douglas Bennett, 'Work and occupation for the mentally ill', in Hugh Freeman and German E. Berrios (eds), *150 Years of British Psychiatry. Volume II: The Aftermath* (London: Athlone, 1996), pp. 193–208, 200.
10 Denis V. Martin, 'Institutionalisation', *The Lancet*, 266:6901 (1955), pp. 1188–90, 1189.
11 On the development of this system of rehabilitation see Julie Anderson, *War, Disability and Rehabilitation in Britain: 'Soul of a Nation'* (Manchester: Manchester University Press, 2011), pp. 72–101.
12 Report of the Interdepartmental Committee on the Rehabilitation and Resettlement of Disabled Persons (1943), Cmd. 6415.
13 W. L. Buxton, 'Industrial rehabilitation units: A British experiment', *International Labour Review*, 67:6 (1953), 535–48; 537–38.
14 Ibid., pp. 535–48; J. A. L. Vaughan Jones, '"Back to work": The industrial rehabilitation units of the Ministry of Labour and national service', *British Medical Journal*, 2:4731 (1951), 601–3.
15 Maxwell Jones, *Social Psychiatry in Practice: The Idea of the Therapeutic Community* (Harmondsworth: Penguin Books, 1968), p. 17.

16 Maxwell Jones, B. A. Pomryn and Eileen Skellern, 'Work therapy', *The Lancet*, 267:6918 (1956), pp. 343–4, 343.
17 Jones, *Social Psychiatry*, p. 17.
18 British National Archives, Kew, Richmond, Surrey (hereafter BNA), Lab 20/33, Ministry of Labour and National Service, 'Liaison with Sutton Emergency Hospital: Special Psychiatric Centre', note of a meeting held 19 August 1946.
19 Jones *et al.*, 'Work therapy', p. 344.
20 See Vicky Long, 'Rethinking post-war mental health care: Industrial therapy and the chronic mental patient in Britain', *Social History of Medicine*, 26:4 (2013), 738–58, 756.
21 Maxwell Jones, 'Industrial rehabilitation of mental patients still in hospital', *The Lancet*, 268:6950 (1956), pp. 985–6.
22 BNA, FD 1/433, Occupational Psychiatry Research Unit, letter from Aubrey Lewis to A. Landsborough Thomson, 29 November 1947.
23 *Ibid.*
24 BNA, FD 1/433, Occupational Psychiatry Research Unit, memorandum sent from Aubrey Lewis to Dr Martin Ware, 'MRC Occupational Psychiatry Research Unit', 13 December 1949.
25 BNA, FD 1/433, Occupational Psychiatry Research Unit, 'Progress Report 1949–50 of the Occupational Psychiatry Research Unit', typescript.
26 *Ibid.*
27 BNA, FD 1/433, typescript, 'Research on the Employability of Defectives', 20 December 1951.
28 *Ibid.*
29 BNA, FD 1/433, Occupational Psychiatry Research Unit, HPH, 'Occupational Adaptation Unit: Visit to the Maudsley Hospital 28.2.1952'.
30 Jack Tisard and Neil O'Connor, 'The employability of high-grade mental defectives – I', *American Journal of Mental Deficiency*, 54 (1950), pp. 563–76; Jack Tisard and Neil O'Connor, 'The employability of high-grade mental defectives – II', *American Journal of Mental Deficiency*, 55 (1950), 144–57; Jack Tisard and Neil O'Connor, 'The occupational adaptation of high-grade mental defectives', *The Lancet*, 260:6735 (1952), pp. 620–3.
31 David H. Clark and R. M. Hoy, 'Reform in a mental hospital: A critical study of a programme', *International Journal of Social Psychiatry*, 3 (1957), 211–33.
32 World Health Organization, 'The Community Mental Hospital', *Third Report of the Expert Committee on Mental Health* (Geneva: WHO, 1953), pp. 19, 22–3.
33 George M. Carstairs, Neil O'Connor and K. Rawnsley, 'Organisation of a hospital workshop for chronic psychotic patients', *British Journal of Preventive Social Medicine*, 10 (1956), pp. 136–40, 136.
34 *Ibid.*, p. 139.
35 National Archives of Scotland, Edinburgh (hereafter NAS), ED 12/27, Ministry of Labour, 'Employment projects in hospitals', 1961. Figures for hospitals in England and Wales only.
36 National Association for Mental Health (NAMH), E. P. H. Charlton speaking in session on 'Work as therapy and occupation in hospital', in *The Place of Work in the*

Treatment of Mental Disorder: Proceedings of a Conference (London: NAMH, 1959), p. 29. This figure referred to the number of hospitals which provided industrial work for patients.
37 Nancy Wansbrough and Agnes Miles, *Industrial Therapy in Psychiatric Hospitals: A King's Fund Report* (London: King's Fund, 1968), p. 5.
38 Discussed in Long, 'Rethinking post-war mental health care', pp. 748–50.
39 Wellcome Library (hereafter WL), archives of Rudolf Karl Freudenberg, PP/RKF/C.2, 'Research in industrial therapy: Appendix A – Memorandum from Dr J. Denham', typescript.
40 On the financial constraints facing hospitals, see Long, 'Rethinking post-war mental health care', p. 753.
41 Wansbrough and Miles, *Industrial Therapy*, p. 37.
42 WL, archives of Rudolf Karl Freudenberg, PP/RKF/C.3, R. V. Wadsworth, B. W. P. Wells and R. F. Scott, 'The state of industrial therapy in the mental hospitals of England and Wales', typescript.
43 Ibid.
44 NAS, ED 12/27, Ministry of Labour, 'Employment Projects in Hospitals'.
45 WL, archives of Rudolf Karl Freudenberg, PP/RKF/C.7, 'Revised draft. Hospital building note: Rehabilitation centre for psychiatric patients', typescript, 1964.
46 Ibid.
47 Ibid. On factory design and layout see Vicky Long, *The Rise and Fall of the Healthy Factory: The Politics of Industrial Health in Britain, 1914-60* (Basingstoke: Palgrave, 2011), pp. 57–68.
48 Nancy Wansbrough and Philip Cooper, *Open Employment after Mental Illness* (London: Tavistock, 1980), p. 32.
49 Ibid., p. 38.
50 Ibid., p. 34.
51 Mark Hewitt, 'The unemployed disabled man', *The Lancet*, 254:6577 (1949), pp. 523–6, 523.
52 Donal F. Early and Ralph V. Magnus, 'Industrial Therapy Organisation (Bristol) 1960–65', *British Journal of Psychiatry*, 114 (1968), 335–6.
53 Donal F. Early, 'The Industrial Therapy Organisation (Bristol): A development of work in hospital', *The Lancet*, 281:7278 (1963), 435–6.
54 Early and Magnus, 'Industrial Therapy Organisation', pp. 335–6.
55 Wansbrough and Cooper, *Open Employment*, pp. 48–9.
56 Ibid., p. 47.
57 Norman Imlah, *Work is Therapy: The History of the Birmingham Industrial Therapy Association 1963-2003* (Studley: Brewin Books, 2003), p. 7.
58 Anne Pattie, Anne Williams and David Emery, 'Helping the chronic psychiatric patient in an industrial therapy setting: An experiment in inter-disciplinary co-operation', *British Journal of Psychiatry*, 126 (1975), pp. 30–3, 30.
59 Bennett, 'Work and occupation', p. 201.
60 John K. Wing, 'Trends in the care of the chronically mentally disabled', in John Wing and Rolf Olsen (eds), *Community Care for the Mentally Disabled* (Oxford: Oxford University Press, 1979), pp. 1–13, 3.

61 *Ibid.*, p. 4.
62 Bennett, 'Work and occupation', p. 203.
63 See Long, 'Rethinking post-war mental health care', pp. 738–58.
64 Bennett, 'Work and occupation', p. 203.
65 John Burnett, *Idle Hands: The Experiences of Unemployment, 1790–1990* (London and New York: Routledge, 1994), p. 276.
66 Formerly known as the Ministry of Labour Industrial Rehabilitation Units.
67 Bennett, 'Work and occupation', p. 204.
68 *Ibid.*, p. 205.
69 Peter Barham and Robert Hayward, *Relocating Madness: From the Mental Patient to the Person* (London: Free Association Books, 1995), p. 14.
70 Gerald Midgley, 'The social context of vocational rehabilitation for ex-psychiatric patients', *British Journal of Psychiatry*, 156 (1990), 272–7.
71 See Feargal McGuinness and Aliyah Dar, Remploy: House of Commons Standard Note, SN00698, 5 August 2014, www.parliament.uk/briefing-papers/sn00698.pdf.
72 Hewitt, 'The unemployed disabled man', p. 525.

17

The hollow gardener and other stories: Reason and relation in the work cure

Jennifer Laws

> Some years ago, a patient much afflicted with melancholic and hypochondriacal symptoms was admitted by his own request. The patient was by trade a gardener, and the superintendent immediately perceived the propriety of keeping him employed ... .[1]

It was by serendipity rather than planning that the opening of the Oxford symposium for which I first drafted a version of this paper fell almost to the day on the two hundredth anniversary of Samuel Tuke's *Description of the Retreat Near York*, published June 1813, in which it is declared that of all methods to coax the melancholic patient back to reality and reason, work was to be regarded both the most effective and efficacious.

As is well known in the history of psychiatry, the *Description of the Retreat: An Institution Near York for Insane Persons of the Society of Friends*, is the detailed and often lively account of the enigmatic Quaker Retreat in North Yorkshire, England, at which moral treatment – and thus work therapy by association – is widely credited to have had its English origins. Written by Samuel Tuke, grandson of the Retreat's founder William Tuke, the text has been celebrated as one of the most significant records in the history of psychiatry. Produced with the intention of promoting moral treatment to a wider audience of practitioners and reformers, the text is imbued with glimpses into early nineteenth-century ideologies of work – from the therapeutic work of patients in the asylum's farm and gardens, to the meticulous 'workings out' of the *methods* of moral treatment so that they might be developed and adopted more broadly.

Today, opinion about the Retreat and its significance to a broader history of psychiatry is mixed, with critiques ranging from questions about how innovative Tuke's interventions really were, to doubts over whether further attention to this site can continue to add to previous discussions.[2] Yet the Retreat at York, as an establishment local to my own institution at Durham and to the sites of my own research (a reflexive ethnography of contemporary spaces of work therapy) remains an evocative starting point for this chapter with some sympathetic resonances to the contemporary material that I shall discuss below.

In this chapter, then, rather than offer a further analysis of the Retreat and its general relevance to the work cure, I pause simply to consider this most quoted idea as it appears in the *Description* – that work is, first, a servant of *reason* and *rationality,* and, second, the most *efficacious* treatment for mental disorder. Elsewhere I have explored how ideas about the curative potential of work have varied across time and space, and yet how, across such history, numerous recurring tensions appear – tensions, I argue, that betray something of our greater human connectedness to work, or to what in contemporary terminology might be thought of as the 'occupational view' of humanity.[3] (Although I will unpack this position later, for now we might consider such an occupational viewpoint as one that sees the human in his or her fullest form as a uniquely working creature, and that emphasises the need for meaningful work and occupation for a happy and healthful existence.)

In this chapter, as Tuke helps me to articulate, I want to develop this argument – to explore how this characteristic framing of work therapy through the lenses of reason and rationality has become a hallmark in the way that work therapy (historic and contemporary) is understood and is advocated; but also how such framing might be curiously at odds with a richer and equally fundamental occupational perspective. Through the telling of two short encounters in the history of work therapy (the first taken from Tuke's original *Description of the Retreat* and the second from my contemporary ethnographic material), I will explore how, while the themes of rationality and reason constitute a dominant account of the therapeutics of work, a much livelier narrative can be found that steps *beyond* such a rational and rationalised framework. Through attending more closely to these *petits récits* or 'smaller narratives', I explore what becomes lost or missing when the rational and furthermore rationalised attributes of work therapy become the only lens through which to understand therapeutic encounters with work – and, as suggested above, how such a focus on the rational and reasoned might simultaneously be at odds with a greater view of the human as a more fundamentally 'occupational being'.

The two case studies I have selected for this chapter both take as their focus the curious relationships that emerge between staff and patients in 'working' therapies (pleasingly, for our purposes, in the psychotherapeutic literature such client/therapist relations are termed 'the working alliance'). Coincidentally, both cases also involve gardening – a facet which, while not essential to the argument, may nonetheless help to create focus on the vital and visceral and soily characteristics of therapy which emerge beyond the realm of the rational.

After providing a brief sketch of the ways in which the work cure has been framed through the ages by reason and rationality, the trajectory of the remainder of this chapter will be to interrogate how the qualities of the working alliance – often deeply personal and affective – can display few of the characteristics of planned reason and rationality that *in principle* descriptions of the work cure advocate. Moreover, despite an undertone of what 'rationally' might be considered *failure* in the gardening tales I tell, I consider how such peculiarities (perversions, even) of a more formal model of therapeutic relation reveal a different and stronger account of the occupational nature of humankind.

Readers will notice that methodologically and stylistically this chapter departs from some earlier contributions to this book. This reflects the interdisciplinary nature of the chapter and its blending of primary historical and contemporary resources. However, through the practices of storytelling and attendance to the incidental and affective, this also indicates a methodological point about the kinds of knowledge that are understood as permissible in considering what makes for an 'effective' therapeutics of work, and the ways in which notions of 'evidence' and 'efficacy' are themselves reasoned and rationalised in the production of an evidence base for work therapy.

***

> In moral treatment work possesses a constraining power superior to all forms of physical coercion, in that the requirements of attention and obligation detach the sufferer from a liberty of mind that would be fatal … through work, man submits his liberty to laws that are those of both morality and reality.[4]

There are a good many reasons for thinking that a focus on reason, on rationality, on *rationalisation* is interesting for a contribution to a volume on work and psychiatry. As is often cited, in moral treatment, Tuke declares, 'of all the modes by which the patients may be induced to restrain themselves, regular employment is the most generally efficacious'.[5] Yet it is in the alliance between work and rationality that the otherwise insular history of work therapy makes its contribution to a broader philosophy of social science. Famously, in what would later become his 'governmentality' thesis, in Madness and Civilisation, Foucault finds in the Retreat a motif to illustrate not just an episode of history but an *episteme* of governance. Of similar renown, preceding those iconic remarks about work and love and the cornerstones of humanity, Freud states that of all activities – psychoanalysis included – it is *work* that most readily binds the individual to reality and reason.[6] Yet a focus on reason and efficacy is justified because, of all the ways in which work therapy has changed in the last two centuries, we find this fascination with reason and rationality to retain no less of its relevance than the context in which the *Description* was first written.

Although it is not my intention to tie this chapter to the Retreat, it is nevertheless interesting to consider the characteristics of reason and rationality as adopted in moral treatment. To the moral therapists, rationality was both the prized goal and innovative means of treating the lunatic. In preceding ideologies, madness was seen as an absolute loss of rational faculty and madmen, accordingly, as wholly incurable (and in some accounts, scarcely human).[7] The abandonment of this view heralded moral treatment as a new means of imagining insanity, envisioning instead a creature who, while injured in the mind, retained an underlying capacity for reason that with the right encouragement could be bolstered and returned to him or her. Within such a framework, work – that most rational of activities – held a unique place, and patients were set to employment wherever possible.

At least two mechanisms of work to induce reason in patients were identifiable at the Retreat. Work therapy was in the first instance a form of operant conditioning that encouraged rational conduct through the presence of reinforcements (an early behavioural therapy of sorts – or better, *cognitive-*behavioural therapy – since it was hoped that the process would not only govern the patient's behaviour from the outside but reform him from the inside out). Partly a result of the kinds of agrarian work offered at the Retreat, some rewards came directly from the produce of labour itself, with sane (sustained and regular) behaviour resulting in healthier crops and bigger harvests, thus leading the madman to 'natural' conclusions about the consequences of his actions.[8] (This was somewhat akin to Freud's later 'reality principle', whereby an individual was considered to mature through the realisation that pleasure was better ruled by long-term interests rather than the fancies of immediate gratification – and, like the moral therapists, Freud saw a particular role for work in this regard.)[9] Yet 'regular employment' also provided a means to mobilise that other great force in the patient – the 'desire for esteem' or to 'feel oneself of consequence'.[10] In providing a way for the patient to belong and become useful (and not forgetting here the strength of the Quaker work ethic), work therapy thus accomplished its battle against unreason not only through the patient's recovering rational faculties but his emotional energies.

However, the Retreat revealed its faith in rationality not only through its reconceptualisation of madness, but through the broader philosophy of its own working practice (what has been described by various authors as both a rationalisation and rationalism of mental health practice).[11] Famously, in that revisionist movement, Foucault's objection to Tuke was that the apparently philanthropic dismissal of physical restraint in favour of psychological interventions simply replaced the disciplining of bodies with the disciplining of minds.[12] However, for Tuke and associates this was exactly the point – that while the requirement to contain the unfettered wilderness of madness was unavoidable, a psychosocial approach was not only more humane than corporeal management, it was also more efficient. In seeking the most *rational* way to treat the madman, it is thus significant that in the preface to the *Description* Tuke presents his work as 'the superior *efficacy* … of a mild system of treatment'[13] – and the remainder of the book might sensibly be understood as a handbook of methods upon how to most rationally (efficaciously) treat the lunatic patient.

***

In a particular reading, then, *The Description* is a thoroughly modern text (by which we mean here 'modernity' in its senses of both early nineteenth-century capitalist industrialisation and the high modernity of the late twentieth and twenty-first centuries), rooted and preoccupied in a set of socioeconomic and intellectual concerns that are widely analogous with our own.

Although an interesting trajectory would analyse this lineage further, addressing perhaps, as other commentators have done, the links between rationality at the Retreat and the emerging logics of capitalism and industrialism,[14] this chapter is not primarily a historical analysis and I want now instead to take from the Retreat some narratives that extend to current-day ideas of a therapeutics of work and its rational credentials. To explore just four such narratives that will help us in our discussion (and I posit these both as stories locatable in the *Description* and histories of the present day), I identify:

1 A continued preoccupation with the connectedness of work to the 'real world' and to 'rational' conduct, and the importance of therapeutic practice to re-establish such links between the patient and his or her occupation. Increasingly in such narratives there appears an emphasis on paid employment as the primary or only form of such work, alongside intensifying discourses of reasoned and responsible citizenship (rather than mere personal conduct) through participation in work activities.
2 A rationalisation of professional knowledge and systematisation of the 'evidence base' within contemporary therapeutic professions.[15] A common tale here concerns the uneasy relation between occupation-based therapies and biomedical interventions with regards to their differing engagements with theory and evidence (as if the kinds of explanations and evidences for the work cure could ever be the same as those of pharmacological intervention; although the idea that they should do is prevalent in the literature).[16] Significantly for some of my later comments, an important theme here is not just the collection of evidence but a rationalisation of the kinds of

knowledge that can themselves be counted as evidence in a rationalistic professional discourse – and while the patient case history has always been and remains an important source of learning for the occupational therapy professions, it is here we see, too, the roots of our current infatuation with 'best evidence': the randomised controlled trial or meta-analysis as the professional acme of rational evidence-gathering.

3 An intensifying economic rationalisation within therapeutic practice, i.e., what might commonly be described as a concern not just with efficacy (the power to achieve a result) but efficiency (the power to do so with the least resource wastage possible).[17] From a historical perspective we might highlight any of several transitions here – the material shortages experienced in both World Wars, the UK recession of the 1980s, or contemporary contractions and restructuring of public and third sector care institutions – although concern with the financial operation of the Retreat was apparent in the *Description* too (see also Tuke's *Practical Hints on the Construction and Economy of Pauper Lunatic Asylums*).[18]

4 An emerging understanding of the therapeutic relationship (what at the opening of this chapter I introduced as the 'working alliance') as itself an object for scientific inquiry and methodological adjustment.[19] Within such a story, we might draw attention to the professionalisation of occupation-based therapies – i.e., the idea of a professional relationship governed by attributes of a different order to the more intuitive persuasions of friendships or other less clearly delineated relationships.[20] Yet to pull together the above narratives, we might also reference here an interest in method more broadly across a range of social institutions (therapy, education, management studies, etc.): that is, following the legacy of modernity left by Bacon and Descartes, the search for a series of standardised techniques and instruments that could be employed, regardless of the intricacies of the particular, with expectation of positive results. It is thus significant that Tuke references John Locke's treatise on education, in which he sees the perfect 'methods book' for educating the young: explicitly, Tuke aspires to provide an equivalent for the treatment of the insane (although it is important to note that he understands the *Description* as just the starting point for such an endeavour).[21] For the purpose of this chapter, such changing ideas about relationship shift emphasis from the temperaments of individual actors to the methods and techniques of a standardisable therapeutic process. They also shift understandings of the nature of recovery from something mysterious and unknowable to a mechanical, predictable and wholly rational affair.

It is my intention to argue that these stories (about work, evidence, rationalisation, relation) are both empirical (that is, descriptions of things that have actually happened), and *historiographical* – i.e., important ways in which the history of work and psychiatry is told and tells itself. (I have illustrated this elsewhere through analysis of twentieth-century occupational therapy training manuals and textbooks to demonstrate the preponderance of such themes in the initiation narratives of the profession.)[22]

However, for the remainder of the chapter I want to focus instead on what happens beyond or outside of these narratives and how such narratives themselves can occlude a more nuanced reading of the lived relations of work therapy. In taking the first of my stories from the *Description*, I signal what I understand to be Latour's provocation that we 'have never been modern'[23] (or put differently, that the stories of reason and rationality we tell are neither inventions of high modernity nor what we 'really' (intuitively) believe to be the only modes of understanding the world). Rather, through these smaller stories of garden work and therapeutic encounters, the chapter will push forward the idea that at the edges of any grand narrative of modernity are the seeds of its unravelling: the understories, the therapeutic failures, the everyday unreasons of human foible.

***

My first vignette then is taken from the *Description* itself, positioned towards the end of the chapter entitled 'Moral Treatment':

> Some years ago, a patient much afflicted with melancholic and hypochondriacal symptoms was admitted by his own request. He had walked from home, a distance of 200 miles, in company with a friend; and upon his arrival found much less inclination to converse on the melancholy and absurd views of his own state than he had previously felt. The patient was by trade a gardener, and the superintendent immediately perceived from the effect of this journey, the propriety of keeping him employed. He led him into the garden, and conversed with him on the subject of horticulture, and soon found that the patient possessed very superior knowledge of pruning, and of the other departments of his art. He proposed several improvements in the management of the garden, which were adopted, and the gardener was desired to furnish him with full employment.[24]

In relation to the greater body of Tuke's chapter, this anonymous case is introduced, among other things, to illustrate the utility of the work cure and importance of meaningful occupation to a patient's recovery. In a detailed footnote, Tuke cites the patient directly in his melancholic fantasies, 'I have no soul, no heart, nor liver, nor lungs, nor anything at all in my body, nor a drop of blood in my veins'[25] – feelings of hollowness, which, as if triggered directly by the patient's deprivation from some wholesome vocation, subside when he is put to the gardens. At first glance, the story is thus a success story. The patient grows with and through the gardens he tends, and as the superintendent sees to grant him a permanent position on the grounds, our wandering labourer is turned from hollow to whole and from patient to worker.

To quote from Tuke again, however, things are rather different. Soon after the patient is allocated to this labour, he begins to display 'a reluctance to regular exertion and a considerable disposition to wandering, which had been one of the previous features of his complaint'. Tuke records that the 'gardener' (by whom he means here the staff gardener in charge of the patient workers) was 'repeatedly charged to encourage him in labour, and to prevent his leaving the premises. But unhappily, the superior abilities of the patient had excited a jealousy in the gardener's mind, which made him dislike his assistance, and it may therefore be presumed that he obeyed his instructions very imperfectly.'

Tuke goes on to explain how from this point on, the wandering escapades of the patient increased and, unable to encourage any more fruitful relationship between the staff gardener and his charge, and despite all efforts of the superintendent – who was clearly greatly distressed by such failure – the Retreat became ultimately unable to keep the gardening patient at his work.

> The poor man rambled several times from the grounds of the Institution; which, in his state of mind, excited considerable anxiety in the family. Of course it became necessary to confine him more within doors. He frequently, however, walked out; and the superintendent took many opportunities to attend him into the fields or garden, and to engage him for a time in steady manual labour. As his disorder had increased, it became difficult to induce him to exert himself; but even in this state, when he had been some time employed, he seemed to forget his distressful sensations and ideas, and would converse on general topics with great good sense.
>
> In this truly pitiable case, the superintendent several times tried the efficacy of long walks, where the greatest variety and attraction of circumstances were presented; but neither these, nor the conversation which he introduced, were able to draw the patient so effectually from the 'moods of his own mind', as regular persevering labour in the garden. It is not improbable, however, that the superior manner in which the patient was able to execute his work, produced a degree of self-complacency which had a salutary effect; and that, had his education enlarged his curiosity, he might have derived much greater advantage, as many patients obviously do, from variety of conversation and scenery ... .[26]

Tuke concludes the case study by remarking that the superintendent 'has frequently expressed the strong feelings of regret which were excited in his mind by the unsuccessful treatment of this patient', and at the end of the section we read that this nameless man lives out the rest of his years within the walls of the asylum before dying of an acute inflammation of the bowel – an ironic affliction indeed for a man who once believed himself to have no organs at all.

Examination of the case records reveals this man to have been Thomas Wellington, married, aged forty-eight, from Shrewsbury in Shropshire, admitted to the Retreat 4 May 1799 until his death 10 June 1809. (It is meaningful to recount these biographical details since, poignantly, given the comments I will make about the evidence base later, heretofore in the historical record this man has lost both his gardens and his name.) Tabulation with probate records show this almost certainly to be the same Thomas Wellington, parish gardener of Holy Cross and St Giles, Shrewsbury, who died in the same year. Although brief, the hospital records tell of the rich relation between the patient's work and his supervisors, and the utility of occupation to draw him out of his introspective preoccupations. ('This patient had a good ear for music, he sang well and played on the violin. When he was walking, he often held his head between his hands, complaining of much pain and saying, "Oh dear! My head will come off and I shall want a new head."')[27] Yet despite the case of the hollow gardener forming one of the most detailed and affective in Tuke's account of the Retreat, and despite the very frequent appearance of the *Description* in later historical analyses, it is interesting that with the exception of just a few brief references in studies of nineteenth-century hypochondrias,[28] the story of Thomas Wellington remains largely forgotten among those greater stories of kindly efficacy.

The second vignette is from my own ethnographic work located some eighty miles north of the Retreat at York – a contemporary therapeutic work project that I refer to as the 'Plumtree Centre' (all names and locations are pseudonyms), comprising a mixture of traditional sheltered employment activities for people with long-term mental health problems, a life skills programme and – like the Retreat – a therapeutic gardening project in which members learn the skills of gardening and grow food for themselves. The research takes place during a period of radical restructuring for the Centre, in response to several generations of social policy reform. In the ethnography I talk about what I call the 'magical' qualities of the therapeutic encounters that take place at the Centre, by which I mean the helping relationships that emerge in the Plumtree project quite independently of the formal languages of therapeutic efficacy and accountability.

> Among the permanent workers at the Centre is Trish, the full-time support worker with boots and dyed hair who heads off on a motorbike each night with a helmeted boyfriend. To collate some comments made about Trish: 'Trish will tell it to you straight'; 'She'll keep lip'; 'Trish will come out for a tab break with you'. For many, Trish is a magical person. Two stories support this description: one comes from a conversation with Lizzie, a younger attendee at the work programme. Lizzie is on 'last warnings' from Plumtree about her self-harming behaviour and is threatened with exclusion if incidents continue. After a family argument, Lizzie turns up at the Project with a stomach full of painkillers, having

overdosed at her parents' house earlier that day. Trish, 'scraping the truth from [her]' invents a reason for them both to leave and takes Lizzie to hospital before anyone can find out and put sanctions in place. The second evidence was Trish's constant, protective, defensive modifications of the Project's rules to help avoid upsets in the community. For members on attendance-based contracts, Trish would 'tweak' sign-in sheets for miscreants who had turned up late (provided she was pacified by their apology, that is). In mid-January snow, Trish could be found running down the street in house slippers to chase after a participant on the skills course, after they had stormed out saying they had quit; in another incident (of which I only really caught the second half), Trish appeared to have personally replaced a packet of cigarettes that one of the users had stolen from another. 'You'll fucking pay me back for those,' she was yelling at him – who despite a long relationship with the criminal justice system was looking pretty scared at this outpouring.

For others, Bill was a magical person. Bill worked on the allotment project; he knew about gardens and he knew about the neighbourhood. He had worked through each of the changes to day services in successive governments; he knew a lot of people. He was a good gardener and a good listener. People commented on both, regularly. Bill had little in common with Trish. Trish challenged, bullied, got under people's skin in order to help. Bill waited. His approach with the users was one of almost apparent indifference. Frequently workers would disappear from the work project, allotted tea breaks turning to a longer kick around with a ball or an early departure. Sometimes service-users (Bill called them 'volunteers') would disappear for longer periods of time – for a hospital admission or a prison sentence perhaps, or most often just into some unknown world beyond the reach of service provision where time and occupation didn't seem to be accounted for in the same way. It didn't seem to matter to Bill whether users had been gone twenty minutes or four months. He never asked and he never chastised. Work began and ended with whoever was there in the gardens at the time. And whenever the person came back up to the allotments – the current front between cultivation and scrubland – he would just start off, 'now that you're here, can you ...' and the user would be back in the world of the garden and the current task at hand.

I don't think it is true to imagine that Bill was unaware of the programme's broader philosophy of 'nurturing a work ethic' in its labour-disengaged members. Rather, Bill simply left accountability to those in the management of the Centre – to those who kept the records and made decisions about people's lives. People would make mistakes and people would be answerable to others. But Bill was just there to garden and to let other people garden with him where possible. And in a sense that was about the extent of Bill's involvement with the therapeutic programme of work at the Project – and for many of the service-users at the work programme, it was this quietness and unassumingness which were exactly the qualities which drew them to him.[29]

In the ethnography I go on to explore the sharp divide between the formal paper-based understanding of the organisation (which is couched in the language of audit trails and employability goals) and these real, emergent, richly therapeutic alliances that emerge through the work and activity of the Centre. I also explore what happens when the project is called upon to increase the visibility and accountability of its processes and outcomes – its efficacy if you will – and when the creative and intuitive but often unorthodox and unpredictable kinds of working relation that are nurtured by Bill and Trish meet head-on with such rationalised modes of working.

To tell here just a portion of this story, through the timescale of the ethnography Plumtree becomes transformed from a 'therapeutic work project' to a back-to-work 'rehabilitation programme', with activities in the gardening project and sheltered workshop replaced largely with classroom-based courses in employability and life skills. Conceptions of 'work' shifted from the in-the-moment work of digging and planting to a future-facing notion of paid employment, to which all activity became orientated. Notions of *relationship* also changed from ones that were based largely on the organic properties of rapport (a working alliance in both literal and therapeutic terms) to a workload model of staff/client contact time – specifically, the introduction of a rationalised 'caseloads' system, in which new users would simply be allocated a caseworker on arrival at the Centre.

For the purposes of this discussion, a particular concern among Plumtree managers became the necessity to demonstrate (for reasons of 'funding capture') evidenceable rationales for resources spent (a reference back to those legacies of rationality I sketched in my discussion above). As the gardening project became increasingly charged with being 'divorced from reality' (with 'reality' a metonym for paid work here), a first obvious challenge involved how best to imagine an evidence trail for the small and personal victories that unfolded at the allotments – let alone how attributes such as building a friendship or redeeming a dying raspberry plant or learning to be more patient with oneself might be *evidenced* to speak to external ends such as 'employability targets'.

At a level of on-the-ground relationship (so to speak), such concerns about evidence took their toll. In a context in which both knowledge and work had been rationalised, as Trish explained while talking me through the paperwork jungle that had overtaken the staffroom, under new auditing and inspection routines not only did the participation of service-users at Plumtree have to be accounted for much more closely than in previous systems (the sign-in registers in the above extract), *staff time* had also become scrutinised on an unprecedented scale. The recording and monitoring of each therapeutic interaction became not only a matter of tracking a *client's* progress, but a means of monitoring the caseload and productivity of individual support workers. The boundaries of the 'caseload' thus rendered work outside of client/caseworker relationships invisible, since any such informal encounters lacked a mechanism through which to be counted. Given my comments previously about the relation of caseworker relationships to 'magical relationships', the therapeutic encounters with Trish and Bill – which sat poignantly beyond the caseload allocation – like the tale of the hollow gardener thus acquired a delicate invisibility to any broader project of 'evidence building' about the value of therapeutic work.

***

What can be said, then, in response to these stories about the nature of the work cure and of Tuke and others' insistence upon the value of work for restoring *reason* and *rationality* in its patients? In the first instance, both stories demonstrate fully what we might think of as the 'occupational view' of the human – that is the human in his or her fullest form as a uniquely working creature.

However, what interests me most in Tuke's story about the hollow gardener is not necessarily the clinical details of the case (for all the intimate details of moral treatment they reveal), but rather the obvious fondness for the patient as shown by the superintendent and Tuke himself. By Tuke's account this patient was the one who *most often* haunted the superintendent (a statement not to be underestimated if we consider some of the extremities of early nineteenth-century asylum care that the superintendent would likely have witnessed) and it seems that this affective connection occurs simultaneously because the two men had worked together and alongside one another, and because the superintendent – a man in his own right recorded as talented and committed to his vocation – found particular distress in a case where another, equally talented and called-upon person was unable to fulfil such vocation in himself. In the gentle narration of the case, Tuke similarly addresses his readers as if 'from worker to worker'. We are not *instructed* to understand the gardener's strange fantasies as a result of his disturbed relation to his work. The effect is more that Tuke is able to trust us to know instinctively that this hollow yearning is for a garden lost or separated – some two hundred miles away, as we are told, or from wherever the imaginations of Thomas Wellington have travelled.

In the work project with Trish and Bill, similarly, everyone is working. While the formal articulation of the Centre's therapeutic intervention occurs through the rehabilitative values of life skills and employability training, therapy is a much broader notion whereby members work through difficulties through their working relations with one another (and I should say that this effect is achieved neither through relegating work to just a mode for building relations nor relationship-building as a means only to encourage working; rather both such processes work together on the person). While notions of 'work readiness' in the gardening project are perhaps only weakly relevant to how staff and users narrate their activities, notions of the therapeutic *value* of work are embraced actively and reflexively, as part of the therapeutic process.

That the more formal 'back to work' programme in the classroom *fails* (which it does) is thus in part because ironically it emphasises the worklessness and rolelessness (irreality) of the project's attendees. In the gardens are fruits and thorns and roots and dirt that necessarily ground participants not only in the 'real world' but in the unending commitment that care of a garden necessitates ('I wasn't going to come back,' says one of the participants about his first trip to the allotment, 'but the soil needed me'). In the classroom, by contrast, in the work of role-*plays* and employment *simulations* in which members rehearse interview skills or workplace interactions – now phrased in terms of competitive ('real') employment – appears a literal absence of reality: a purposeful descent into the fantastical realm of the future conditional.

While embracing wholeheartedly an occupational view of the human, then – and accepting at large the notion that there is something profoundly important about the propensity of work to bring a person to reality – what I *do* want to do in these stories is to question the idea that the ability of work to bring the madman/patient/service-user/client into the real world has any necessary relation to the characters of reason and rationality described earlier in this chapter; or to put it otherwise, if Tuke and Freud are correct in their assertion that work brings us out of ourselves and into the world, then as suggested by these case studies this might better be understood as bringing us into a world of richness and relation ordered not by calculated rationality but by moral ambiguity and the vulnerabilities of sentiment and friendships.

To tend first to the hollow gardener, we might speak initially of resource *rationalisation* (a foretaste of moral treatment's eventual demise into moral management, perhaps) as the cost of a particular rationalised way of working: the gardener relapses (we might say) as a result of insufficient resources to afford him a private attendant to support a fuller occupational recovery. Yet, moreover, the story reveals a fault in thinking of the real world as purely a *reasonable* and *rational* one (especially where reason and rationality are positioned against affect and intuition). In the *Description*, Tuke asks of his attendants, 'Be rational!', 'Let not your own emotions get in the way of the therapy that is happening!'[30] Yet the treatment of Tom Wellington fails precisely at the moment at which the realisation of his skills in his work excite the (unreasonable, irrational) jealousies of the other gardeners, who feel envious and insecure and can no longer attend to him kindly and wisely. This is not to make any crude statement therefore that the world is irrational and that moral treatment must fail (and, indeed, if we are to believe Tuke about the talents of this particular patient, the staff gardeners may well have had reason to feel threatened and uncomfortable). Yet still it is not failure of technique but fallibility of the human spirit through which the story of the hollow gardener ends: in reuniting the patient with his occupation, he re-joins that great community of human being – yet simultaneously, in joining that community and becoming accepted in the workaday world, he must leave the protective milieu of rational, planned 'therapy', and enter a less reasoned and less predictable community of human relations that include all of what is muddled and painful about being human.

To become part of fully human relations, then, to acquire through work what Marx might describe as a 'species life' – that is, membership to a community of humans working and acting together – is also simultaneously to move away from the carefully delineated relations we might think of as befitting for formally professional working alliances. In rendering relations as working relations (which work therapy must do), relations move away from the rational and prescribed relations sanctioned by professional articulations of 'therapy' into therapeutic *adventures* – adventures in which concepts such as 'success' and 'failure' (the backbones of efficacy and efficiency) themselves become matters to be worked through or upon rather than simply measured or evaluated. It is therefore inevitable that Tuke's gardener (by whom we mean Tuke's *patient* – for Tuke elides the terms 'gardener' and 'labourer', and 'worker and patient') succeeds in his recovery at the moment in which he fails; that is in inspiring the jealousies of his keepers that eventually lead to his relapse, his membership has been confirmed to that great and real sphere of human relationship whereupon he and his work can be evaluated not only as symptoms of disease but as signs of skill and workmanship – inspiring care and esteem but also jealousy and hostility.

At the Plumtree Centre, likewise, therapeutic practice takes place among a rationalised discourse of 'service delivery', yet despite pressure to evidence efficiency and efficacy the lived realities of the gardens nonetheless evidence a continuing space for the beyond-the-evidential, the wonderful, the magical. In the rationalised/rationalistic framework of the audit trail, it is true that these therapeutic adventures fare poorly, impervious as they are to targets and measurement. Yet despite my remarks about the gulf between the lived and the recorded, it is interesting to note that – like the recalcitrant tale of Mr Wellington in that other handbook of rational modernity – traces of such magic nevertheless appear at the margins of the formal record. To quote briefly from one of the final reports from the governors of Plumtree:

> We are struck by the work that happens in the work teams, especially on the horticultural programme, in dealing with hard to help clients ... Although it is felt that [the gardening activities] do not always reflect the core strategic goals of the organisation as it moves forward, the ability of the staff and volunteers

to build extraordinary rapport with vulnerable or long-term clients should be recorded as a matter of excellence.

The report ends with recommending that the organisation might explore ways to capture this 'extraordinary' work of the garden in its formal measured outputs, and to consider ways in which it might ground its practice in methods that will further benefit the 'evidence base'. For some, this will offer an olive branch to an organisation that does not easily fit the organisational discourses in which it has found itself; to others this will fail to see the ways in which extraordinary rapport exists in forms that are inexorably *beyond* the rationalistic, the methodical, the measurable.

***

I suggested at the beginning of this chapter that the turn toward *petits récits* and to storytelling, and to embracing the sentimental and affective in my writing, indicates a broader methodological point about the ways in which we understand notions of evidence and efficacy of therapeutic relations (in occupation-oriented therapies or elsewhere). To conclude this chapter by reflecting on this briefly: in systematised, rationalised forms of knowledge, stories like those of Thomas Wellington or the encounters at Plumtree fit awkwardly in the 'evidence base', partly because in their entanglement with the specific and the particular they resist conversion into any more general therapeutic recommendations (other than a general call to attend to the particular), and partly because the kinds of matter they deal with – the intuitive, the affective, the sentimental, the 'magical' – sit outside of the dominant languages of rationality and efficacy in which professional helping relationships have come to be articulated.

To turn to Tuke's *Description* one final time, it is interesting that Tuke mentions just two 'indulgences' at the Retreat, both of which he relates to writing: an indulgence in providing quality writing materials to patients, and an apology for his own writing of the *Description*, which he suggests may be considered by some as turning too often to poetry and literary sources to be suitable for a 'proper' evidence base. The first I think references the therapeutic work of writing, which has not been the focus of this chapter, but which remains an interesting and enduring theme across the history of work and psychiatry. The second signifies what I believe to be Tuke's own reservations about the way in which the regular languages of evidence building encounter the personal and affective relations of work therapy. As I have it in this chapter, the language of reason and rationality is a language that tells a powerful story about the importance of work to human health and happiness. The challenge (for historians, for philosophers, for contemporary social scientists, for practitioners) is to prevent it becoming the only one.

Acknowledgements

In memory of Thomas Wellington, patient at the York Retreat from 1799 until his death in 1809.

With many thanks to Kath Webb, Borthwick Institute (University of York), for archival support.

Notes

1. Samuel Tuke, *Description of the Retreat, an Institution near York, for Insane Persons of the Society of Friends* (York: W. Alexander, 1813), p. 153.
2. Anne Digby, *Madness, Morality and Medicine: A study of the York Retreat, 1796–1914* (Cambridge: Cambridge University Press, 1985), p. xiii.
3. Jennifer Laws, 'Crackpots and basket-cases: A history of therapeutic work and occupation', *History of the Human Sciences*, 24 (2011), 65–81.
4. Michel Foucault, *Madness and Civilisation: A History of Insanity in the Age of Reason*, trans. R. Howard (London: Tavistock, 1967), p. 247.
5. Tuke, *Description of the Retreat*, p. 156.
6. Sigmund Freud, *Civilisation and Its Discontents*, trans. David McLintock (London: Penguin, 2002).
7. Andrew Scull, 'Moral treatment reconsidered: Some sociological comments on an episode in the history of British psychiatry', *Psychological Medicine*, 9 (1979), 421–8, 423.
8. Chris Philo, *A Geographical History of Institutional Provision for the Insane from Medieval Times to the 1860s in England and Wales* (Lampeter: Edwin Mellen Press, 2004).
9. Nancy Scheper-Hughes, *Saints, Scholars, and Schizophrenics: Mental Illness in Rural Ireland* (Berkeley: University of California Press, 2001), p. 163.
10. Tuke, *Description of the Retreat*, p. 158.
11. Gary Kielhofner, *Conceptual Foundations of Occupational Therapy* (Philadelphia, PA: F. A. Davis Company, 2004); Clare Hocking, 'The way we were: The ascendance of rationalism', *British Journal of Occupational Therapy*, 71 (2008), 226–33.
12. Foucault, *Madness and Civilisation*, p. 247
13. Tuke, *Description of the Retreat*, p. vi.
14. Scull, 'Moral treatment reconsidered'.
15. Karen Serrett, *Philosophical and Historical Roots of Occupational Therapy* (London: Haworth Press, 1985), p. 3.
16. Kielhofner, *Conceptual Foundations*, ch. 3.
17. Clare Hocking, 'The way we were: Thinking rationally', *British Journal of Occupational Therapy*, 71 (2008), 185–95.
18. Samuel Tuke, *Practical Hints on the Construction and Economy of Pauper Lunatic Asylums* (York: W. Alexander, 1815).
19. Digby, *Madness, Morality and Medicine*, p. 140.

20 Anne Wilcock, *Occupation for Health: A Journey from Self Health to Prescription* (London: British Association and College of Occupational Therapy, 2001), vol. 1, p. 459.
21 Tuke, *Description of the Retreat*, p. 150; John Locke, *Some Thoughts Concerning Education* (Cambridge: Cambridge University Press, 1693).
22 Jennifer Laws, 'Working Through: An Inquiry into Work and Madness' (PhD thesis, Durham University, 2012).
23 Bruno Latour, *We Have Never Been Modern*, trans. Catherine Porter (Cambridge, MA: Harvard University Press, 1993).
24 Tuke, *Description of the Retreat*, pp. 152–3.
25 *Ibid.*, p. 152.
26 *Ibid.*, pp. 154–5.
27 Borthwick Institute for Archives, York, RET 6/5/1/1A, case book – annotation to entry 10 June, 1809 (undated).
28 Wilcock, *Occupation for Health*, vol. 1, p. 459.
29 Laws, 'Working Through', pp. 206–8.
30 Paraphrased from Tuke's *Description of the Retreat* (see, for example, pp. 107, 161, 175).

Index

Note: Page numbers in *italic* refer to figures, those in **bold** to tables.

action 1–5
activities
   arts and crafts 12, 26, 70, 123, 325
   at Japanese inns 187–9
Adam, James 279–82, 289
Adamson, Edward 321
Addison, Joseph 35
administration 315–16
age, *see* patients, age of
agriculture 150
   increasing involvement in 225–6
   in Romania 200–2
   as treatment 110
   see also farm (agricultural) colonies
Akimoto, Haruo 172
alienation 3–4, 27, 94, 196
alienists 59, 95, 239, 277–8, 281, 288–90, 300
Allen, Nathaniel, trial of 84
Allen, Thomas 146–8
Altscherbitz Asylum 204
America 55–76
   New Jersey 77–98
amusement(s) 92–3
   and class 150
   and gender 108
   in India 119, 123
   and moral treatment 34, 37, 39, 44, 58–60
   and self-injury 280
   withholding of 129

Aristotle 2
Arnold, Thomas 39
art therapy 321
Association of Medical Officers of Asylums and Hospitals for the Insane 315
Association of Occupational Therapists 325
Astley Ainslie Hospital, Edinburgh 325
asylums
   administrative framework of 315–16
   annual reports of 102–3, 106
   birth of 56–7
   for chronics 60–3
   in the First World War 228–9
   Irish district 298–313
   populations 144–5
   in Romania 198–9
   rural 220–37
   as safe places 251–3
   self-sufficiency of 105, 123–4
   in South Asia 118
   superintendents of 58, 102
   West Indian 142–62
   work in 91–3
Austria 22, 262–76

'back to work' programme 363
Bacon, Francis 35
Baliff, Leon 205
Banstead Hospital 340–1
Barron, John, trial of 81
Barton, Russell 322

Index

bath treatment (*Dauerbad*) 240–3
Battie, William 32, 36
Beard, George 64–5
bed rest (*Bettbehandlung*) 240–3
Beers, Clifford 319
Bentham, Jeremy 6
Bentley, Richard I., report of 103–4
Berkeley-Hill, O.A.R. 133–4
Bertholf, John, trial of 81–2
Bethel (Gehring) Asylum 67–9
   women sawing *69*
Bethlem Hospital 38, 278–80, 282–3, 288, 315, 317
Biraud, Dr Yves M. 120
Bischoff, Ernst 270–1
Blyth, Edith Mary Ellen 288–90
Board of Control 316–20, 322, 326–7
Board of Lunacy 315–16
Bodington, George F., reports of 104–5, 112
Boerhaave, Hermann 34
Bond, Sir Hubert 315–16
Boston Lunatic Asylum 58–9
Brăescu, Alexandru 19, 197, 203–5
Brânzei, Petre P. 205
Britain 22–8, 277–97
   psychiatric care in 334–50
   transfer of methodologies from 154
   work and moral treatment in 31–54
   see also England
British Columbia 13–14, 100
   mental institutions in 100–2
   patient work in 99–116
British Guiana 148–51
British West Indies 14–15, 142–62
Bruteanu, Mircea 199
Bucharest, patient work in 199–203
Bucknill, John Charles 281–2
Burrows, George Man 46
Buttolph, John 79, 92–3, 95

Cabanis, Pièrre-Jean-Georges 35
Cabot, Richard 65–7
Calicut Mental Hospital 126, 130–1
   embroidery *132*
   rope making *131*
   tailoring *133*
   weaving *134*
Call, Annie Payson 65
Canada 13–14, 99–116
Cardiazol 318
Carson, Daniel, guardianship of 85–7

case studies
   Bill, Trish and Lizzie (the 'Plumtree Centre') 359–62, 364–5
   Mathilde S. 262, 265, 271
   Miss M. 290
   Paula E. 270
   Thomas W. (the hollow gardener) 357–9
caseloads 361–2
Casson, Dr Elizabeth 172, 323, 327–8
Central Psychiatric Hospital, Bucharest 199–203
Cheyne, George 35
Chiarugi, Vincenzo 31, 34, 41–2
Child Guidance Clinics 319, 329
Chinese patients, and work 110–12
chlorpromazine 318
civil trials, process of 79–81
Clancarty, [William] Lord 308
Clark, David 323, 335–6, 340–1
Clarke, Dr Charles K. 107
class 9, 12, 47–9
   and diet 127
   and occupation 279, 281
   in Romania 198
   and treatment quality 127–8
Collie, Sir John 286
colonialism 127–8, 136, 143
colour, in West Indies 155
Commission for Forced Labour Facilities and Borstals (CFLFB) 262–3, 268
committal, in West Indies 144–5
community, care in 346
Connaught District Lunatic Asylum, Ballinasloe 23–4, 298, 305, 307
Connolly, John 300
Constantinescu, George 207
convulsions 318
cooking 124–5
Cork Lunatic Asylum 42–3
court trials, lunacy 12
Cox, Joseph Mason 38–9
Craiova, patient work in 205–8
creative therapies 25–6, 321–2
Crichton Royal Institution 279–80

Daiunji-Temple 182–3
d'Alembert, Jean 35
Danvers State Hospital 70
Daquin, Joseph 34, 39–40
Darenth Park 339
deinstitutionalisation 26, 73, 334
   psychiatric 335–6, 343–5

Delhi Asylum 119–20
Denham, John 342
Department of Employment 344
dependence (*amae*) 16, 175
Dhunjibhoy, Dr Jal E.
  reports of 119
  use of OT 129–30
  views on work 120–3
Dickens, Charles 58–9
Diderot, Denis 35
Diefenbach, Lorenz 4
diet 5, 34, 309–10
  and class 127
  as discipline 9, 124
  minimalist 120, 124
  poor 249
  supplemented 222
  as treatment 36–7, 40, 280
dietetics 221, 239
Disabled Persons (Employment) Act (1944) 337
discipline 7, 33, 37, 43, 122–6, 263, 270
  self- 45, 49
  teaching 61
  work as 91, 142, 342
discrimination 346
disease 64–5, 226, 229–30, 271
  feigned 285–6, 288
Dix, Dorothea 59
Dorset House, Bristol 323–4
drugs 134–5
  abandonment of 44
  alkaloid 206
  psychotropic 318
  sedative 242, 317–18
Drummond, Peter, trial of 90–1
Dundas-Grant, Sir James 287

Earle, Pliny 59
Early, Dr Donal 343–4
economic rationalisation 28, 356
Eforia Spitalelor Civile 195–6
Egham Rehabilitation Centre 337
Eikichi, Tsuchiya 185, 187
Eldridge, Aaron, legal agreement by 85–7
Ellis, Sir William Charles 46–7, 142, 300, 304
Elser, Andreas 222
embroidery *132*, 245–6, *246*
  as therapy 55
employability 21, 27–8, 241–2, 250, 336, 361–2

employment 21–2, 27, 142, 150, 298
  diversity in 124
  function of 5, 278, 334–50
  and gender 108
  industrial 153
  in Irish asylums 308
  and moral treatment 41–2, 44–5, 49
  and race 127
  in Weimar Republic 20, 243
England
  policies of professionalisation in 314–33
  reason and relation in 351–67
  see also Britain
English Association of Occupational Therapists 316
epileptics 203, 269, 310
Epsthein, Dr M. 209
ergotherapy 199, 203
  scientific 19, 210
Esquirol, Jean-Étienne Dominique 47–8, 240
Essondale Hospital 102
ethnicity, in West Indies 155
eugenics 269
European Hospital at Ranchi 133–4
euthanasia 20, 230, 247
exercise 5–6, 10–11, 40–2, *189*
  attitudes towards 34–6
  bodily 36, 44, 65, 300
  and class 58, 166
  and gender 130, 146
exploitation 13–16, 99, 103–4, 112, 172, 200, 207, 220–37, 248

family care 20, 226–8
  and local economy 189–90
  and mental hospitals 190, 202–3
  and patient work 182–93
  in Transylvania 208–10
family host system 17–18
farm (agricultural) colonies 20, 59, 211, 239
  at Golia asylum 203–5
  at Hamburg-Langenhorn 239–40
  at Sibiu 209
  in Zwiefalten 221, 226–8, 231–2
Faulkner, Benjamin 37
fear
  as control 37–9, 41, 44–5, 57, 286
  of joblessness 253
Ferriar, John 37–8
Fidler, Gail S. 173

Index 371

Fidler, Jay W. 173
finances
  in India 121
  and work 120–1, 150, 152
First World War, and healing 240–3
fishery 147–8
food
  restriction of 122, 124, 247
  wartime shortages 229
forced labour 22
  facilities (*Zwangsarbeitsanstalt*) 262–76
Forel, Auguste 4
forgetfulness 88–9
Fort Canje Asylum 149
Foucault, Michel 32–3, 353–4
France
  early authors in 39–41
  work and moral treatment in 31–54
Freud, Sigmund 318, 353–4
Freudenberg, Rudolf 342–3
Freudianism 72
Fulbourn Hospital 340
Fulton, Margaret 323

Gǎnescu, Nicolae 196
Gartnavel Royal Hospital, Glasgow 319
Gavin, Hector 285–7
Gehring, John G. 67–8
gender 47
  and amusements 108
  and labour 128
  and lunacy trials 80–1, 83
  and moral looseness 131–4
  and occupation 279
  and training 329
  and work 103–4, 108, 168, 239, 303–4
Georget, Étienne-Jean 47
Germany 19–21, 220–37
  Weimar 4, 20, 229–30, 238–61
Gheel, Belgium 17, 200, 202–3, 207, 209
  'Japanese' 18, 182, 186–7, 190
Glenside Hospital, Bristol 343
Golia Asylum 203–5
Griesinger, Wilhelm 241
Grieve, Dr Robert 15, 149–51
Gross, Robert 227
Gütersloh model 8, 242, 320

habit training 68, 171–2, 340
Hall, Herbert 69–70
Hallaran, William 31–2, 42–3
Hamburg-Langenhorn Asylum 21, 238–61

Hanselman, Nicolae 206
Hanwell Asylum 46–7
Hanyu, Ritsu 171
Haslam, John 34, 38, 44–5
healing, concept of 240–3
healthcare, Western model of 16
Henderson, Dr David 319
Higgins, Daniel, trial of 82
Higgins, Lewis 82
Hill, Adrian 321
Hirata, Janet M. 174
Hogland, Lukas, trial of 89–90
Hospital Bonifazio 41–2
hospitals
  legal standards for 73
  for the mentally ill 60–3
  in Romania 195
  see also mental hospitals
Hoyojo (guest house) 186–7
human activity 1–5
Hume, George Boughton 280
humoralism 10–11, 34–6, 41–2, 77
hydrotherapy 15, 106, 117, 135–6, 318

Iasi, patient work in 203–5
idiocy 241, 269, 301, 310
  and work 83–4
idleness
  discouragement of 112–16
  as a vice 241
Imai Inn *183*
imprisonment 267–8
improvement 264–5
India 14, 117–41
  and race 9, 126–9, 136, 155
indolence 44, 48, 130
industrial employment 153
Industrial Therapy Association 344
industrial therapy (IT) 25–7, 321, 334, 346
  after 1975 344–6
  origins of 337–40
  for psychiatric patients 340–4
Industrial Therapy Organisation 343
industrialisation 10–11
industriousness 265–7
inns 183–6
  work and activities at 187–9
insane
  as children 44
  chronic 60
  and class 278, 281
  humane treatment of 15, 34, 37, 57, 146

insane (*cont.*)
  jailing of 40, 101, 151, 194
  labour of 13, 78
  management of 8, 33, 36, 142
  trials of 79–89
insanity
  medicalisation of 195–7
  moral treatment of 31–54
institutional framework, in England 315–16
institutionalisation 5–6, 18, 21, 239, 250, 282
  and OT 336
insulin coma therapy 318
insurance 248, 285, 287
internment 262–3
Ionaşiu, Liviu 210
Ireland 23–4, 298–313
Irren-Colonie, Langenhorn 239–40
Iwakura 17, 182–93
  Mental Hospital 185, *186*, 189–90
Iwama, Michael K. 16, 176

Jacob, Sarah 288
Jacobi, Maximilian 240
jails, in British Columbia 101
Jamaica 145–8
  Lunatic Asylum 145–6
James, William 65–6, 68
Japan 16–18, 163–93
  inns 183
  post-war 170–2
Jarvis, Edward 60
Johnson, Samuel 35
Jones, Maxwell 338
Jung, Carl Gustav 318

Kálmán, Pándy 19, 209
Karasuyama Byōin 172
Katō, Fusajirō 167–70
kawa model 16, 175–6
Kimori Guest House 187
Kingston Asylum 145
Kirkbride, Thomas 58–60, 63
Kobayashi, Hachiro 16, 170
Koch, Julius Ludwig August 222, 226
Kokuritsu Musashi Ryōyōjō 170–2
Kraepelin, Emil 241
Kure, Shūzō 164–6
Kyoto Tenkyōin 164, 184–5

labour 1–5
  domestic 3

plantation 155
and race 126–8
unpaid 73
unproductive 78, 94
useful 93
Lake, Charles 146
Langegg, Ferdinand Adalbert Junker von 164, 184
Langenhorn Asylum 21–2, 238–61
Large, Rebecca, trial of 82–3
Lazar, Erwin 270–1
leucotomy 318
Lewis, Aubrey 338–40
life therapy 16, 170–2
local economy, and family host care 189–90
Long Grove Hospital, Epsom 342
lunacy
  investigation law 77–98
  trials 12, 77–98
Lunatic Asylums Act (1845) 315

McInnes, Thomas R., report of 103
McIntire, John, trial of 81
McMullen, Walter James 284
McPherson, Phebe, trial of 83
madness
  management of 36
  relationship with work 13
  treatment of 56–7
Madona-Dudu Asylum 205–8
Madras Asylum, recreation hall *124*
Maeda, Norizō 167–8
malingering 23, 277, 284–7
  discouragement of 112–16
  motiveless 287–91
Manchester, Dr George H. 101, 106–8
  reports of 112
manufacturing, and competition 245
Marblehead, Massachusetts 69
Mărcuţa 196
  Lunatic Asylum 199–203
Marek, Lawrence 72
Martin, Denis 336
Martin, Dr Alfred 151
Marx, Karl 3–4, 78, 364
mass murder 230
Matsuzawa Byōin 166, 168–9
Maudsley, Henry 290
Maudsley Hospital 317, 324
  Occupational Psychiatry Research Unit 338–9

Index

medical influence 322–3
medical paradigms 5–10
Medical Research Council 339
  Social Psychiatry Research Unit 341
medical superintendents, presentation of patient work by 99
medical treatment 134–5
medical witnesses 88
medicalisation 268–71
Medico-Psychological Association 315
melancholia 35, 288, 290, 310, 318
mental decline, and work 84–9
Mental Deficiency Act (1913) 316
mental health, new ideas in 318–19
Mental Health Act (1959) 329, 335
Mental Health (Scotland) Act (1960) 335
mental hospitals
  Banstead Hospital, Surrey, England 340–1
  Bethel (Gehring) Asylum, Maine, USA 67–9
  Bethlem Hospital, London 38, 278–80, 282–3, 288, 315, 317
  Boston Lunatic Asylum, Massachusetts, USA 58–9
  Calicut Mental Hospital, India 126, 130–1
  Central Psychiatric Hospital, Bucharest, Wallachia 199–203
  colonial 117–41
  Connaught District Lunatic Asylum, Ballinasloe, Ireland 23–4, 298, 305, 307
  Cork Lunatic Asylum, Ireland 42–3
  Crichton Royal Institution, Dumfries, Ireland 279–80
  Danvers State Lunatic Asylum, Massachusetts, USA 70
  Delhi Lunatic Asylum, Punjab, India 119–20
  development of occupation in 327–30
  English 314–33
  Essondale Hospital, British Columbia 102
  and family host care 190
  Fort Canje Asylum, British Guiana 149
  Fulbourn Hospital, Cambridgeshire, England 340
  Gartnavel Royal Hospital, Glasgow, Scotland 319
  Glenside Hospital, Bristol, England 343
  Golia Asylum, Moldavia, Romania 203–5
  Hamburg-Langenhorn Asylum, Germany 21, 238–61
  Hanwell Asylum, London, England 46–7
  Hospital Bonifazio, Tuscany 41–2
  Iwakura Mental Hospital, Japan 185, *186*, 189–90
  Jamaica Lunatic Asylum, British West Indies 145–6
  in Japan 163–81
  Kingston Asylum, British West Indies 145
  Long Grove Hospital, Epsom, England 342
  Madona-Dudu Asylum, Craiova, Wallachia, Romania 205–8
  Madras Lunatic Asylum, India *124*
  Maudsley Hospital, London, England 317, 324, 338–9
  Marcuta Lunatic Asylum, Bucharest, Wallachia 199–203
  Metropolitan District Asylum, Caterham, England 279, 282
  New Jersey State Lunatic Asylum, USA 92–3
  New Westminster Asylum, British Columbia 102, 104, 107
  Pennsylvania Hospital for the Insane, USA 57–8
  Ranchi European Mental Hospital, Bihar, India 133–4
  Ranchi Indian Mental Hospital, Bihar, India 118
  Rasapagla Asylum, Bengal, India 119–20
  rural 220–37
  St Andrew's Hospital, Northampton, England 320, 325
  St Luke's Asylum, London, England 36
  Sibiu Mental Hospital, Transylvania, Romania 208–10
  Socola Psychiatric Hospital, Iași, Moldavia, Romania 203–5
  Southern Counties Asylum, Dumfries, Scotland 279
  Trinidad Lunatic Asylum, British West Indies 151–4
  Victoria Lunatic Asylum, British Columbia 101
  Weissenau Asylum, Württemberg, Germany 227
  Willard Asylum, New York State, USA 60–3
  York Retreat, England 7–8, 28, 43, 281, 351–2

mental hospitals (cont.)
  Zaragoza Asylum, Aragon, Spain 33, 40
  Zwiefalten Asylum, Württemberg, Germany 19–20, 221
mental hygiene movement 319
mental illness
  Romanian ideas on 195–7
  in the USA 55–76
mental nurses 322–4, 326
Mental Patients' Custody Act (1900) 185
Mental Treatment Act (1930) 319
Mercier, Charles 290
Mercurialis, Hieronymus 34–5
Metropolitan District Asylum, Caterham 279, 282
Meyer, Adolf 71, 172, 319, 324, 327
Midgley, Gerald 346
migration
  of doctors 143
  transnational 145
Mileticiu, George 19, 206–8
Ministry of Health, England and Wales 318
Ministry of Labour 337–8, 343
Mitchell, S. Weir 64–5
Moldavia 18–19, 194
moral management 142
moral therapy 15
  and asylums 56–7
  eclipse of 63–4
  and management 10–11
moral treatment 7, 10–11, 351
  and creation of 'useful members of society' 281–3
  early treatises on 31–54
  emergence of 32–4
  English publications on 36–9, 42–7
  French publications on 39–41, 47–8
  Tuscan publications on 41–2
more active therapy (*aktivere Krankenbehandlung*) 240–3
mortality 106, 229, 335
  rates of 20, 107, 120, 122, 125, 305
Mukherji, A.K. 129
Muramatsu Guest House *187–9*, 189
Murray, Dr Thomas 151
music 25, 48, 119, 127, 130, 165, 201, 209, 321, 359

Nagayama, Yasumasa 169
Nakamiya Byōin 168–9
Nanzenji-Temple *185*

National Health Service (NHS) 322–3, 329
National Socialism, and psychiatry 20, 230, 247
Neisser, Clemens 241
neurologists 64–5
neurosis 65, 69, 338, 342
New Jersey 12–13
  lunatic trials in 77–98
  State Lunatic Asylum 92–3
New Poor Law 315
New Westminster Asylum 102, 104
  cost of 107
nitrogen inhalation 318
non compos mentis judgements 79–80
North Wales Hospital, Denbigh 326

Obregia, Alexandru 197, 199, 201–3, 211
occupation 277, 280
  clinical objectives of 327
  development issues in England 327–30
  and identity 283
  in the late nineteenth century 278–81
  new ideas in 319–20
  in Romania 194–219
  suitability of 43
  at Zwiefalten 221–5
occupational therapists 174–5, 314
  definition of 326
occupational therapy (OT) 11–12, 15, 25–6, 70–1
  early stages of 164–6
  in Indian asylums 128–31
  and institutionalisation 336
  in Japan 163–4, 167–70
  kawa (river) model of 175–6
  regulation of 329–30
  rhetoric of 327
  training in 323–6, **324**
Okayama Guest House 188
open care 241

Pacheco, Dr J.N.J. 130
pain
  infliction of 36, 41
  self-inflicted 287
Pargeter, William 37
Parhon, Constantin I. 197, 204–5
patient work 1–2
  in America 11–12
  in British Columbia 99–116
  in Bucharest 199–203
  economic advantages of 244

Index

emergence of 32–4
English publications on 42, 46–7
and family care 182–93
French publications on 47–8
monetary value of 106–7
in New Jersey 91–3
in practice 243–5
remuneration for 199, 203
in rural asylums 220–37
in South Asia 117–41
in Transylvania 208–10
in the USA 55–76
patients
  achievements of 121
  activities for 61
  age of 6, 83, 94, 198, 302, 309, 336
  autonomy of 107
  Chinese 110–12
  chronic mentally ill 60–3
  crafts of 250–1
  curriculum vitae of 249
  decline in long-stay 345
  employment of 124
  escaped 166, 169
  European 127–8
  external control of 39
  Indian *131–4*
  Irish 59–60
  Japanese *184, 187–9*
  labelling of 263, 301–2
  lack of motivation in 252–3
  long-term 231
  motivation of 63
  non-working 309–10
  occupations and amusements for 58–60
  productivity of 303–**4**
  rewarding of 125
  self-funded 165–6
  treated like children 40–1, 44, 242
  view of work therapy 238–61
  voluntary 251–2
  weak-minded 282
Paton, Dr G. 119–20, 122–4
Pennsylvania Hospital for the Insane 57–8
Perfect, William 36–7
physical therapists 174
Pinel, Philippe 31–4, 40–1, 240
Plaxton, Joseph 148
'Plumtree' project 359–62, 364–5
pocket money 247

politics
  of professionalisation 329
  and work 307–8
Powell, Enoch 335
Preda, Gheorghe 209–10
Prince, Morton 65
prison 6, 22, 148, 262, 265, 305
private settings 328
productivity, cult of 12
professionalisation, policies of 314–33
Professions Supplementary to Medicine Act (1960) 329
profiteering 120
property
  fitness to govern 80
  wasting of 81–3
Protici, Petre 199, 211
Prouty, Olive Higgins 71–2
Provincial Mental Hospitals, BC 13–14
psychiatric care, employment in 334–50
psychiatrists, English 327
psychiatry 64
  British asylum 277–97
  motiveless malingering in 287–91
  and National Socialism 20, 230, 247
  Romanian 194–219
psychoanalytic theory, in OT 172–5
psychological paradigms 9–10
psychological treatment 57
psychosurgery 171
psychotherapy 65
  psychodynamic 319
puerperal maniacs 309–10
punishment 122–6, 267–8
Putnam, James Jackson 64–5, 68

race 12, 145
  and labour 126–8
  in West Indies 155
racial hygiene 230
racism 110–12
Ranchi Indian Mental Hospital 118
  agriculture at 122
  occupational therapist at 129
  work at 121
Rasapagla Asylum 119–20
rationalisation 353
  economic 356
  of resources 363–4
  of therapeutic professions 355–6
rationality 351–67
Ray, Isaac 63

reality principle 354
reason 351–67
recompense in kind 247–8
recovery, working towards 89–91
rehabilitation 27–8, 173, 250
　industrial units 338
　military 321, 337–8
　multi-disciplinary 322
　OT as 170
　psychiatric 334–6
relationships, notions of 361
Remploy 343, 346
resource rationalisation 363–4
rest cures 65–7
Ricklingen 249
Riggs, Austin 68–9, 71
Rihabiriteshon Gakuin 173–4
Robbins, Dr George, testimony of 86
Rogers, Abraham, trial of 84–7
Rogers, Elizabeth, legal agreement by 85–6
Roller, Christian Friedrich Wilhelm 239–40
Romania 18–19, 194–219, *195*
Roretz, Albrecht von 164
Rousseau, Jean-Jacques 35
Roy, William, medical evidence of 88
Royal Medico-Psychological Association (RMPA) 315–16, 320, 327–8
　Certificate in Occupational Therapy for Mental Nurses 324
Rush, Benjamin 57
Russell, Dr Iveson 322, 324

St Andrew's Hospital, Northampton 320, 325
St Luke's Asylum 36
Sakaki, Hajime 165
Savage, George Henry 278–9, 281–3, 290
Schäffer, Carl von 222, 224–5
schizophrenia 318, 341, 344
Schreiber, Narciss 222
scientific ergotherapy 19, 210
Scull, Andrew 7
Seccombe, George 152–4
Second World War, impact of 320–3
segregation
　in Japan 166
　of sexes 131–4, 201
Sekine, Shin'ichi 171
self-consciousness 279–80
self-injury 280–1
self-mutilation 287–91

selfhood 279
sheltered working groups 344
sheltered workshops 345
shock therapies 230
shoemaking 250–1
Sibiu Mental Hospital 208–10
Siemen, Hans-Ludwig 241
Simon, Dr Hermann 8, 135, 240–3, 320
six non-naturals 34–6
　see also humoralism
Slagle, Eleanor Clarke 129, 171–2
slavery 143
Smith, Adam 2–3
Snell, George 151
society, useful members of 277–97
Socola Psychiatric Hospital 203–5
sodium amytal 318
South Asia 117–41
Southern Counties Asylum 279
Spain, work treatment in 33
sport 35, 48
sterilisation 230
Strong, F.P. 119–20
supercedas retrial 80
Sutzu, Alexandru 18–19, 196–7, 200–1, 211
swinging 38, 57
Sydenham, Thomas 34
Sykes, William 284
Szabo, Ştefan 19, 208
Szasz, Thomas 8

Tajima, Akiko 175–6
Tanzi, Dr Eugenio 109
Tavistock Clinic 319
Tebbitt, Constance 323
techniques, standardisation of 356
temples, and the mentally ill 182
Tennent, Dr Thomas 324–5, 328
therapeutic professions, rationalisation of 355–6
therapeutic relationship 356
therapy
　medical 300–3
　more active 240–3
　physical 299–300
　psychiatric 197–9
　and work 118–19, 154
　work as 334–50
　and working life 249–51
　at Zwiefalten 221–5
Thorpe, George 287
Tokyo Fu Sugamo Byōin 165–6

Tokyo Fu Tenkyōin 165
Tomescu, Petre 197
training
  colleges 25–6, 175
  courses 320, **324**–6, 328–9
Transylvania 18–19, 194
  patient work in 208–10
travel 41
treatment
  change from in- to out-patient 335
  work as 45, 108–10, 142–62
  at Zwiefalten 221–5
trials, in lunacy 77–98
Trinidad Lunatic Asylum 151–4
Tuke, Daniel Hack 38, 281, 287
Tuke, Samuel 31–2, 42–4, 351–2, 354–5, 357–9, 363–5
Tuke, William 32, 44, 351
Tuscany, work and moral treatment in 31–54

unemployment 345
usefulness 23

Valsalva, Antonio Maria 34
Van Auken, Daniel, trial of 87–9
Van der Scheer, Professor [W.M.] 320
Victoria Lunatic Asylum 101
Vincent, George 154
violence 90

wages, and work 245–8
Wallachia 18–19, 194
Wandel, William H. 173
Ward, Mary Jane 55
Watanabe Guest House 188
Weber, Max 6
Weimar Republic 4, 20, 229–30, 238–61
Weissenau Asylum 227
Wellington, Thomas (the hollow gardener) 357–9
Wesley, John 35
Westernisation, challenges of 184–7
Willard Asylum 60–3
  men working outside 62
  sewing room 62
Willis, Francis 7, 9, 33–4
  catching the eye 37
Wing, John 344
Winslow, Forbes 286–7
Wood, Jacob, trial of 83–4

work 1–5
  ability to 12–13
  as absolute necessity 106–8
  in asylums 91–3
  benefits of 102–5
  and Chinese patients 110–12
  connectedness of 355
  economic value of 304–7
  for Europeans 127–8
  in factories 339
  the failure to 284–7
  and finances 120–1, 201
  and freedom 4
  and gender 103–4, 108, 133–4, 168, 239, 303–**4**
  and idiocy 83–4
  in Irish district asylums 298–313
  at Japanese inns 187–9
  laundry 111
  as medical therapy 300–3
  and mental decline 84–9
  in outside world 251–3
  by patients, *see* patient work
  as physical therapy 299–300
  and politics 307–8
  as privilege 310–11
  productive 3
  as punishment 6
  relationship with madness 13
  remuneration for 224–5
  as a right and duty 243
  role of 31–54
  in Romania 194–219
  satisfaction 3–4
  science-based 19
  sheltered 344
  and 'species life' 364
  therapeutic 66, 70–3
  as therapy 118–19, 334–50
  as treatment 45, 108–10, 142–62, 201
  unproductive 3–4
  usefulness of 245
  and wages 245–8
  at Zwiefalten 221–5
work cures 65–7
  in practice 67–70
  reason and relation in 351–67
work therapy
  in Japan 164
  patient's view of 238–61
  in practice 243–5
workhouses 315

working alliance 352–3, 356
working life 249–51
workshyness 22, 262–76
Württemberg 19, 220–37

York Retreat 7–8, 28, 43, 281, 351–2, 354
   narratives of 355–6

OT school at 325
role of work at 32–3

Zaragoza Asylum 33, 40
Zwiefalten Asylum 19–20, 221
   carpenter's workshop *223*
   cobbler's workshop *223*

EU authorised representative for GPSR:
Easy Access System Europe, Mustamäe tee 50,
10621 Tallinn, Estonia
gpsr.requests@easproject.com

www.ingramcontent.com/pod-product-compliance
Ingram Content Group UK Ltd.
Pitfield, Milton Keynes, MK11 3LW, UK
UKHW021850210426
5322IPUK00022B/583